ANKYLOSING SPONDYLITIS AND THE SPONDYLOARTHROPATHIES

Coming soon.......additional companion titles to *Rheumatology*

ANKYLOSING SPONDYLITIS AND THE SPONDYLOARTHROPATHIES

Michael H. Weisman, MD
Director, Division of Rheumatology
Cedars-Sinai Medical Center
Professor of Medicine
UCLA School of Medicine
Los Angeles, California

Désirée van der Heijde, MD
Professor of Rheumatology
Department of Medicine
Division of Rheumatology
University Hospital Maastricht
Maastricht, The Netherlands

John D. Reveille, MD
George S. Bruce Professor of Arthritis
Department of Medicine
The University of Texas
Houston, Texas

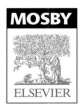

ELSEVIER

1600 John F. Kennedy Blvd.
Ste 1800
Philadelphia, PA 19103-2899

ANKYLOSING SPONDYLITIS
AND THE SPONDYLOARTHROPATHIES
ISBN-13: 978-0-323-03104-2
ISBN-10: 0-323-03104-8

Copyright © 2006 by Mosby, Inc., an affiliate of Elsevier Inc.

Notice

Knowledge and best practice in this field are constantly changing. As new research and experience broaden our knowledge, changes in practice, treatment, and drug therapy may become necessary or appropriate. Readers are advised to check the most current information provided (i) on procedures featured or (ii) by the manufacturer of each product to be administered, to verify the recommended dose or formula, the method and duration of administration, and contraindications. It is the responsibility of the practitioner, relying on his or her own experience and knowledge of the patient, to make diagnoses, to determine dosages and the best treatment for each individual patient, and to take all appropriate safety precautions. To the fullest extent of the law, neither the Publisher nor the Editors assume any liability for any injury and/or damage to persons or property arising out or related to any use of the material contained in this book.

The Publisher

Library of Congress Cataloging-in-Publication Data

Ankylosing spondylitis and the spondyloarthropathies / [edited by] Michael H. Weisman,
   John D. Reveille, Désirée van der Heijde.
      p. ; cm.
   Includes bibliographical references and index.
   ISBN 0-323-03104-8
      1. Spondyloarthropathies. 2. Ankylosing spondylitis. I. Weisman, Michael H.
   II. Reveille, John D. III. Heijde, Désirée van der.
   [DNLM: 1. Spondylarthropathies. 2. Spondylitis, Ankylosing. WE 725 A6113 2006]
   RC935.S67A55 2006
   616.7′3—dc22

200506148

Acquisitions Editor: Kim Murphy
Developmental Editor: Denise LeMelledo
Text Direction: Jayne Jones
Cover Design: Jayne Jones
Marketing Mananger: Laura Melsky

Printed in the United States of America

Last digit is the print number: 9 8 7 6 5 4 3 2 1

Contributing Authors

Nurullah Akkoc, MD
Professor of Medicine
Chief, Division of Rheumatology and Immunology
Department of Medicine
Dokuz Eylul University School of Medicine
Izmir, Turkey

Dominique Baeten, MD, PhD
Department of Rheumatology
Ghent University Hospital
Ghent, Belgium

Susan A. Baker
Attending Physician
Department of Rheumatology
Cedars-Sinai Hospital
Los Angeles, California

Xenofon Baraliakos, MD
Department of Rheumatology
German Rheumatology Research Center
Berlin, Germany

Jan Brandt, MD
Professor
Rheumazentrum Ruhrgebiet
Herne, Germany

Juergen Braun, MD
Professor
Rheumazentrum Ruhrgebiet
Herne, Germany

Matthew A. Brown, MD
ARC Senior Research Fellow
Clinical Reader in Musculoskeletal Sciences
Institute of Musculoskeletal Sciences
University of Oxford
The Botnar Research Centre
Nuffield Orthopaedic Centre
Headington, United Kingdom

Rubén Burgos-Vargas, MD
Professor of Medicine
Universidad Nacional Autónoma de México
Rheumatology Department
Hospital General de México
Mexico City, Mexico

John C. Davis, Jr., MD, MPH, FACR, FACP
Assistant Professor of Medicine
Associate Director, Clinical Trials Center
Director, Lupus Clinic
University of California, San Francisco
San Francisco, California

Filip De Keyser, MD
Department of Rhuematology
Ghent University Hospital
Ghent, Belgium

Maxime Dougados, MD
Professor of Rheumatology
René Descartes University
Hospital Cochin
Paris, France

Laure Gossec, MD
Hospital Cochin
Paris, France

Sandra Guignard, MD
Hospital Cochin
Paris, France

Robert D. Inman, MD
Professor of Medicine and Immunology
University of Toronto
Department of Medicine/Rheumatology
Toronto Western Hospital
Toronto, Canada

Muhammad Asim Khan, MD, MACP, FRCP
Professor of Medicine
Case Western Reserve University
Cleveland, Ohio

Robert Landewé, MD, PhD
Associate Professor of Rheumatology
University Hospital Maastricht
Department of Internal Medicine/Rheumatology
Maastricht, the Netherlands

Marjatta Leirisalo-Repo, MD
Professor of Rheumatology
Division of Rheumatology
Department of Medicine
Helsinki University Central Hospital
Helsinki, Finland

Walter P. Maksymowych, MD, FRCPC
Senior Scholar Alberta Heritage Foundation
    for Medical Research
Professor of Medicine
Department of Medicine
University of Alberta
Edmonton, Canada

Tammy M. Martin, PhD
Research Assistant Professor of Ophthalmology
Molecular Microbiology and Immunology
Casey Eye Institute
Portland, Oregon

Herman Mielants, MD
Department of Rheumatology
University Hospital
Ghent, Belgium

Shirley W. Pang, MD
Department of Rheumatology
University of California, San Francisco
San Francisco, California

John D. Reveille, MD
Professor and Director
Division of Rheumatology
University of Texas Medical School
Houston, Texas

James T. Rosenbaum, MD
Professor of Ontology, Medicine and Cell Biology
Chief, Division of Arthritis and Rheumatic Diseases
Director of the Uveitis Clinic
Casey Eye Institute
Portland, Oregon

Sebastian Schnarr
International Trainee Member
Hannover Medical School
Hannover, Germany

Joachim Sieper, MD, PhD
Medical Department I, Rheumatology
Charitè, Campus Benjamin Franklin
Berlin, Germany

Millicent A. Stone, MD
Research Member
St. Michaels Hospital
Toronto, Canada

Filip van den Bosch, MD, PhD
Department of Rheumatology
University Hospital
Ghent, Belgium

Désirée van der Heijde, MD
Professor of Rheumatology
University Hospital Maastricht
Maastricht, the Netherlands

Michael M. Ward, MD
Investigator
National Institute of Arthritis and Musculo-Skeletal
    and Skin Diseases
National Institutes of Health
Bethesda, Maryland

Michael H. Weisman, MD
Division of Rheumatology
Department of Medicine
Cedars-Sinai Medical Center
Los Angeles, California

Michael S. Wertheim, MD
Specialist Registrar in Ophthalmology
Bristol Eye Hospital
Bristol, United Kingdom

Henning Zeidler, MD, PhD
Director, Department of Rheumatology
Center of Internal Medicine
Medizinischen Hochschule Hannover
Hannover, Germany

Foreword

Spondyloarthritis in its multiple forms represents an important family of diseases that causes significant pain, disability, and societal burden around the world. Although recently shown to have afflicted ancient peoples, their recognition as clinical entities only began in the late nineteenth and early twentieth centuries, with clinical descriptions of ankylosing spondylitis by Marie and Strumpell and descriptions of distinctive radiologic features by early roentgenologists such as Forrestier. Even then, these diseases were considered "variants of rheumatoid arthritis" by early rheumatologists. Two seminal events in the early 1970s, however, catapulted these diseases squarely into prominent focus for modern clinical and basic scientific investigation. First, elegant clinical, epidemiologic, and family studies by Moll et al. demonstrated that ankylosing spondylitis; reactive arthritis (then termed Reiter's syndrome or disease); psoriatic arthritis; and arthritis related to the inflammatory bowel diseases, ulcerative colitis, and Crohn's disease, were intimately related to each other and were distinctly different than rheumatoid arthritis. Moll et al. called the diseases *spondylarthritis* (they were later termed *spondyloarthropathies* and, more recently, *spondyloarthritis*). Second, the discovery that the human leukocyte antigen (HLA)-class I allele, HLA-B-27, was a major genetic susceptibility factor for all of these disorders, albeit to variable degrees, led to an explosion of discovery. The clinical spectrum of spondyloarthritis was broadened significantly by the application of this genetic marker, and soon juvenile-onset, incompletely expressed, overlapping, and undifferentiated forms were recognized. Basic investigations into the pathogenetic mechanisms underlying these diseases also exploded and continue to provide new insights, leading to more targeted and effective therapies.

This book, edited by Drs. Weisman, van der Heijde, and Reveille, brings together a talented and productive group of clinical investigators and thought leaders in the field of spondyloarthritis, who comprehensively and critically review the current state of knowledge regarding the clinical features, epidemiology, pathogenetic mechanisms, and current treatments for each member of the spondyloarthritis family of diseases. To my knowledge, it represents the first such focused compendium on this subject in more than 20 years. It includes the most current information relevant to recognizing and treating these disorders, as well as the most recent and relevant basic scientific findings from modern molecular genetics, immunology, and microbiology studies. Therefore, it will be a valuable resource to specialists and primary-care physicians, researchers, students, residents, and fellows. While spondyloarthritis remains a significant health problem, this book shows that progress is being made at every level and is a valuable contribution to the dissemination of modern medical and scientific information.

Frank C. Arnett, MD
Professor of Internal Medicine,
Pathology and Laboratory Medicine
Elizabeth Bidgood Chair in Rheumatology
The University of Texas Health Science
Center at Houston
Houston, Texas

Preface

Spondyloarthritis and its main characteristic disease, ankylosing spondylitis (AS), finally have received the attention of the medical and rheumatologic community in a major way. Long isolated in the backwaters of academic research and pharmaceutical industries, and largely relegated to descriptive concepts, they have become key players in the fast- and forward-thinking lanes of genetic, environmental, and pathogenetic links. It was our feeling that these new ideas needed to be presented and documented, and that belief was the genesis behind the current volume.

The chapters that follow address historical concepts and the evolution of the terminology used for these diseases, the epidemiology of AS and related conditions, clinical features, childhood forms of the disease, and treatment considerations. The editors have supplied critical and up-to-date chapters on the pathogenesis and genetics of AS (or *pathogenetics*), in addition to information about outcome measures now commonly used in clinical trials and in the clinic. Furthermore, we have brought imaging for AS and related diseases into the twenty-first century; imaging issues and considerations for early diagnosis are addressed in this volume. The impact of AS and spondyloarthritis on society in general and on the patient in particular is prominently displayed.

It is clear that AS and related diseases will become hot topics of research and therapeutic interest. We hope that this volume will provide a foundation for that effort.

Contents

ANKYLOSING SPONDYLITIS AND THE SPONDYLOARTHROPATHIES

COLOR PLATES

PLATE 1

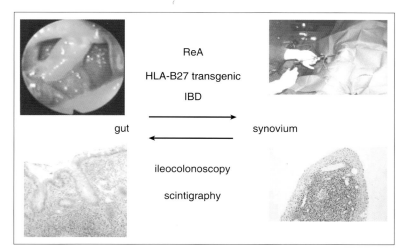

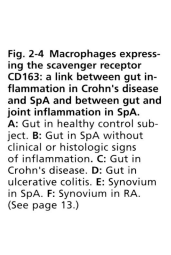

ReA

HLA-B27 transgenic

IBD

gut → synovium

synovium ← gut

ileocolonoscopy

scintigraphy

Fig. 2-3 Relationship between gut and joint inflammation in SpA is suggested by clinical observations (reactive arthritis), animal models (HLA-B27 transgenic rats), the overlap with IBD, as well as by histologic and scintigraphic studies indicating subclinical gut inflammation. The accessibility of gut and joint for biopsy sampling allows immunopathologic studies to unravel this relationship. (See page 11.)

Fig. 2-4 Macrophages expressing the scavenger receptor CD163: a link between gut inflammation in Crohn's disease and SpA and between gut and joint inflammation in SpA. **A:** Gut in healthy control subject. **B:** Gut in SpA without clinical or histologic signs of inflammation. **C:** Gut in Crohn's disease. **D:** Gut in ulcerative colitis. **E:** Synovium in SpA. **F:** Synovium in RA. (See page 13.)

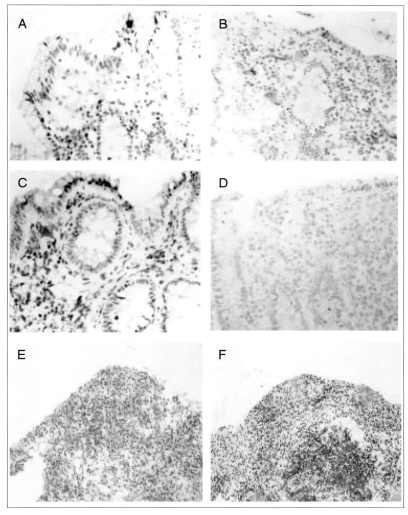

PLATE 2

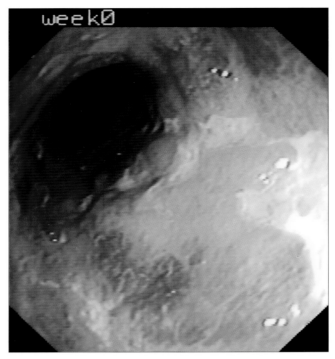

Fig. 6.1 Ileocolonoscopy in Crohn's disease. A: Before treatment with infliximab: presence of important ulcerations. **B:** After treatment with infliximab: disappearance of inflammation and ulcerations. (See page 69.)

PLATE 3

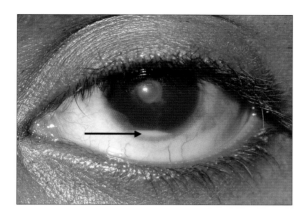

Fig. 9.1 Collection of white cells in the inferior anterior chamber known as a hypopyon *(arrow)* **seen in a patient with severe uveitis associated with ReA.** (Courtesy of Roger George, MD.) (See page 107.)

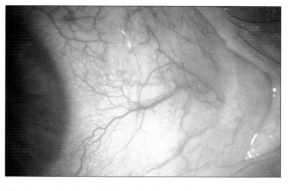

Fig. 9.4 Injection of the scleral vessels in a patient with scleritis. (See page 109.)

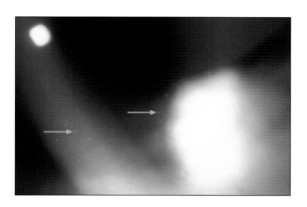

Fig. 9.2 Fine keratic precipitates (KPs) on the endothelial layer of the cornea *(arrows).* These KPs are typical in the uveitides associated with the spondyloarthropathies. (See page 108.)

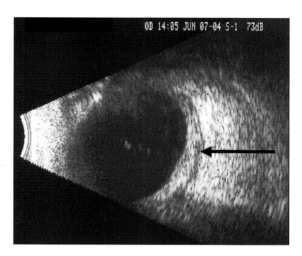

Fig. 9.5 B-scan ultrasound of the right eye showing thickened sclera and fluid behind the sclera *(arrow)* **in a patient with posterior scleritis.** This is called the T-sign. (See page 111.)

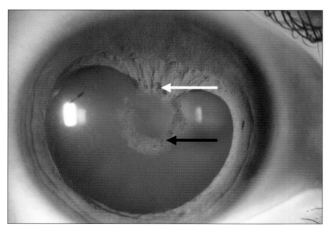

Fig. 9.3 Iris adhesions to the lens. These are known as posterior synechiae *(white arrow)* and pigment deposition on the lens epithelium *(black arrow)* can both be signs of current or previous intraocular inflammation. (See page 108.)

PLATE 4

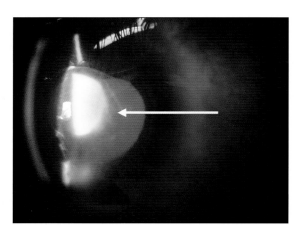

Fig. 9.6 Cataract. The *white arrow* indicates a cataract (opacification of the lens) due to inflammation in a patient with ReA associated uveitis. (Courtesy of Roger George, MD.) (See page 112.)

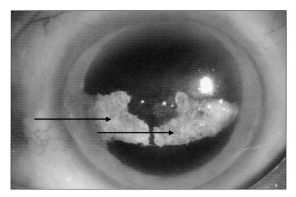

Fig. 9.8 Corneal band keratopathy, deposition of calcium under the corneal epithelium *(arrows).* This sign is most commonly found in chronic eye inflammation. (See page 113.)

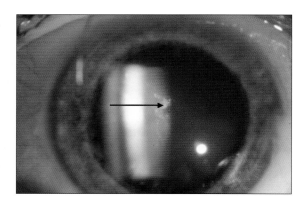

Fig. 9.7 Posterior subcapsular cataract. This is a lens opacity forming on the back surface of the lens, commonly seen in chronic ocular inflammation and with chronic topical steroid application to the eye. (See page 113.)

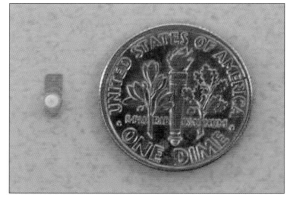

Fig. 9.9 Sustained release steroid implant next to a dime. This particular implant is a fluocinolone acetonide intravitreal implant (Retisert) manufactured by Bausch and Lomb. (See page 114.)

1

Introduction to the Unifying Concepts of Spondyloarthropathy, Including Historical Aspects of the Disease

Susan A. Baker and Michael H. Weisman

DEFINITION OF THE SPONDYLOARTHROPATHIES AS WE KNOW THEM TODAY

The spondyloarthropathies (SpAs) are a group of chronic inflammatory rheumatic disorders that share distinctive pathophysiologic, clinical, radiographic, and genetic features. Inflammatory back pain with or without arthritis of the peripheral joints together with certain extraskeletal features are characteristic signs and symptoms of these disorders.[1] The traditional clinical profiles defining this group include ankylosing spondylitis (AS), considered the prototype of the SpAs, reactive arthritis (ReA), psoriatic arthritis (PsA), arthropathy of inflammatory bowel disease (IBD), undifferentiated spondyloarthropathy, and juvenile chronic arthritis.[2] The term *Reiter's syndrome* is no longer used as an eponymous distinction; ReA is now generally considered a sufficient descriptive term.[3–6] Although some of the triggers for these conditions have been explored and identified, the causes of these disorders have yet to be determined. However, major clues to finding a cause such as a strong association with human leukocyte antigen (HLA)-B27 have led to dramatic advances in our understanding of the SpAs.[7] Treatment paradigms are currently undergoing very significant changes as we gain a more comprehensive understanding of the disease process and outcome, refine our diagnostic imaging techniques and classification criteria, and take advantage of advances in understanding molecular mechanisms of chronic inflammation. This chapter includes a review of the historical background of the SpAs from antiquity to the present, a discussion of the replacement of the term *rheumatoid variants* with the concept of SpA, and an examination of the heredity of these disorders that has characterized the SpAs as a class of diseases.

THE HISTORY OF THE DISEASES

Antiquity

An appreciation of where we are today depends on understanding the history of these disorders. The exact antiquity of the SpAs remains controversial and continues to be debated. It is generally accepted that AS is an ancient disease that occurred in animals and man in prehistoric times.[8] Lesions characteristic of SpA were found in Rothschild's survey of fossil and modern skeletons of perissodactylae from North America. These findings led to the conclusion that there was a progressive increase in SpA throughout geologic time in Equidae and Rhinocerotidae and raised the question as to whether or not SpA conferred an evolutionary advantage.[9] Other studies have demonstrated spinal lesions thought to be characteristic of AS in prehistoric and modern animals as varied as crocodiles from the Miocene and Pliocene periods, dinosaurs, cave bears, saber-toothed tigers, and modern primates. However, the findings in animals are considered by some investigators more likely to represent normal development or perhaps degenerative changes.[8]

Paleopathologic and paleoepidemiologic studies have demonstrated changes characteristic of SpA dating back to several thousand years B.C.[10] Nevertheless, large numbers of pathologic specimens have been re-examined from the 21st dynasty Egyptian mummy to mid-19th century skeletons for evidence of AS. This paleopathologic material underwent anthropologic, demographic, paleopathologic, radiologic, and rheumatologic assessment. The investigators concluded that the previously high frequency of AS in pathologic material reported in the literature is unreliable and that the findings more likely represent cases of diffuse skeletal hyperostosis (DISH) or possibly other cases of spinal fusion such as the spondylitis of psoriasis or ReA. With the paucity of convincing cases and the presence of other explanations for the paleopathologic specimens reported in the literature, they speculated that AS may be of more recent origin and the antiquity of AS reported in the earlier literature needed reappraisal.[11]

AS was described in many Egyptian pharaohs including Amenhotep II, Ramses II, and his son Merenptah, through paleoradiographic research in France in 1976.[12] However, a reappraisal of the x-ray films of Ramses II was recently conducted by Chhem et al.[12] who used paleoradiologic, clinical, and historical data to conclude that a diagnosis of AS is unlikely and that, again, the findings are more consistent with a diagnosis of DISH or spondylosis deformans. They cite limitations in x-ray techniques, lack of established radiographic criteria, and lack of a differential diagnosis generated as the reasons for misinterpretation of the data.[13]

Many argue that there appear to be a few convincing cases of AS or other SpAs in ancient remains. The counter arguments cite the incomplete collection of skeletal remains, lack of radiographic confirmation, and inconsistent terminology that often resulted in misinterpretation of data. Reappraisal with modern scientific techniques such as HLA typing and computed tomography studies may provide additional and perhaps invaluable clues leading to proof of the prehistoric existence of SpA.[14]

The First Clinical Descriptions

The first clinical description of AS is credited to Bernard Conner (1666–1698), an Irish physician. In 1691, Dr. Conner summarized the clinical features of AS in his M.D. thesis entitled, "Une Dissertation Physique sur la Continuite de Plusiers Os, a l'Occasion d'une Fabriue Suprenante d'une Tronc de Squelette Humain, oui les Vertebres, les Cotes, l'Os Sacrum, et les Os des Iles, qui Naturellement sont Distiner et Separes, ne font qu'un Seul Os Continu et Inseparable." In his thesis, he describes fusion of the thoracic vertebrae down to and including the sacroiliac joints and ribs.[8,15]

Despite a number of isolated medical reports, there appears to be no clearly identifiable clinical descriptions of SpA over the next century.[8,16] Early in the 19th century Carl Wenzell of Frankfurt provided the first thoughtful comparison between AS and hyperostotic spondylosis, thereby recognizing, in 1824, the anatomical differences between these two entities. In 1830, Lyons is thought to have been the first to describe what is now called reactive arthritis or psoriatic arthritis.[17] In 1850 Sir Benjamin Brodie published a report associating iritis with AS in his famous book, *Diseases of the Joints* (1850); thus, Brodie is recognized as one of the first to contribute descriptions of the extraaxial manifestations of the disease.[8]

In 1877, Charles Fagge, an English physician, correlated his clinical observations with his own autopsy findings on the same patient, a traditional English pedagogical approach. In his report, he describes a male, ". . . age 34 with a cough, ridged curved spine and fixity of the ribs, breathing exclusively with his abdomen. . . . Autopsy revealed ankylosis of vertebral bodies, apophyseal joints, ribs and right hip joint but also upper lobe fibrosis, bronchiectasis and a cardiac lesion—possibly an endocarditis."[16]

The second half of the 19th century marked a great period of clinical descriptions of AS, the most important of which were made by three notable neurologists of the time, A. Strumpell of Leipzig, Vladimir Bechterew of St. Petersburg, and Pierre Marie of Paris.[8,16] In 1884, Strumpell described two cases in his textbook and later went on to report his own clinical observations in his paper, *The Classic*, published in 1897.[18] Although Bechterew recognized similar cases of spinal stiffness and deformity in 1893, he would point out that there were clear differences in his observations from those of Marie and Strumpell.[19] Chief credit has been given by some authors to Marie for his full account of the anatomic and clinical features of AS, which he accurately described in 1898 in his famous presentation to the Societe Medicale des Hopitaux de Paris, "La Spondylose Rhizomelique" (a term derived from Greek roots, *spondylosis* = vertebra, *rhiza* = root, and *melos* = extremity). In this report, he emphasized the peripheral joint involvement of the shoulders and hips in AS. In the years between 1899 and 1906, Marie and his student, Andre Leri, supplied the pathologic-anatomical observations needed to complete the clinical description of *ankylosing spondylitis,* the term that would eventually replace *rhizomelique spondylitis* and the number of other eponyms that preceded it. Their contributions mark one of the landmarks in the modern-day history of AS. In 1890, Bernard Sachs, a New York neurologist, echoed Marie's observations in publishing "progressive ankylotic rigidity of the spine," which provided the first American statement.[20]

Modern Times

The 20th century marked a prolific phase in the history of AS. It was characterized by important clinicopathologic observations that ultimately led to the modern-day concept of inflammatory SpA. Wilhelm Roentgen in 1895 made the breakthrough discovery of the x-ray, permitting the pathology of the disease to be observed during the lifetime of the patient. In 1930 with the recognition of sacroiliac radiology, Forresteir, Drebs, and Scott described sacroiliitis and Robert and Forresteir described syndesmophytes.[17] Major contributions were also made in Scandinavia by Romanus and Yden with their description of "shiny corners."[20–22] As MRI becomes the standard diagnostic and investigative approach for patients with inflammatory back pain, descriptions of pathology in the thoracic spine (long known by clinicians to be an important part of early disease) now find their way into the literature.[23] The presence of lesions up, down, and scattered throughout the spine in patients with early disease calls into question the theory that AS ascends progressively upward via microbial spread in the veins of Batson from an initial infection in the most caudal parts of the skeleton.

Etiology and Treatment

Despite a clearer understanding of the clinical manifestations of AS, there were few clues to the causation of the SpAs before the end of the 19th century. At that time two major concepts, diathesis and infection, dominated the medical literature. Direct infection with bacteria such as gonococcus or tuberculosis, among others, was hypothesized to play an inciting role. Although no specific bacterial organism was ever consistently recovered, the idea of focal sepsis evolved, which resulted in the use of vaccines and the removal of a number of different organs as treatment.[16]

These concepts gradually fell from favor, and in their place other limited and potentially harmful treatments emerged. X-ray therapy to the sacroiliac joints and spine was popularized in the United Kingdom by Gilbert Scott in the 1930s but has been abandoned in modern medicine because of the high risk of leukemia and aplastic anemia.[16,17,22] In 1948 the therapeutic effects of corticosteroids were discovered, and they have dominated the treatment of arthritides including SpA until recent times. Dr. Philip Showalter Hench, a founding member of the American Rheumatism Association and its president from 1940 to 1941, discovered this "new cure" that was applied to many patients with AS. For his pioneering work in the treatment of rheumatoid arthritis (RA) with cortisone and adrenocorticotropic hormone, he won the Nobel Prize in Physiology or Medicine, which he shared with Dr. Edward Kendall, his friend and collaborator, and Dr. Tadeur Reichstein of Switzerland.

TERMINOLOGY AND CLASSIFICATION

"Rheumatoid Spondylitis"

Before the 1950s there were two uses of the term *rheumatoid arthritis*. First, it was used to describe a disease unto itself that is recognized today as typical RA. Second, it was used to refer to those diseases that shared certain similar disease characteristics but deviated sufficiently to be termed *rheumatoid variants* or *rheumatoid spondylitis* and included AS, PsA, ReA, and the arthritis of IBD. Two schools of thought dominated at that time, affectionately nicknamed "lumpers" and "splitters."[24] The European opinion that the SpAs were a disease entity separate from RA had long been entered into the debate. However, practitioners in the United States continued to view AS and associated diseases as expressions of RA because of their similar synovial pathologic characteristics and peripheral joint involvement.

The U.S. description of *rheumatoid spondylitis* is well documented in the monograph entitled *Rheumatoid Arthritis* written by Dr. Charles Short, Dr. William Bauer, and Dr. William Reynolds and published in 1957 for the Commonwealth Fund by Harvard University Press.

In it, they reviewed the historical background of the disease and concluded that rheumatoid spondylitis represented spinal localization of RA. The differences between the two disorders were, however, fully recognized. Those patients with spondylitis had a greater male sex distribution, an earlier age of onset, increased occurrence of uveitis, absence of subcutaneous nodules if peripheral joints were involved, favorable response to x-ray therapy, and lack of response to gold. Their misconceptions were due in part to minimal histopathologic information available at the time.[25] With the recognition of rheumatoid factor in 1940 by Waaler, its reintroduction into the scientific literature in 1948 by Rose, and improved radiographic techniques that allowed better skeletal resolution, it became clear that the two diseases were separate entities.[8] In 1963 the American Rheumatism Association officially approved the name *ankylosing spondylitis*.[20]

Classification Criteria

The need to develop classification criteria for epidemiologic purposes became increasingly apparent with the growing awareness of the disorders through the screening of young men during the two World Wars. In Bethesda, Maryland, an initial meeting was held at the National Institutes of Health for the purpose of establishing a set of criteria. In 1960 a symposium sponsored by the World Health Organization and held in Rome established the first set of diagnostic criteria for AS. These criteria were subsequently revised in 1966 and became known as the New York Criteria and subsequently as the Modified New York Criteria. Because these criteria were felt to be too restrictive and were not suited for early diagnosis, the European Spondyloarthropathy Study Group (ESSG) Criteria were developed to help identify patients with undifferentiated SpA.[2]

HEREDITY

HLA-B27

Before the 1970s, little was known about the etiology or genetic characteristics that predispose individuals to these disorders or other inflammatory rheumatic diseases.[17,22] This changed with the simultaneous and independent discovery of HLA-B27 association in 1973 by Schlosstein et al. in Los Angeles and Brewerton et al. in London.[26–28] This reporting of the very high incidence of B27 (W27) antigen in AS was a significant advance in the understanding of the disease and immediately served to clarify several important issues. First, it clearly established that the SpAs were separate disorders from RA and paved the way for appropriate classification. It also strengthened the concept of the familial nature of the disease that could now be attributed to a genetic marker.[26,29]

During that period, the possible links between certain diseases and specific HLA types were hypothesized, but no striking correlations had yet been found.[29] Dr. Seymour White, a dermatologist, was the first to discuss HLA typing and rheumatic disease in his work on psoriasis with Dr. Paul Terasaki. They reported a threefold increase in the frequency of HLA-13 and HLA-17 among patients with psoriasis in 1972. This began the search for HLA associations in all rheumatic diseases.[30–32]

Personal accounts of the experiences of those early investigators provide important insights into the type of novel thinking needed to generate scientific advances. Brewerton, in his personal account of his involvement in the study later recounted in 2003, wrote "I immediately proposed tissue-typing for people with ankylosing spondylitis because it was a common inflammatory disease with an unexplained genetic component. . . . We learned that B27 was present in eight of eight patients with ankylosing spondylitis, a chance of less than one in a million. Imagine the excitement of the moment!"[22] The credit of the moment, however, would have to be shared, because simultaneously in Los Angeles, Bluestone and Terasaki and their colleagues had also uncovered the same association while studying HLA typing in patients with gout. As Bluestone wrote in his own account of their discovery in 1988, "The way the whole thing happened was rather remarkable. We wanted control groups, and one of the selected control groups was patients with ankylosing spondylitis, i.e., patients with another well-defined rheumatic disease, the majority of them male. The first 20 patients that we typed from this control group came back with a 95% incidence of HLA-B27. . . ."[26,33]

This was a landmark discovery not only for its obvious pathogenetic implications but also because it became an important diagnostic and prognostic tool. Since that time, many other studies have confirmed the same association, and it is now believed that 90% to 95% of Caucasian patients with AS carry the B27 antigen, compared with approximately 8% of the general Caucasian population (of Western European extraction).[34] This association showed the highest relative risk of any disease with a major histocompatibility complex (MHC) gene.[29,35] The strength of the association was found to show considerable variation among different races and ethnic groups.[34,36] It has been hypothesized that the inheritance of B27 may have conferred a selective advantage to the host, but no effect has yet been shown.[8]

Genetics

The heredity of the SpAs remains a genetic puzzle. There is strong evidence that B27 is not the only MHC gene involved in susceptibility, but probably operates in combination with other genes to determine the true susceptibility to the disease.[28] To date, 24 allelic variants or subtypes of HLA-B27 have been reported, but whether or not they confer susceptibility is unknown. It is expected that many more genes and how they contribute to the disease will be discovered in the future.[7,34]

UNIFYING CONCEPTS

Seronegative Spondyloarthropathies

The unifying concept of the SpAs was enormously strengthened by the realization that these clinical syndromes are all strongly associated with HLA-B27. However, the actual concept of the *seronegative spondyloarthropathies* was formulated almost a decade earlier by Wright et al. who later published an excellent review of the relationships among these disorders in 1974.[2] The term *seronegative spondyloarthropathies* was used to include an interrelated yet heterogenous group of disorders sharing many common clinical, radiologic, and serologic features in addition to familial and genetic relationships.[36] These diseases initially included AS, PsA, Reiter's syndrome, the arthropathies of ulcerative colitis and Crohn's disease, Whipple's disease, and Behçet's syndrome. Inclusion of these disorders rested on a number of different points of similarity that included rheumatoid factor negativity, the absence of subcutaneous nodules, radiographic sacroiliitis with or without inflammatory peripheral arthritis, certain skin and mucous membrane symptoms, and a tendency for familial aggregation.[37]

In addition, the nature of the inflammatory process of the SpAs differs from that of RA with much of the clinical and radiographic manifestations being seen predominately but not entirely at the entheses, where ligaments attach to bone. Unlike RA, the main target of the initial inflammatory process of the SpA appears to be the so-called hard tissues of bone and cartilage and to a lesser extent the synovium. The inflammatory process has a tendency to heal with new bone formation in fibrous scar tissue, resulting in ankylosis and irreversible ossification of axial and peripheral joints.[38–41]

With the recognition of the association of B27 and AS, similar research in HLA typing soon confirmed that all of these diseases carried a significantly increased association with the B27 antigen.[29] The same groups of investigators in Los Angeles and London undertook similar studies with HLA typing and confirmed similar B27 antigen frequencies between AS and ReA.[42,43] In their studies on patients with IBD, their observations supported the concept of two distinct arthropathies of IBD with different pathogenic mechanisms. These investigators noted that the peripheral arthropathy of IBD occurring as an extraintestinal manifestation showed no increased association with the B27 antigen and responded to treatment of the underlying bowel disease. However, it was observed that the spondylitis occurring in the same patient with IBD was associated with the B27 antigen 75% of the time. These findings suggest that pathogenetic mechanisms in this latter group are similar to those operating in the idiopathic variety of AS and that patients with IBD and HLA-B27 are at higher risk of developing AS.[42,43]

Similar but more complicated relationships exist between psoriasis and its associated arthropathies. Patients with psoriasis alone were found to have no increased occurrence of HLA-B27 but did show an increased association with HLA-13 and HLA-17. Patients with peripheral PsA also had no evidence of increased B27 antigen occurance, although 45% of patients with psoriatic spondylitis have the B27 antigen, an association that was significantly less than that seen in idiopathic AS and ReA. Nevertheless, these observations confirmed that PsA should be included among the other seronegative SpAs. These data also revealed that other factors must play a role in the pathogenesis of inflammatory arthritis of the spine.[43,44]

As a result of later observations, it became obvious that certain forms of juvenile chronic arthritis should also be included under the umbrella of the SpAs. Children with pauciarticular disease have an increased frequency of the B27 antigen. Whipple's disease and Behçet's syndrome, however, are no longer included in the SpAs owing to the lack of association with HLA-B27 and their possession of other additional features.[45,46]

Terminology

Difficulties have arisen over the years in deciding on accepted terminology. The term *seronegative spondylarthropathies* was abandoned because of difficulties in pronunciation, as well as the unnecessary presence of prefix, *seronegative*. This terminology was viewed as redundant and created confusion with seronegative RA.[2]

CONCLUSION

Modern medical management of the SpAs has clearly benefited from recent advances in the use of biologic agents in rheumatic diseases. Although their short-term effectiveness in relieving symptoms has been established, the effect on long-term sequelae for the SpAs has yet to be determined. With the inception of the biologic agents as useful treatment modalities, additional methods are being sought to improve patient outcome, limit disability, and ultimately achieve remission. Some of these methods include early disease detection. Efforts to accomplish these goals are underway and include redefining disease classification, reassessing the histopathology of early disease, and understanding the value of newer imaging techniques such as magnetic resonance imaging and ultrasound in the detection of early disease. Preclinical disease findings may also become a realizable goal with the anticipation of the identification of biomarkers in the near future. The ever-changing concepts of the SpAs are illustrated well in its history and, as Bywaters wrote more than 20 years ago, ". . . there's a lot more history still to be made, and (what) a wonderful challenge."[16]

REFERENCES

1. Khan MA. Clinical features of ankylosing spondylitis. In: Hochberg M, et al., eds. Rheumatology. Section 9: Spondyloarthropathies. Spain: Elsevier; 2003;1161–1181.
2. Van Der Linden S, Van Der Heijde D. Classification of spondyloarthropathies. In: Hochberg M, et al., eds. Rheumatology. Section 9: Spondyloarthropathies. Spain: Elsevier; 2003;1149–1151.
3. Wallace DJ, Weisman MH. Should a war criminal be awarded with eponymous distinction? The double life of Hans Reiter (1881-1969). J Clin Rheumatol. 2000;6:49–54.
4. Panush RS, Paraschiv D, and Dorff RE. The tainted legacy of Hans Reiter. Semin Arthritis Rheum. 2003;32(4):231–236.
5. Gross HS. Changing the name of Reiter's syndrome: a psychiatric perspective. Semin Arthritis Rheum. 2003;32(4):242–243.
6. Gottlieb NL, Altman RD. An ethical dilemma in rheumatology: should the eponym Reiter's syndrome be discarded? Semin Arthritis Rheum. 2003;32(4):207.
7. Brown MA, Wordsworth BP, Reveille JD. Genetics of ankylosing spondylitis. Clin Exp Rheumatol. 2002;20(6 suppl 28): S43–S49.
8. Spencer DG, Sturrock RD, Buchanan WW. Ankylosing spondylitis: yesterday and today. Med Hist. 1980;24:60–69.
9. Rothschild BM, Prothero DR, Rothschild C. Origins of spondyloarthropathy in Perissodactyla. Clin Exp Rheumatol. 2001; 19(6):628–632.
10. Ramos-Remus C, Russell AS. Clinical features and management of ankylosing spondylitis. Curr Opin Rheumatol. 1993;5: 408–413.
11. Rogers J, Watt I, Dieppe P. Paleopathology of spinal osteophytosis, vertebral ankylosis, ankylosing spondylitis, and vertebral hyperostosis. Ann Rheum Dis. 1985;44:113–120.
12. Chhem RK, Schmit P, Faure C. Did Ramesses II really have ankylosing spondylitis? A reappraisal. Can Assoc Radiol J. 2004;55: 211–217.
13. Rothschild BM. Paleopathology, its character and contribution to understanding and distinguishing among rheumatologic diseases: perspectives on rheumatoid arthritis and spondyloarthropathy. Clin Exp Rheumatol. 1995;13:657–662.
14. Copeman WS. Historical notes on rheumatology. Rheumatol Phys Med. 1971;11:145–155.
15. Bywaters EG. Historical perspectives in the aetiology of ankylosing spondylitis. Br J Rheumatol. 1983;22(4 suppl 2):1–4.
16. Bywaters EG. Historical aspects of ankylosing spondylitis. Rheumatol Rehabil. 1979;18:197–203.

TABLE 2.1 EVIDENCE OF GUT INFLAMMATION IN SpA

	Evidence	Reference
Clinical	Reactive arthritis	1, 4
	Overlap with IBD	
	Progression to IBD	11
Animal	HLA-B27 transgenic rats	2, 3, 36
Histologic	Subclinical inflammation in 30%–70%	5–8
	Association with persistent arthritis	9, 10, 12–14
Prehistologic immune alterations	Lymphoid follicles	15
	CD11a, CD11c, VCAM-1	15
	CD163+ macrophages	16

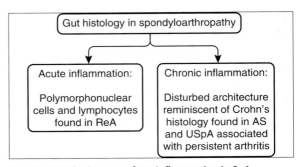

Fig. 2.1 Histologic types of gut inflammation in SpA.

not effective.[4] Taken together, these findings suggest that gut inflammation and the microbial triggering of the gut-associated immune system rather than the bacterial infection itself are important for the initiation of the inflammatory arthritis.

Gut inflammation in other spondyloarthropathy subtypes

In humans, there is now compelling evidence that gut inflammation and increased gut permeability play a role not only in ReA but also in other types of SpA.[5–7] Subclinical gut inflammation revealed by ileo-colonoscopy in patients with different forms of SpA has been confirmed in multiple studies (reviewed in reference 8). In USpA, the prevalence of macroscopic gut lesions at ileocolonoscopy varies from 24% to 38% and microscopic lesions are found in 24% to 72% of patients. A similar prevalence of gut lesions was described in patients with AS. Gut inflammation was also described in other diseases included in the SpA concept: enterogenic and urogenital ReA, pauciarticular late-onset juvenile arthritis, and PsA presenting as axial and/or pauciartic-ular disease.

Histology of gut inflammation in spondyloarthropathy

Two histologic types of gut inflammation can be distinguished in SpA: acute and chronic inflammation[9] (Fig. 2.1). Importantly, this classification refers to the morphologic characteristics and not to the onset or duration of the disease. The acute type resembles acute bacterial enterocolitis. The mucosal architecture is well preserved. The ileal villi and crypts are infiltrated by polymorphonuclear cells. In the lamina propria, there is an increased number of inflammatory cells, consisting of a mixture of granulocytes, lymphocytes, and plasma cells. The chronic type resembles chronic ileocolitis, mostly indistinguishable from Crohn's disease. In this type, the mucosal architecture is clearly disturbed. The villi are irregular, blunted, and fused. The crypts are distorted, and the lamina propria is edematous and infiltrated by mononuclear cells. Basal lymphoid follicles occur. In some patients with chronic lesions, aphthoid ulcers, branching of the crypts, the ulcer-associated cell lineage (pseudo-pyloric metaplasia), and sarcoid-like granulomas are present. Whereas acute lesions are mainly seen in patients with ReA, chronic lesions are slightly more prevalent than acute lesions in USpA and AS.[10]

Clinical overlap between spondyloarthropathy and inflammatory bowel disease

Although the presence of chronic gut lesions with a histologic resemblance to Crohn's disease in an important fraction of patients with SpAs was already suggestive for a pathogenic relation with classical Crohn's disease, these findings awaited further evidence to link them more formally with Crohn's disease. On the one hand, in a prospective study involving 123 patients with SpA who had undergone initial endoscopy, the clinical evolution of SpA and the evolution of the intestinal inflammation were studied.[11] Evolution to clinically overt IBD was observed in 7% of patients. Patients with initial chronic inflammation were mainly the ones at risk. Other risk factors included persistent high C-reactive protein levels and radiologic sacroiliitis in the absence of HLA-B27. On the other hand, a significant proportion of patients with IBD demonstrated clinical and radiologic signs compatible with SpA, as is discussed in a separate chapter of this book. Taken together, the histologic and clinical data strongly suggest that gut inflammation in SpA and Crohn's disease may be closely related. In the third section of this chapter, we review the immunologic and genetic data supporting this concept.

Clinical evidence of a relationship between gut and joint inflammation in spondyloarthropathy

Several lines of clinical evidence also point to the fact that gut and joint inflammation are related in SpA and thus that the gut could have an important pathogenic role. First, in AS the prevalence of gut inflammation was higher in patients with associated peripheral arthritis than in patients without arthritis.[12] Second, chronic lesions seen on gut histologic studies were associated with more advanced radiologic signs of sacroiliitis and spondylitis and with more erosive and destructive peripheral articular disease.[9] Third, upon follow-up of patients with SpA in whom a second ileocolonoscopy was performed, remission of joint inflammation was associated with a disappearance of the gut inflammation, whereas persistence of locomotor inflammation mostly was associated with the persistence of gut inflammation, confirming the strong relationship between gut and joint inflammation.[13] Most patients with normal histologic results or acute intestinal lesions exhibited transient arthritis, whereas the majority of those with chronic intestinal lesions had persistent inflammatory joint symptoms.[10,14] In the fourth section of this chapter, we will focus on the histologic and immunopathologic data supporting a link between the gut and joints in SpA.

Evidence That Gut Inflammation in Spondyloarthropathy Is Pathogenetically Related to Crohn's Disease

Early, prehistologic immune alterations in spondyloarthropathic gut mucosa

The question has been asked whether gut mucosa in patients with SpA may display changes that cannot be observed solely at a classical histologic level (Fig. 2.2). The answer requires immunohistochemical analysis applying specific antibody probes or tools looking at gene expression. Such approaches are reviewed hereunder and confirm, together with other evidence, the relationship between immunologic alterations in the gut of patients with SpA and overt Crohn's disease.

Demetter et al.[15] investigated the presence of lymphoid follicles and the expression of leukocyte adhesion molecules in gut mucosa of patients with SpA. Histologic evaluation and immunohistochemical analysis were performed on the ileum and colon of 14 patients with SpA who did not have macroscopic or microscopic gut inflammation and 21 control subjects. Lymphoid follicles were counted and immunohistochemical staining results for leukocyte adhesion molecules, lymphocyte subtypes, macrophages, and plasma cells were scored. The number of lymphoid follicles was increased in both the ileum and colon of patients with SpA. Spondyloarthropathic ileum showed an increase in leukocytes expressing CD11c, whereas cells expressing CD11a and vascular cell adhesion molecule-1 (VCAM-1) were increased in spondyloarthropathic colon. Macrophages, characterized by the expression of CD68, were more numerous in colonic mucosa from patients with SpA. The amounts of lymphoid follicles and lamina propria mononuclear cells expressing CD11a, CD11c, and VCAM-1 were increased in noninflamed gut mucosa from patients with SpA. These findings clearly demonstrate the presence of preinflammatory changes of the gut-associated immune system in SpA and suggest increased antigen handling and presentation and augmented maturation of naïve T cells toward memory T cells in spondyloarthropathic gut.

Investigating further the immune cells involved in antigen handling and presentation, the same authors analyzed macrophages and other antigen-presenting cells in gut mucosa from patients with SpA and Crohn's disease using a similar approach.[16] Biopsy samples from patients with SpA (again without macroscopic or microscopic signs of gut inflammation), Crohn's disease, and ulcerative colitis and from control subjects were immunohistochemically stained with different markers

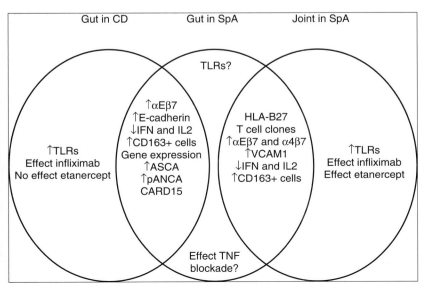

Fig. 2.2 Overlap in cellular and molecular disease mechanisms in gut and joint inflammation in SpA and in gut inflammation in Crohn's disease.

for macrophages and dendritic cells. SpA and Crohn's disease were associated with large numbers of CD68[+] macrophages. The colons of patients with both SpA and Crohn's disease, but not ulcerative colitis, showed increased numbers of macrophages expressing the scavenger receptor CD163. These findings again highlight the presence of early immune alterations in spondyloarthropathic gut mucosa, which are reminiscent of those in Crohn's disease and bring up a strong argument for a role of macrophages in this group of diseases.

Immune features in the gut mucosa of patients with spondyloarthropathy reminiscent of Crohn's disease

Besides these immune features preceding the occurrence of microscopic bowel inflammation, a number of histologic alterations related to inflammation also appeared to be common in SpA and Crohn's disease. E-cadherin mediates homotypic, homophilic intercellular adhesion in epithelial cells. It is a transmembrane glycoprotein, mainly localized to the zonula adherens junctions of all normal epithelia. An up-regulation of E-cadherin and its associated catenins was demonstrated in clinically overt IBD.[17] In SpA, expression of the proteins of the E-cadherin-catenin complex in acute and chronic subclinical gut inflammation was found to be increased as well,[18] especially at the sites of active inflammation. E-cadherin is not only involved in epithelial cell-cell adhesion but it is also a ligand for the $\alpha_E\beta_7$ integrin on intraepithelial T cells. We observed an up-regulated $\alpha_E\beta_7$ expression among interleukin (IL)-2 expanded T-cell lines (CD3 as well as CD8) from mucosal biopsy specimens from patients with AS,[19] a finding that has also been documented for patients with Crohn's disease.[20]

Mucosal T lymphocytes in SpA and Crohn's disease resemble each other not only phenotypically but also functionally. On T-cell activation, distinct lymphocyte populations can be distinguished: Th1 lymphocytes are characterized by the production of interferon (IFN)-γ and IL-2; Th2 lymphocytes secrete IL-4, IL-5, and IL-10. Our group studied T-cell cytokine profiles in the gut mucosa of patients with SpA and Crohn's disease.[21,22] There is a predominance of Th1-producing mucosal T cells in both conditions. However, in lamina propria lymphocytes in the colon in both SpA and Crohn's disease, a proportional decrease of IFN-γ and IL-2 producing CD3 and CD3[+]CD8[−] lymphocytes was observed.

Gene expression profiles in the gut in spondyloarthropathy and Crohn's disease

To elucidate the biologic dysregulation underlying gut inflammation in SpA, Laukens et al.[23] examined global gene expression in the gut mucosa and identified about 1500 expressed sequence tags that are up- or down-regulated in gut mucosa in SpA and Crohn's disease. These clones, together with the appropriate controls, were selected and used for designing a dedicated microarray. Gut biopsies of 17 patients with SpA, 14 patients with Crohn's disease, and 11 control subjects were analyzed by these microarray chips. Discriminant analysis was used to successfully distinguish gut biopsies from the three groups studied, suggesting that gene modification in the gut of patients with SpA is a biologically relevant concept. Also, the authors identified a set of genes that are candidates for early Crohn's disease markers in individuals with SpA who have subclinical gut inflammation.

Common gut-related serologic markers in spondyloarthropathy and Crohn's disease

An interesting new serum marker in the field of IBD is the anti-*Saccharomyces cerevisiae* antibody (ASCA). These antibodies were first described in patients with Crohn's disease (both immunoglobulin G [IgG] and immunoglobulin A [IgA] antibodies), and IgA ASCA levels were recently reported to be elevated in patients with AS.[24] Hoffman et al.[24] investigated whether ASCAs are present in SpA and in its subgroups AS, USpA, and PsA, in comparison with healthy control subjects or patients with RA. ASCA IgA and IgG levels were measured in 26 patients with Crohn's disease, 108 patients with SpA, 56 patients with RA, and 45 healthy control subjects. ASCA IgA levels were significantly higher in SpA, and more specifically in AS, than in healthy control subjects and patients with RA. No correlation between the presence of subclinical bowel inflammation and ASCA IgA levels was noted (although the relevant study groups were small). These data were recently confirmed by Torok et al.[25] These authors found that ASCA IgA but not ASCA IgG levels were significantly increased in patients with SpA compared with those in control subjects. Also in this study, IBD-associated perinuclear antineutrophil cytoplasmic antibodies (pANCAs) were often found in patients with SpA. Neither antibody, however, was associated with gastrointestinal symptoms. It remains speculative whether these IBD-related antibodies in SpA are associated with development of IBD.

Common gut-related genetic polymorphisms in spondyloarthropathy and Crohn's disease

A correlation has been reported between polymorphisms in the *CARD15* gene and an increased susceptibility for Crohn's disease.[26,27] Three independent single nucleotide polymorphisms (SNPs) in *CARD15* are associated with Crohn's disease in about 30% to 46% of patients (one frame-shift mutation, 1007fs [SNP13], and two missense mutations, R702W [SNP8] and G908R [SNP12]). These variants increase the risk for

Crohn's disease with factor 3 for heterozygous and factor 38 or 44 for, respectively, homozygous or compound heterozygous individuals. CARD15 encodes for an intracellular protein, which is expressed in monocytes, granulocytes, dendritic, epithelial, and Paneth cells and has binding affinity for bacterial cell wall components such as muramyl dipeptides. The CARD15 protein is involved in nuclear factor-κB activation and in apoptosis by two N-terminal caspase recruitment domains (hence the term CARD), although the precise pathogenetic role in Crohn's disease remains to be determined.

Several studies have been performed to investigate the role of CARD15 polymorphisms in SpA. These studies did not demonstrate an association with SpA or AS in particular.[28–32] In view of the apparent correlation between gut inflammation in SpA and clinical evolution to Crohn's disease, Laukens et al.[33] investigated the relationship between the presence of polymorphisms in this susceptibility gene for Crohn's disease and gut inflammation in patients with SpA. This study included 104 patients with SpA who underwent an ileocolonoscopy with histologic evaluation, and the prevalence of three SNPs in the CARD15 gene (R702W, G908R, and 1007fs) were identified by restriction fragment length polymorphism–polymerase chain reaction. The carrier frequencies of R702W, G908R, or 1007fs variants in the SpA populations was similar to those in the control population but was increased in the subgroup of patients with SpA who had chronic gut inflammation, being significantly higher than in the other SpA subgroups and in the control group, with no significant difference from the prevalence in patients with Crohn's disease. These findings demonstrate that the presence of CARD15 polymorphisms in patients with SpA is associated with a higher risk for development of chronic gut inflammation.

Evidence That Gut Inflammation in Spondyloarthropathy Is Pathogenetically Related to Peripheral Joint Inflammation

Relationship between gut and joint inflammation in animal models of spondyloarthropathy

As reviewed in the previous paragraphs, there is increasing genetic and immunologic evidence supporting the clinical and histologic overlap between gut inflammation in SpA and Crohn's disease. A second major issue suggested by the clinical findings is that gut inflammation is linked to peripheral joint disease in SpA, raising the question of common immunologic and inflammatory pathways in these two distinct organ manifestations of SpA (Fig. 2.3).

Several rodent models have illustrated that the induction of gut inflammation, essentially by influencing the normal gut flora, could lead to associated peripheral arthritis. A transient peripheral arthritis could be induced in rodents by bacteria from a patient with Crohn's disease[34] and by bacteria from gram-positive normal enteric flora.[35,36] Similarly, feeding pigs with a protein-rich diet, which resulted in an abnormal intestinal microbial flora with increased numbers of Clostridia perfringens and increased antibody titers to this organism, led to peripheral joint inflammation in these animals.[36] The best animal model illustrating the link between gut and joints is the transgenic HLA-B27/human β_2-microglobulin rat.[37] Rats from two of the transgenic lines (LEW 21-4H and 33-3) spontaneously developed a multiorgan inflammatory disease analogous to the human disorders related to HLA-B27

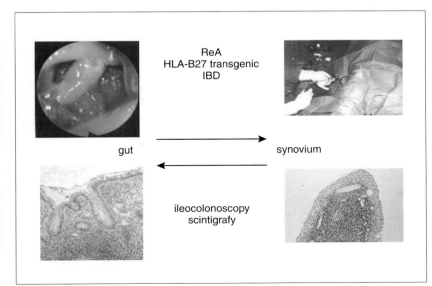

gut → synovium

ileocolonoscopy
scintigrafy

ReA
HLA-B27 transgenic
IBD

Fig. 2.3 Relationship between gut and joint inflammation in SpA is suggested by clinical observations (reactive arthritis), animal models (HLA-B27 transgenic rats), the overlap with IBD, as well as by histologic and scintigraphic studies indicating subclinical gut inflammation. The accessibility of gut and joint for biopsy sampling allows immunopathologic studies to unravel this relationship.

and involving the gastrointestinal tract, peripheral and axial joints, male genital tract, skin, nails, and heart. The most prevalent site of inflammation in the transgenic rats appeared to be the gastrointestinal tract, suggesting that the events initiating the disease process occur in the gastrointestinal tract. This was confirmed by the fact that the animals did not develop gut and joint inflammation when kept in a germ-free state.[2,38] Whereas this model illustrates well the link between gut and joint, it was surprising that the disease was not critically mediated by CD8+ T lymphocytes, but rather resulted from a failure of tolerance involving specific T-cell populations.[39,40] Alternatively, recent data suggest that T-cell–independent mechanisms contribute to the disease pathogenesis.[41]

T lymphocytes and the gut-joint axis in spondyloarthropathy

Based on the animal models, the role of bacterial antigens, and the major histocompatability complex (MHC) class I linkage, it has been proposed that HLA-B27 is involved in both the priming and the reactivation of cytotoxic CD8+ T lymphocytes by presenting either specific bacterial peptides or arthritogenic self-peptides cross-reacting with bacterial antigens. Supporting this hypothesis, the inflammatory infiltrate of the intestinal mucosa, the synovium, and the enthesis in SpA is rich in T cells, more particularly CD8+ T cells.[42–44] Moreover, recent studies have identified HLA-B27– restricted CD8 epitopes from the *C. trachomatis* and the *Y. enterocolitica* proteome in patients with ReA.[45,46] However, the T-cell response appears not to be restricted to CD8+ cells triggered in a MHC class I context, because CD4+ T cells specific for *Yersinia* and *Chlamydia* antigens were also raised from the synovial fluid in ReA.[46–48] Of interest, some of the CD4+ T-cell epitopes were nearly identical to the HLA-B27–restricted cytotoxic T-lymphocyte epitopes. In line with these findings in ReA, T-cell oligoclonality was demonstrated in both CD8+ and CD4+ T-cell subsets in AS.[49] Taken together, these data fit with the findings in the animal models and suggest the following hypothesis: specific T-cell populations (not restricted to CD8+) are primed by bacterial antigens at the place of the primary encounter with the bacterial antigens, the gut, and subsequently recirculate between the gut and the peripheral joint where they could be reactivated by bacterial antigens or by cross-reacting self-peptides.

The gut-joint recirculation of lymphocytes, which could at least partially explain the linkage between both disease localizations in SpA as well as in Crohn's disease, is supported by several immunologic studies looking at adhesion molecules involved in the homing of T lymphocytes to gut and synovium. In a recent study, gut-derived lymphocytes from patients with IBD were demonstrated to be able to bind to synovial vessels using multiple homing receptors and their corresponding endothelial ligands, including vascular adhesion protein-1.[50] As mentioned before, another series of studies highlighted the role of the β_7 integrins and their ligands, mucosal addressin cell adhesion molecule-1 (MadCAM-1), VCAM-1, and E-cadherin, in the gut inflammation in SpA. Of interest, there is also differential expression of the integrins $\alpha_E\beta_7$ and $\alpha_4\beta_7$ on synovium-derived T-cell lines in SpA, and one of the ligands of $\alpha_4\beta_7$, VCAM-1, is highly expressed in spondyloarthropathic synovium.[51,52] A formal proof of concept for the recirculation hypothesis has been put forward by the identification of identical T-cell expansions in the colon mucosa and the synovium of a patient with enterogenic spondyl-oarthropathy.[53]

As for the gut-derived lymphocytes, subsequent studies focused on the functional characterization of the T-cell cytokine profiles in the spondyloarthropathic joint. Paralleling the observations in the gut, low secretion of IFN-γ, IL-2, and/or tumor necrosis factor-α (TNF-α) and an increase of the IL-10 production by T cells was also reported in peripheral blood of patients with ReA,[54] AS,[55] and other types of SpA[56] compared with both healthy control subjects and patients with RA. Moreover, analysis of synovial fluid T cells and synovial membrane specimens in SpA and RA confirmed that the decreased Th1 (IFN-γ)/Th2 (IL-4) ratio also extended to the joints of patients with SpA.[57,58] These findings fit into the concept that a defective Th1 response, certainly at the mucosal site, may impair the immune defense against intracellular bacteria and thereby contribute to a decreased immune tolerance against bacterial antigens. To illustrate this theory, it was demonstrated that low secretion of TNF-α, but not of other T-cell cytokines, correlated with chronicity in ReA.[59] In conclusion, similar expression of T-lymphocyte adhesion molecules and their ligands and a similar functional behavior (impaired Th1/Th2 profile) further underscore the immunologic link between joint and gut in SpA and Crohn's disease. However, it remains unclear why the Th1 response is decreased and, by default of a Th1 response, how bacterial persistence might drive the inflammation. Studies on macrophages and the innate immune system may lead to new insights in this process.

Macrophages and the gut-joint axis in spondyloarthropathy

Beside antigen uptake and presentation by antigen-presenting cells to T lymphocytes leading to a T-cell–mediated inflammation, bacterial persistence can also lead to tissue inflammation by direct stimulation of inflammatory cells such as monocytes, macrophages, and neutrophils, but also intestinal epithelial cells (the so-called innate immune system). A group of molecules that plays a central role in the innate immune recognition of bacterial products are the macrophage scavenger receptors. The macrophage receptor with collagenous structure (MARCO), which plays a role in the defense against gram-negative bacteria, is up-regulated on peripheral blood mononuclear cells (PBMCs) of patients developing ReA but is low in the synovial compartment in SpA compared with RA, thus suggesting a defective host defense mechanism in the spondyloarthropathic joint.[60] Another scavenger receptor, CD163, was investigated in the gut and the joint of patients with SpA (Fig. 2.4). As previously mentioned, macrophages expressing CD163 are increased in the gut in Crohn's disease and SpA.[16] The same subset of macrophages was demonstrated to be selectively increased in spondyloarthropathic synovium, especially in HLA-B27+ SpA, compared with rheumatoid arthritic synovium and appeared thus to be another candidate for a role in the gut-synovium axis.[61] Functional studies on these CD163-positive macrophages indicated different possible roles in the disease pathogenesis. First, they appeared to produce high levels of soluble CD163 locally in the joint.[62] This soluble CD163 downregulated the activation of synovial T lymphocytes, which provides a second mechanism of impaired T-cell function beside the defects in antigen-presenting cells. Second, functional analysis in vitro has shown that these macrophages have a specific cytokine profile, with production of TNF-α but not IL-10 after lipopolysaccharide stimulation.[61,62] This is surprising because stimulation with the natural CD163 ligand, haptoglobin-hemoglobin complexes, usually leads to an anti-inflammatory response of these cells, suggesting that other receptors are involved.

In general, innate immune cells such as macrophages recognize microbial pathogen-associated molecular patterns through their Toll-like receptors (TLRs) and

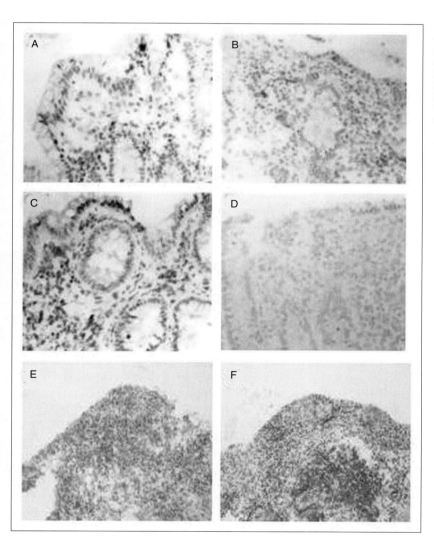

Fig. 2.4 Macrophages expressing the scavenger receptor CD163: a link between gut inflammation in Crohn's disease and SpA and between gut and joint inflammation in SpA. A: Gut in healthy control subject. **B:** Gut in SpA without clinical or histologic signs of inflammation. **C:** Gut in Crohn's disease. **D:** Gut in ulcerative colitis. **E:** Synovium in SpA. **F:** Synovium in RA.

initiate a rapid and quite nonspecific innate immune response upon TLR triggering. After binding of bacterial lipoproteins (TLR2), endotoxins (TLR4), flagellin (TLR5), bacterial CpG dinucleotides (TLR9), or bacterial heat shock proteins, the TLRs in association with the adaptor molecule MyD88 initiate a signaling cascade that results in the activation of nuclear factor-κB and the induction of oxidative stress, the production of inflammatory cytokines, apoptosis, and so on. Although these mechanisms have not yet been studied thoroughly in IBD and SpA, there is evidence of an abnormal expression of TLRs on gastrointestinal epithelial cells in IBD.[63] Of interest, we recently found that both TLR2 and TLR4 are also significantly increased in spondyloarthropathic synovium compared with rheumatoid arthritic synovium, which appeared to be at least partially related to the increased expression of these two TLRs on the CD163-positive macrophages (unpublished data).

Taken together with the previously mentioned role for NOD2/CARD15 in SpA, these data support the concept that the combination of microbial triggering and an abnormal inflammatory response of the innate immune system in genetically susceptible hosts can lead to a breakdown of the normal immunologic tolerance and to a pathogenic cellular immune response to specific bacterial species and/or cross-reacting self-molecules. As indicated, this may lead to a disturbed balance between pro-inflammatory cytokines such as TNF-α and anti-inflammatory cytokines such as IL-10, which may ultimately result in inflammation in the gut and the joint. Indeed, TNF-α has been demonstrated in the sacroiliacal joint of patients with AS and in synovium of patients with PsA.[64,65] Increased serum levels and stool concentrations of TNF-α and an elevated number of TNF-α–secreting mucosal cells were observed in patients with Crohn's disease,[66] and chronic exposure to high TNF-α levels can contribute to the impairment of a normal Th1 response, which plays an important role in the clearance of intracellular bacteria. Therefore, targeting pivotal cytokines involved in the innate immune balance such as TNF-α and IL-10 may be valuable strategies for immunotherapy of both gut and joint inflammation in SpA. Studies on TNF-α blockade have recently provided a proof of concept for this hypothesis.

Therapeutic and Biologic Implications
Infliximab therapy: from Crohn's disease to spondyloarthropathy

Patients with Crohn's disease were among the first to profit from anti-TNF-α therapy. The first multicenter, randomized, double-blind, placebo-controlled trial in patients with Crohn's disease included patients with moderate to severe disease.[67] The treatment produced a rapid and profound benefit for all response variables measured. Clinical improvement was also directly associated with endoscopic improvement.[68] A placebo-controlled study in patients with fistulizing Crohn's disease demonstrated a significant reduction in the number of open fistulae and complete remission in a significant number of patients.[69] Recent data from the ACCENT I (A Crohn's Disease Clinical Trial Evaluating Infliximab in a New Long Term Treatment) trial demonstrated that patients who respond to an initial dose of infliximab are more likely to be in remission at weeks 30 and 54, to discontinue corticosteroids, and to maintain their response for a longer period of time if infliximab therapy is maintained every 8 weeks.[70]

The pathogenetic link between SpA and Crohn's disease and the efficacy of infliximab in the latter disease, together with other rationales including the efficacy of infliximab in RA and increased expression of TNF-α in serum and at the sacroiliac joints in patients with AS, led to development of a clinical trial program with this compound in patients with AS and other forms of SpA. In the first pilot trial, Van den Bosch et al.[71] treated 4 patients with refractory Crohn's disease associated with SpA in an expanded access program of infliximab (5 mg/kg intravenous regimen). In all 4 patients, infliximab induced not only gastrointestinal remission but also remission of articular symptoms. The onset of effect was shortly after infliximab infusion. This pilot experience raised hope for efficacy of this new compound in the treatment of patients with SpA not associated with overt inflammatory bowel disease. The effect of infliximab in SpA associated with Crohn's disease was also confirmed in another open study.[72] These authors treated 24 patients affected by SpA associated with Crohn's disease for a period varying from 12 to 18 months. Infliximab improved both gastrointestinal and overall articular symptoms.

Shortly after the described pilot trial, two open studies with infliximab in SpA were concluded almost simultaneously in two European centers, namely Ghent and Berlin. The Ghent group engaged in a monocenter open study involving 21 patients fulfilling the European Spondyloarthropathy Study Group (ESSG) SpA classification criteria.[73] Patients with active treatment-resistant disease, including different subtypes, received three infusions of infliximab 5 mg/kg at weeks 0, 2, and 6. Spinal pain as well as peripheral symptoms improved significantly. The Berlin group treated 11 patients with AS and active disease with three infusions of infliximab (baseline and weeks 2 and 6; 5 mg/kg).[74] One patient withdrew because of urticarial xanthoma. Significant improvement was documented in 9 of the 10 patients and lasted for 6 weeks after the third infusion in 8 of 10 patients. In a later phase, they also treated 6 patients with undifferentiated SpA with infliximab at dosages of 3 or 5 mg/kg (baseline and weeks 2 and 6) over a 12-week period.[75]

Fast significant improvement lasting until week 12 was reported in 5 of 6 patients, with the 5 mg/kg dosage regimen having a superior effect. Spinal and peripheral symptoms responded equally. Several other groups further reported good results in open studies with infliximab in patients with AS or other types of SpA.

Based on the data of the open proof of concept studies, two double-blinded, placebo-controlled trials were again conducted simultaneously in Ghent and Berlin. Van den Bosch et al.[76] randomly assigned 40 patients with active SpA to receive a loading dose (infliximab 5 mg/kg at baseline and weeks 2 and 6) or placebo in a monocenter 12-week clinical trial. The primary end points were improvement in patient and physician global assessments of disease activity (visual analog scale). Both end points improved significantly in the verum group compared with baseline values, with no improvement in the placebo group. Braun et al.[77] assigned 70 patients with active AS to infliximab (5 mg/kg at baseline and weeks 2 and 6) or placebo in a multicenter 12-week study, with regression of disease activity of at least 50% as primary outcome. A highly significant effect of infliximab was achieved compared with placebo. A more recent 24-week multicenter, randomized placebo-controlled trial (ASSERT [Ankylosing Spondylitis Study for the Evaluation of Recombinant Infliximab Therapy] trial) confirmed the efficacy of infliximab in patients with AS.[78] Different questions remain open, including optimal dosing, long-term safety, and efficacy of this new treatment on the structural level. However, a therapeutic breakthrough like the one currently reviewed has seldom occurred in arthritis care.

Infliximab and etanercept act differentially on the gut inflammation in Crohn's disease and spondyloarthropathy

Although the efficacy of etanercept was later also confirmed in AS, the medical community has become aware of some important differences in specific disease situations between different TNF-α blockers such as infliximab and etanercept. In this sense, the differential effect of infliximab and etanercept for the treatment of chronic arthritis on the one hand and IBD on the other hand is striking. A clear benefit has been seen with infliximab treatment in patients with Crohn's disease. In contrast, in an 8-week randomized, double-blind, placebo-controlled trial, etanercept did not prove effective for this disease.[79] Also, Marzo-Ortega et al.[80] reported on two patients with SpA and associated Crohn's disease treated with etanercept whose arthritis showed an excellent response with complete resolution of spinal pathologic conditions, whereas their Crohn's disease persisted or flared. These findings suggest that the effect of TNF-α blockade with etanercept in SpA differs between the joint and the bowel.

Although it is still speculative at this point to try to explain the differences in biologic responses induced by the two anti–TNF-α compounds, several data deserve particular attention. Lügering et al.[81] reported that infliximab induced apoptosis in monocytes from patients with chronic active Crohn's disease. Peripheral blood monocytes from healthy volunteers and patients with chronic active Crohn's disease were isolated and apoptosis was determined by annexin V staining, DNA-laddering, and transmission electron microscopy. Activation of capases and mitochondrial release of cytochrome c was determined by immunoblotting. Treatment with infliximab at therapeutic concentrations resulted in monocyte apoptosis in patients with chronic active Crohn's disease in a dose-dependent manner. This was determined by annexin V binding and caspase-3 activation as soon as 4 hours after treatment with infliximab. Van den Brande et al.[82] investigated the differences in TNF-α–neutralizing capacity, human lymphocyte binding, and apoptosis-inducing capacity of infliximab and etanercept. They used a nuclear factor-κB reporter assay and a cytotoxicity bioassay to study TNF-α neutralization by both compounds. Lymphocyte binding and apoptosis-inducing capacity was investigated using fluorescence-activated cell sorter analysis, annexin V staining, and cleaved caspase-3 immunoblotting with mixed lymphocyte reaction-stimulated peripheral blood lymphocytes from healthy volunteers and lamina propria T cells from patients with Crohn's disease. Both infliximab and etanercept neutralized TNF-α effectively. Infliximab bound to activated peripheral blood lymphocytes and lamina propria T cells, whereas binding of etanercept was equal to a nonspecific control antibody. Infliximab but not etanercept induced peripheral and lamina propria lymphocyte apoptosis compared with a control antibody. Infliximab activated caspase-3 in a time-dependent manner, whereas etanercept did not. Thus, although both infliximab and etanercept showed powerful TNF-α neutralization, only infliximab was able to bind to peripheral blood lymphocytes and lamina propria T cells and subsequently to induce apoptosis of activated lymphocytes. These data may provide a biologic basis for the difference in efficacy of the two TNF-α–neutralizing drugs.

Other potential targets for immune therapy of gut and joint inflammation

Besides TNF-α blockers such as infliximab, other targeted therapies are in the pipeline for treating IBD and may be of interest for treating SpA, in view of the aforementioned pathogenetic relation between the two disease complexes. These agents include inhibitors of lymphocyte trafficking such as natalizumab or intercellular adhesion molecule-1 (ICAM-1) inhibitors, inhibitors of Th1 polarization such as anti-IL-12, and immunoregulatory cytokines such as IL-10.

Natalizumab is a humanized monoclonal anti-α_4 integrin antibody that blocks leukocyte migration. $\alpha_4\beta_1$ integrin on circulating leukocytes binds to VCAM-1. This allows leukocytes expressing this integrin to move from the peripheral blood into the tissues. Ghosh et al.[83] conducted a double-blind, placebo-controlled trial of natalizumab in 248 patients with moderate-to-severe Crohn's disease. Patients were randomly assigned to receive one of four treatments: two infusions of placebo; one infusion of 3 mg of natalizumab per kg of body weight, followed by placebo; two infusions of 3 mg of natalizumab per kg; or two infusions of 6 mg of natalizumab per kg. The group given two infusions of 6 mg of natalizumab per kg did not have a significantly higher rate of clinical remission than the placebo group at week 6. However, both groups that received two infusions of natalizumab had higher remission rates than the placebo group at multiple time points. The quality of life improved in all natalizumab groups; C-reactive protein levels improved in groups receiving two infusions of natalizumab. The compound is currently in phase III trials for the treatment of multiple sclerosis and Crohn's disease and will be further explored for its potential to treat chronic autoimmune arthritis such as RA. In view of the aforementioned data, it might have potential to treat SpA as well.

Biologic immunomodulation of the gut-synovium axis by tumor necrosis factor-α blockade in spondyloarthropathy

In consideration of the major clinical effect of infliximab in SpA, it was tempting to use it as a human TNF-α knock-down model to study the effect on various components of the gut-synovium axis such as T-cell cytokines, adhesion molecules, specific macrophage subsets, and their products. As mentioned before, patients with SpA have an impaired Th1/Th2 balance, with decreased T-cell production of IFN-γ and IL-2 and increased IL-10 synthesis. The impaired Th1 cytokine production is highly compatible with the clinical efficacy of TNF-α blockade. Treatment with three infusions of infliximab in patients with SpA resulted in a rapid and sustained increase of Th1 cytokines (IFN-γ and IL-2) to levels comparable with those in healthy control subjects.[56] A reduction in IL-10$^+$ T cells was observed in those patients with high baseline values. However, this effect was only observed in the first 4 weeks. No effect was seen on IL-4 production. Together, these data support the view that TNF-α blockade essentially reverses the state of anergy of Th1 cells, whereas no significant effect on Th2 cells is observed.

Further studies were undertaken to analyze the effect on immunopathologic and structural features of SpA.

In the first study, the synovial histopathology was assessed in 8 patients who were included in the Ghent open-label trial: 3 with AS, 1 with USpA, and 4 with PsA. In these patients who were treated with infliximab 5 mg/kg at weeks 0, 2, and 6, synovial biopsies were obtained at baseline, week 2, and week 12.[52] At baseline, the synovial tissue samples depicted the typical characteristics of spondyloarthropathic synovitis: a moderate lining hyperplasia, a strong hypervascularity with endothelial activation, and a moderate and diffuse inflammatory infiltration with macrophages as well as lymphocytes and polymorphonuclear cells. Evaluation at week 2 indicated a significant reduction in numbers of macrophages and polymorphonuclear cells in the sublining layer as well as an impaired expression of VCAM-1, the ligand for the $\alpha_4\beta_7$ integrin, suggesting that infliximab acts on spondyloarthropathic synovitis by reducing the influx of inflammatory cells. The effect on macrophages, neutrophils, and VCAM-1 was maintained at week 12, with an additional trend for reduction of CD4$^+$ lymphocytes. Interestingly, two other effects were observed at week 12. First, there was a decrease of the hypervascularity and a trend to reduction of the synovial lining hyperplasia, indicating that infliximab modulates the structural synovial characteristics of the disease. Second, there was a significant increase in the number of B cells and plasma cells in the synovium of the infliximab-treated patients suggesting that, at least in SpA, infliximab does not affect B-cell homing and/or maturation.

The histopathologic observations were extended to a second cohort of 15 patients included in the Ghent double-blind, placebo-controlled trial.[84] Twelve of the patients were treated with infliximab 5 mg/kg at weeks 0, 2, and 6, whereas 3 patients were treated with placebo. Biopsy sampling and histopathologic evaluation was performed in exactly the same way as in the first study. In the infliximab-treated group, evaluation at week 12 confirmed the reduction in lining layer hyperplasia, VCAM-1 expression in the lining, and hypervascularity. This was paralleled by a significant decrease of soluble vascular endothelial growth factor, E-selectin, and ICAM-1 in the serum of these patients. As to the inflammatory infiltration, there was a decrease in overall cell infiltration and number of macrophages, polymorphonuclear cells, and CD3$^+$, CD4$^+$, and CD8$^+$ T lymphocytes but no decrease of B cells and plasma cells. These data thus confirm the preliminary observations of the open study, indicating 1) a significant reduction in endothelial activation and inflammatory infiltration, 2) a structure-modifying effect on hypervascularity and lining layer hyperplasia, and 3) a differential effect of infliximab on T and B cells. Of interest, there was also a clear decrease of the specific CD163$^+$ macrophage subset,[62] which was paralleled by a decrease of the expression and function of TLR2 and -4, thereby pointing to a down-modulation of the innate immune inflammation as a fourth effect (unpublished data). More recently, all four effects were also demonstrated in patients with SpA treated with the soluble TNF-α receptor, etanercept (unpublished data).

Similarly, gene microarray experiments on spondyloarthropathic synovial biopsy specimens and normal PBMCs identified three groups of highly expressed genes in spondyloarthropathic synovium. With the pre- and post-infliximab samples, there was no effect on the first group, consisting of some major T-cell cytokines such as IL-2. However, there was a major impact on the group consisting of adhesion molecules such as VCAM-1 and chemokines (metaphase chromosome protein-1 [MCP1]), and on the group with matrix metalloproteinase (MMP)-3 and MMP-11. The effect on the adhesion molecules and the MMPs was confirmed by independent methods such as enzyme-linked immunosorbent assay and immunohistochemistry.[85,86] These results seem to indicate that infliximab acts on upstream pathways of VCAM-1 and MMPs, but does not suppress major T-cell cytokines. This is in agreement on one hand with the histopathologic observations on inflammatory infiltration and structure modification and on the other hand with the previous findings on cytokine profiles of lymphocytes in infliximab-treated patients.

Biologic stratification of patients with spondyloarthropathy for diagnosis and therapy

The growing insights into the pathogenesis and treatment of gut-joint–related diseases also have important clinical implications: Given the growing choice between different therapeutic alternatives, the heterogeneity of clinical expression and disease course, and the cost and safety issue of the new bioengineered therapies, it is mandatory that the best candidates for each given therapeutic option be selected. Thus, new diagnostic and therapeutic challenges arise: Which patient will benefit most from a given therapeutic modality? This choice implies the necessity for early diagnosis, careful evaluation of disease activity and risk factors for more severe disease, and prediction or early assessment of better response to therapy and decreased risk for side effects. Although this field is largely unexplored in SpA, the gut-synovium axis may provide us with a number of candidate biomarkers: genetic markers (HLA-B27 and CARD15), cytokine profiles, serum markers (soluble CD163 and serum MMPs), immunopathology of the disease tissues (gut and joint), and others. As a proof of concept, it has been shown that synovial histopathology can contribute to the diagnostic classification of patients presenting with an undifferentiated arthritis by predicting the diagnosis of SpA based solely on synovial analysis.[87] Furthermore, we recently demonstrated that synovial histopathology and especially synovial

infiltration with innate immune cells such as polymorphonuclear cells and CD163-positive macrophages reflects global disease activity in SpA and may thus be used as an additional surrogate outcome in early-phase clinical trials with new drugs in SpA (unpublished data). Finally, we identified a number of serum proteins (MMP3 and multidrug resistance protein [MRP] 8/MRP14) directly derived from the inflamed tissues as sensitive biomarkers for response to therapy in SpA (reference 85 and unpublished data). Further studies will have to be done to evaluate whether these and other biomarkers may help us to stratify in daily clinical practice our patients with SpA and Crohn's disease who have gut and joint inflammation.

Spondyloarthropathy-Crohn's Disease as a Prototype of Immune-Mediated Inflammatory Disease

In conclusion, we reviewed the ample experimental, clinical, genetic, histopathologic, and immunologic evidence for an important role of the gut in the pathogenesis of SpA and for an overlap between SpA and Crohn's disease. Although further fundamental studies are needed to unravel the cellular and molecular common pathways, with special attention for the innate immune system, these data suggest that SpA and Crohn's disease should be scientifically and clinically considered as distinct phenotypes of common immune-mediated inflammatory disease pathways rather than as separate disease entities (Fig. 2.5). Classification, diagnosis, and therapy based on pathophysiologic insights are likely to become superior to an approach based exclusively on signs and symptoms, as evidenced by the recent evolution in treatment of SpA by TNF-α blockade.

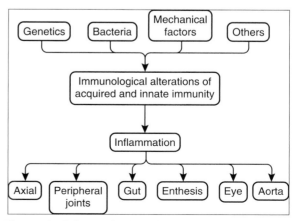

Fig. 2.5 Gut inflammation in Crohn's disease and SpA and joint inflammation in SpA are distinct phenotypic manifestations of common immune-mediated inflammatory disease pathways.

83. Ghosh S, Goldin E, Gordon FH, et al. Natalizumab for active Crohn's disease. N Engl J Med. 2003;348:24–32.

84. Kruithof E, Baeten D, Van den Bosch F, Mielants H, Veys EM, De Keyser F. Histological evidence that infliximab treatment leads to downregulation of inflammation and tissue remodelling of the synovial membrane in spondyloarthropathy. Ann Rheum Dis. 2005;64:529–536.

85. Vandooren B, Kruithof E, Yu DT, et al. Involvement of matrix metalloproteinases and their inhibitors in peripheral synovitis and down-regulation by tumor necrosis factor α blockade in spondyloarthropathy. Arthritis Rheum. 2004;50:2942–2953.

86. Yang C, Gu J, Rihl M, et al. Serum levels of matrix metalloproteinase 3 and macrophage colony-stimulating factor 1 correlate with disease activity in ankylosing spondylitis. Arthritis Rheum. 2004;51:691–699.

87. Baeten D, Kruithof E, De Rycke L, et al. Diagnostic classification of spondyloarthropathy and rheumatoid arthritis by synovial histopathology: a prospective study in 154 consecutive patients. Arthritis Rheum. 2004;50:2931–2941.

3

The Pathogenesis of Ankylosing Spondylitis

John D. Reveille and Matthew A. Brown

INTRODUCTION

Most rheumatic diseases are felt to be the result of the interaction of genes with the environment. Seronegative spondyloarthritis in general and ankylosing spondylitis (AS) in particular have provided some of the best examples of this interaction. The descriptions of the association of human leukocyte antigen (HLA)-B27 with AS more than 30 years ago[1,2] was a landmark in the modern era of genetic analysis, catalyzing a generation of investigators to examine the associations of HLA and other hereditary markers in other rheumatic diseases. In most cases, such studies were less rewarding, and in few other rheumatic diseases has the predictive value of any genetic marker been so robust. HLA-B27 testing is often used in diagnosis by clinicians and the association of AS with HLA-B27 remains one of the best examples of a disease association with a hereditary marker.

Many questions remain unanswered, however. Even after 30 years, the mechanism by which HLA-B27 actually causes AS is not well understood. Moreover, most HLA-B27–positive individuals never develop AS or other spondyloarthritis.[3] Furthermore, approximately 5% to 10% of patients with AS do not have the HLA-B27 gene, although whether AS in these patients has the same etiopathogenesis as AS in HLA-B27–positive patients is uncertain. In some ethnic groups (i.e., those of African extraction), up to half of the patients with AS lack HLA-B27.[4] Finally, very little is known about what triggers the onset of spondylitis in the genetically predisposed individual.

In this chapter, the pathogenesis of AS is reviewed, especially covering the genetic component, the possible roles that HLA-B27 may play in disease susceptibility, genetic studies in families (including genome-wide scans), studies of genes other than HLA-B27, and finally the impact of nongenetic (i.e., infectious and mucosal) factors in susceptibility to AS.

THE GENETIC CONTRIBUTION TO ANKYLOSING SPONDYLITIS

Familial Aggregation

A hereditary predisposition has been shown for most rheumatic diseases, as documented by clustering in family members of patients, especially in twin studies (in which nonidentical twins share a common environment but differ genetically), and in disease associations with hereditary markers. In genetically predisposed individuals, environmental influences such as infections or chemicals can interact to trigger disease onset. These and other genetic factors continue to affect disease pathogenesis, ultimately influencing outcome. Susceptibility to AS is clearly attributable to genetic factors, with a well-documented and long-recognized tendency toward familial aggregation,[5] a concordance rate in identical twins as high as 63% (compared to 23% in nonidentical twins)[6] and a disease heritability exceeding 90%.[7]

Familial aggregation in other types of spondyloarthritis has been less extensively studied. It has been reported that AS and reactive arthritis (ReA), although both associated with HLA-B27, tend to run separately in families, suggesting that they have different genetic risk factors. More recently, in an excellent segregation analysis, Breban et al.[8] investigated the familiality of undifferentiated spondyloarthritis and AS. Families with multiple patients with spondyloarthritis could be clustered into two groups, one having typical disease features of AS and the other having disease features more closely resembling those of undifferentiated spondyloarthritis. These clusters were inherited distinctly, suggesting that they are determined by specific genetic factors.

Basic Genetic Principles

To the nongeneticist, genetic terminology seems like a language unto itself and frustrates attempts to understand the published literature. We introduce some of the basic terminology here.[9] A *gene* is a specific sequence of DNA that encodes a protein. A gene may occur in specific forms or states called *alleles*. The relative frequencies in the population of the difference alleles of a gene are called *gene frequencies*. A *locus* is a general term that denotes a specific place on a chromosome. A *genetic marker* is a specific locus that is variable in the population under study. There are two main types of genetic markers that have been analyzed in recent genetic studies: 1) *single nucleotide polymorphisms* (SNPs) and 2) *microsatellites*. Microsatellites are a type of *variable number of tandem repeat* (VNTR) markers, which are characterized by a core sequence of DNA consisting of a number of identical repeated sequences. Microsatellite loci are found in large numbers and are relatively evenly spaced throughout the genome, like mile markers on a highway.

The expression (or observable result) of a particular gene or genotype is called a *phenotype*. *Penetrance* is the conditional probability of observing the corresponding phenotype given the presence of the specific genotype. *Hardy-Weinberg equilibrium* indicates that the genotype frequencies in a given population depend only on the gene frequencies; in other words, that selective external pressures are not at work. A *centimorgan* (cM) is a measure of genetic distance between two loci; 1 cM is the distance between two loci that will recombine with a frequency of exactly 1% during one meiotic event.

There are two ways to establish whether a gene is involved in susceptibility to a disease: linkage analysis and allele association analysis. *Linkage* describes the phenomenon whereby loci that are close to one another on the same chromosome tend to be transmitted together from generation to generation more often than they would be by chance. *Linkage analysis* is the examination of the probability that two genes or traits are in linkage. There are two different techniques of linkage analysis: *parametric* and *nonparametric*.

In *parametric (model-based) linkage analysis*, the parameters assumed include: 1) Transmission mode of disease (i.e., dominant or recessive); 2) recombination fraction; 3) trait allele frequencies; 4) penetrance values for each possible disease phenotype; and 5) marker allele frequencies. The likelihood of linkage is usually expressed by the term *LOD score*, which is a statistical estimate of whether two loci are likely to lie near each other on a chromosome and are therefore likely to be inherited together as a package. LOD stands for logarithm of the odds (to the base 10). A LOD score of 3 or more is generally taken to indicate that two gene loci are close to each other on the chromosome, with odds of 1000 to 1 in favor of genetic linkage.

Nonparametric (or model-free) linkage analysis focuses on allele sharing, usually in sib-pairs. In nonparametric linkage analysis, allele-sharing methods test whether affected relatives inherited a region *identical by descent* or *identical by sharing* more often than expected under random Mendelian segregation. The principle here is simple: if the marker locus is independent of the trait locus, the probabilities of the affected sib-pairs sharing 0, 1, or 2 alleles identical by descent will remain as 0.25, 0.50, or 0.25, respectively. However, if the marker locus is linked to the trait locus, affected sib-pairs will share on average more alleles identical by descent.

The other type of genetic analysis is *allelic association analysis*. This can be carried out in two ways:

1. *Population-based.* Population-based (case-control) analysis is robust and has been the most widely used to date. The major pitfalls of case-control studies are stratification error and lack of power. In the former, the patient and the control population may be different (mismatched)—this can occur particularly in studies using community-based patients and university-based control subjects in which subjects from a much broader geographic distribution may be included. On the other hand, many, if not most, case-control studies reported thus far are limited by power issues, particularly when the genetic factor under analysis provides only a small contribution to disease susceptibility, such as is seen in complex diseases.

2. *Family-based.* The transmission disequilibrium test (TDT) is a test of both linkage and linkage disequilibrium. The TDT compares the number of times alleles at a locus are transmitted and nontransmitted from heterozygous parents to offspring. Here the clinical status of the parents is irrelevant—what matters is what genes or haplotypes are or are not passed on to the affected offspring. The TDT avoids "spurious" false-positive results that may be seen with case-control study designs.

The Major Histocompatibility Complex

The gene encoding HLA-B27 sits in the class I region of the major histocompatibility complex (MHC), which spans over 3.6 megabases of DNA on the short arm of chromosome 6 (6p) (Fig. 3.1). The MHC contains more than 220 genes, many of which are crucial to immune functioning, especially in the processing and presentation of antigens to T cells.[10] This interaction is critical in combating microbiologic invasions, controlling malignant cell proliferation, and governing transplant success.

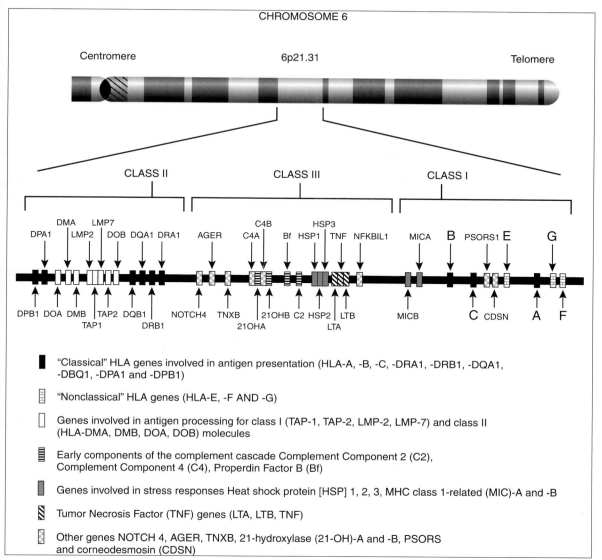

Fig. 3.1

Major histocompatibility complex class I genes

The MHC class I region contains the histocompatibility genes, as well as other genes involved in stress responses (MHC class I associated chain (MIC) genes, see later). MHC class I molecules fall into two groups: "classical" or type Ia molecules (HLA-A, -B, and -C) and "nonclassical" molecules (HLA-E, -F, and -G). In addition to these are a number of HLA class I–like sequences, such as HLA-H and HLA-J, whose expression is doubtful and which are regarded as pseudogenes.[10]

Type Ia (HLA-A, -B, and -C) molecules have widespread expression on most tissues and an extraordinary degree of polymorphism (Table 3.1), especially around the peptide binding groove (Fig. 3.2). HLA-A,

-B and -C molecules play an important role in antiviral immunity, binding viral peptides and conveying them to the cell surface where they are recognized by cytotoxic T cells. They also interact with receptors on natural killer (NK) cells to inhibit lytic activity and cytokine production. As of May 2005, more than 675 alleles have been described at HLA-B alone (www.ebi.ac.uk/imgt/hla/), making it the most polymorphic gene in the human genome (Table 3.1).

MHC class Ib genes include HLA-E, -F, and -G. They have a low level of tissue expression and show limited polymorphism (Table 3.1). HLA-E presents hydrophobic peptides from leader sequences of other class I molecules to CD94/NKG2 receptors on NK and T-cells, although

TABLE 3.1 POLYMORPHISM AT HLA LOCI*	
HLA	Number of Alleles*
Class I	
A	373
B	675
C	190
E	5
F	2
G	15
Class II	
DRA1	3
DRB1	399
DQA1	28
DQB1	62
DOA	9
DOB	9
DMA	4
DMB	7
DPA1	23
DPB1	118

*As of April 2005.

HLA-E–peptide complexes can also be recognized through α:β T-cell receptors (TCRs).[11] HLA-G is a nonclassical MHC class I molecule that is primarily expressed at the fetal-maternal interface, where it is thought to play a role in protecting the fetus from the maternal immune response.[12] HLA-G binds a limited repertoire of peptides and interacts with the inhibitory leukocyte immunoglobulin (Ig)–like receptors LIR-1 and LIR-2 and possibly with certain NK cell receptors. HLA-F is considered to be the progenitor of all MHC class I genes.[13] Its function is unknown, and it has not been demonstrated on the cell surface. HLA-F has a restricted pattern of expression in tonsil, spleen, and thymus, and structural predictions based on the sequence of HLA-F suggest that it may bind peptides and may reach the cell surface under appropriate conditions.

Major histocompatibility complex class II genes

The products of HLA-DR, -DQ, and -DP genes are expressed as α:β heterodimers on the surface of B cells, activated T cells, dendritic cells, and other somatic cells after induction by γ-interferon. They are required for the recognition of foreign (exogenous) antigens by T-helper cells. As with class I genes, there are classical MHC class II genes (HLA-DR, -DQ, and -DP), thought to function primarily in antigen presentation

and the nonclassical group (HLA-DM, HLA-DO, TAP, and LMP), which function more in peptide processing and loading. The classical HLA class II genes have been implicated in many rheumatic diseases (reviewed in reference 14).

Classical major histocompatibility complex class II genes

The HLA-DR region is composed of one nonpolymorphic *DRA* gene whose product combines with the product of numerous *DRB* genes to form the HLA-DR heterodimers. Most of the polymorphism of classic HLA-DR molecules is derived from the *DRB1* gene, where more than 399 DNA polymorphisms are now recognized (Table 3.1). The presence and number of other DRB loci vary on different HLA-DR haplotypes. The HLA-DQ molecule is composed of the product of the two *DQA* and two *DQB* genes, with only one of each (*DQA1* and *DQB1*) encoding a functional product. HLA-DP is the last and most centromeric-lying of the classical class II loci to be described.

Other major histocompatibility complex class II alleles

A number of genes relevant to antigen processing lie between HLA-DQ and -DP. In the MHC class II pathway, HLA-DM functions in the loading and editing of peptides; recent work demonstrated that it is acting not only in late endosomal compartments but also in recycling compartments and on the surface of B cells and immature dendritic cells.[15] The genes encoding the α and β chains of HLA-DM, *DMA,* and *DMB* lie between HLA-DQ and the *TAP-LMP* gene complex. HLA-DO is a nonpolymorphic MHC class II–like heterodimer composed of DOA and DOB. It is expressed in B lymphocytes and modulates the peptide loading activity of HLA-DM in the endocytic pathway.[16] Binding to HLA-DM is required for HLA-DO to egress from the endoplasmic reticulum. Peptides generated mainly by proteasomes in the cytosol are transported into the lumen of the endoplasmic reticulum by transporters associated with antigen processing (TAP) for loading onto MHC class I molecules.[17] The low molecular weight proteosome (LMP)-2 and -7 genes encode two subunits of a multicatalytic proteinase (proteasome) complex whose function is to degrade cytosolic proteins into peptides that are subsequently bound by MHC class I molecules.[17]

Major histocompatibility complex class III genes

This region, located between HLA class I and class II, is densely packed with immunologically relevant genes. In addition to the *TNF* loci (containing the genes *LTA, LTB,* and *TNF*) (Fig. 3.1) and the heat shock protein (HSP) genes (see later), the genes encoding the early components of the complement cascade (complement

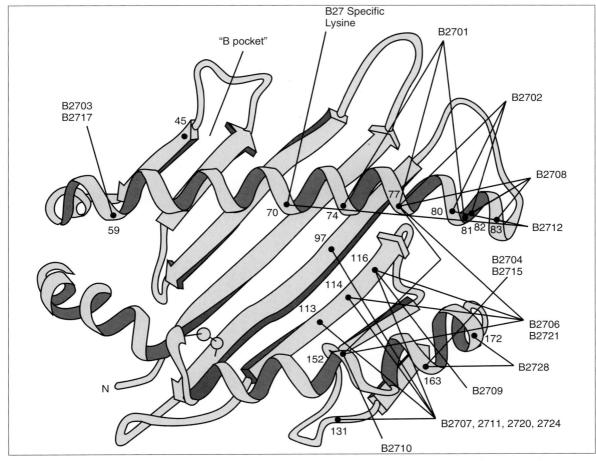

Fig. 3.2 The crystallized HLA-B27 molecule, indicating positions of amino acid substitutions in selected HLA-B27 subtypes.

components C2, C4, and properdin factor B [Bf] and the 21-hydroxylase A and B genes are found here. The relevance of these latter factors to AS susceptibility has not been established. In addition, a number of new genes have been described in the class III region of the MHC that need further study in AS susceptibility,[18] including, among others, the nuclear factor (NF) κB-IL1 (*NFKB-IL1*) gene, which encodes a protein resembling members of the I κB protein family that regulate bioavailability of NF-κB[19]; the *TNXB* gene, which encodes a protein called tenascin X, important in neural development and recently implicated in susceptibility to schizophrenia[20] and mutations of which cause a form of Ehlers-Danlos syndrome[21]; the *NOTCH4* gene, which encodes an oncogenic protein that is important in regulating vascular development and remodeling, and which has recently been implicated in susceptibility to alopecia areata[22]; and the receptor for AGE (advanced glycation end products) (AGER or RAGE), a member of the immunoglobulin superfamily, a specific cell surface interaction site for the products of nonenzymatic glycation/oxidation of proteins/lipids, which accumulate in natural aging and chronic inflammatory disorders.[23]

HLA-B27 and ankylosing spondylitis

HLA-B27, which is encoded in the MHC class I region, confers the greatest known risk for AS and is found in more than 90% of patients of European ancestry with AS (reviewed in references. 24 and 25). Approximately 70% of patients with ReA have HLA-B27, except in Africa, where no association of HLA-B27 is seen in those with human immunodeficiency virus (HIV)–associated ReA and spondyloarthritis.[26] HLA-B27 is found in 60% to 70% of patients with psoriatic spondylitis and in 25% of those with peripheral psoriatic arthritis (PsA). Up to 70% of those with irritable bowel disease (IBD)-associated spondylitis have HLA-B27, although no HLA-B27 association is seen with asymptomatic sacroiliitis. Approximately 50% of patients with acute anterior uveitis (AAU) alone are HLA-B27 positive.[27]

HLA-B27 subtypes

More than 27 molecular subtypes of HLA-B27 have been described thus far (www.ebi.ac.uk/imgt/hla/) (Table 3.2).[24,28] Most of these subtypes differ from each other by only a very few amino acids, which alter the peptide-binding properties of the molecule (Fig. 3.2).

TABLE 3.2 AMINO ACID SEQUENCE OF HLA-B27 SUBTYPES IN THE DIVERSITY REGIONS OF THE FIRST AND SECOND DOMAINS

Position	60	70	80	90	100	110	120	131	151	160	172
B*270502	EYW	DRETQICKAK	AQTDREDLRT	LLRYNQSEA	GSHTLQNMYG	CDVGPDGRLL	RGYHQDAYDG	SSWTA	RVAEQLRAYLEGE	CVEWLRRYL	
B*2701	—	—	—Y—N—	A—	—	—	—	—	—	—	—
B*2702	—	—	—N—I	A—	—	—	—	—	—	—	—
B*2703	-H-	—	—	—	—	—	—	—	—	—	—
B*2704	—	—	—S—	—	—	—	—	—	-E	—	—
B*270503	—	—	—	—	—	—	—	—	—	—	—
B*270504	—	—	—	—	—	—	—	—	—	—	—
B*270505	—	—	—	—	—	—	—	—	—	—	—
B*270506	—	—	—	—	—	—	—	—	—	—	—
B*270507	—	—	—	—	—	—	—	—	—	—	—
B*270508	—	—	—	—	—	—	—	—	—	—	—
B*2706	—	—	—S—	—	—	—	—D-Y—	—	-E	—	—
B*2707	—	—	—	—	—S—	—	—HN-Y—	R—	—	—	—
B*2708	—	—	—S—N	—RG—	—	—	—	—	—	—	—
B*2709	—	—	—	—	—	—	—H—	—	—	—	—
B*2710	—	—	—	—	—S—	—	—HN-Y—	R—	-E	—	—
B*2711	—	—	—S—	—RG—	—	—	—	—	—	—	—
B*2712	—	T——TN	——S—N	—	—	—	—	—	—	—	—
B*2713	—	—	—	—	—	—	—	—	—	—	—

B*2716	---		T-	---	---	---	---	---	---	---
B*2717	-F-	TN		---	---	---	---	---	---	---
B*2718	---		---S-	T—Y—S—N	-RG—	---	---	---	-E	---
		TN								
B*2719	---				---	--II-R--	---	---	---	---
B*2720	---		—S—		---	---	---	HN-Y	R	-E
B*2721	---		—S—		R—	---	---	—D-Y	---	-E
B*2723	---		—N—F-	T—Y—S—	---	---	---	---	---	---
		TN								
B*2724	---		—S—		---	—S—	---	—HN-Y	R	-E
B*2725	---		—S—		---	---	---	---	---	-E—W—L
B*2726	---		—S—	-RG—	---	---	---	---	---	---
	Q									
B*2727	---		---	---	---	---	---	—HN-Y	---	---
B*2728	---		---	---	---	---	---	---	---	-T---H-

HLA-B*2705 is found in all populations and appears to be the original or "parent" HLA-B27 molecule. Most of the other subtypes appear to have evolved from three pathways, defined by the pattern of amino acid substitutions in the first (α_1) and second (α_2) domains and along geographic patterns (Fig. 3.3).[24] One pathway is characterized by substitutions in the α_1 domain and accounts for HLA-B27 subtypes seen in European Caucasians and Africans. The second, which accounts for polymorphisms seen in eastern Asia, involves a specific substitution in the α_1 domain and different patterns of diversity in the α_2 domain. A third pathway appears to have evolved in southern Asia and the Middle East, and includes subtypes identical to HLA-B*2705 in the α_1 domain but differing in α_2. The two exceptions are HLA-B*2713, an Iberian subtype that differs from B*2705 in the signal peptide at the −20 position, resulting in an Ala to Glu substitution, and HLA-B*2718, an Asian B27 subtype that has numerous substitutions in the α_1 domain but is identical to HLA-B*2705 in α_2.

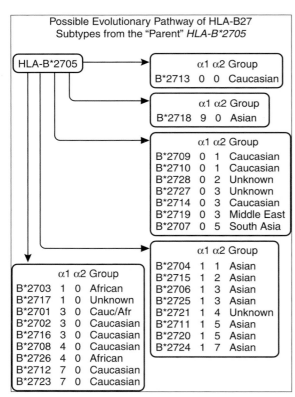

Fig. 3.3 Possible evolutionary pathway of HLA-B27 subtypes from the "parent" *HLA-B*2705*. The three major families of HLA-B27 subtypes (*HLA-B*2713* and *B*2718* are assumed to have evolved separately) are denoted in relationship to the parent subtype *HLA-B*2705*. The number of amino acid substitution from B*2705 in the first (α1) and second (α2) domains are indicated, as well as the predominant ethnic group in which the subtype was described. For example, *HLA-B*2704* differs from HLA-B27 by one amino acid substitution in the α1 and one amino acid substitution in the α2 domain.

The most common subtypes (HLA-B*2705, B*2702, B*2704, and B*2707) are clearly associated with spondyloarthritis.[24] Two subtypes of HLA-B27, HLA-B*2706 and B*2709, found in southeast Asia and Sardinia, respectively, appear not to be associated with AS,[22] possibly due to amino acid differences in the "B" pocket of the HLA antigen-binding cleft, which could alter the composition of peptides presented by these HLA-B27 subtypes. The only difference between the AS-associated HLA-B*2705 and the nonassociated HLA-B*2709 subtypes is the exchange of position 116 from aspartate to histidine, which is located within the peptide-binding groove at the floor of the F pocket and plays a pivotal role in anchoring the COOH-terminal peptide residue, as demonstrated by differences in the repertoires of peptides eluted from HLA-B*2705 and B*2709 molecules.[28] The other subtypes of HLA-B27 are too rare to have had disease associations established, although cases of AS have also been reported in carriers of B*2701, *2703, *2704, *2707, *2708, *2710, *2714, *2715, and *2719.

The exact mechanism underlying the effect of HLA-B27 on disease susceptibility still has not been determined.[29] As an MHC class I protein, the classical function of HLA-B27 is to present endogenous (i.e., viral, bacterial, and tumor) peptides to the α:β T-cell antigen receptor on cytotoxic (CD8[+]) T lymphocytes. However, in addition to their classical antigen-presenting role, HLA class I proteins are recognized by members of the killer immunoglobulin receptor family on NK cells, although how this contributes to disease susceptibility remains to be established.

Unique properties of HLA-B27

Several features of HLA-B27 make it unique among HLA class I molecules and may influence its role in disease susceptibility.[30] One such property of HLA-B27 is that free heavy chains of HLA-B27 can reach the cell surface in the absence of β_2-microglobulin and maintain their peptide-binding groove in vitro. Alternative recognition of different forms of HLA-B27 by leukocyte receptors could influence the function of cells from both innate and adaptive immune systems and may indicate a role for various leukocyte populations in spondyl-oarthritis.

Putative roles of HLA-B27 in the pathogenesis of ankylosing spondylitis

The exact mechanism underlying the effect of HLA-B27 on disease susceptibility still has not been determined. Four different theories exist (Fig. 3.4):

1. *Arthritogenic peptide hypothesis.* This hypothesis suggests that AS results from the ability of HLA-B27 to bind a unique antigenic peptide or a set of antigenic peptides, either bacterial or self.[28–31]

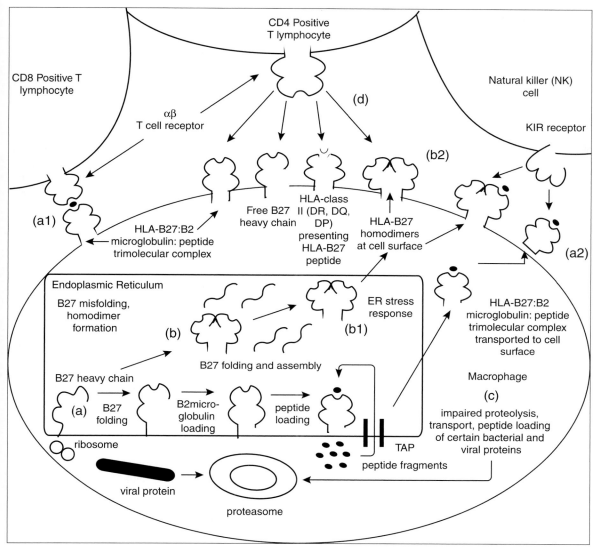

Fig. 3.4 Unique intracellular and extracellular functions of HLA-B27 that may affect susceptibility to spondyloarthritis. a) The HLA-B27 heavy chain is transcribed off ribosomes in macrophages, and folded onto β_2-microglobulin, and antigenic peptide is loaded via the TAP proteins onto it in the endoplasmic reticulum (ER). Thence the trimolecular peptide complex (HLA-B27 heavy chain, β_2-microglobulin and peptide) travels to the cell surface, where the antigenic peptide is presented either to the α:β TCR on CD8+ T lymphocytes or to the killer immunoglobulin (KIR) receptor on NK cells. **b)** The HLA-B27 heavy chain misfolds in the endoplasmic reticulum, forming B27 homodimers and other misfoldings, where it either **b1)** accumulates there, causing an proinflammatory endoplasmic reticulum stress response or **b2)** the B27 homodimers migrate to the cell surface where they either become antigenic themselves or present peptide to receptors on other inflammatory cells. **c)** Intracellular impairment of peptide processing or loading into HLA-B27 by viruses or intracellular bacteria causes a selective impairment of the immune response or **d)** either the trimolecular complex presents processed peptide to the α:β TCR on CD4+ T lymphocytes or free HLA-B27 heavy chains or HLA-B27 homodimers are recognized as antigenic by the TCR thence or processed antigenic fragments of HLA-B27 are presented to the TCR of CD4+ T lymphocytes.

Disease results from an HLA-B27–restricted cytotoxic T-cell response to this (these) peptide(s) found only in joints and other affected tissues. Such a peptide could be bound and presented by all disease-associated HLA-B27 subtypes but not by other HLA class I molecules. Pathogenic T cells then could be primed in the joint or in other sites, such as the genital or gut mucosa,

which could then result in a breakdown of self-tolerance by initial HLA-B27–restricted presentation of a peptide or peptides derived from one of the triggering pathogens. Evidence for this hypothesis comes from the identification of HLA-B27–restricted peptides from the *Chlamydia trachomatis* proteome,[32] as well as from molecular mimicry between endogenous B27 peptides and

TABLE 3.3 GENETIC FACTORS IMPLICATED IN SPONDYLOARTHRITIS				
Factor	Ankylosing Spondylitis	Reactive Arthritis	Psoriatic Arthritis/Spondylitis	Enteropathic Arthritis/Spondylitis
HLA-B27 frequency	90%–95%	70%–80%	24%/60%	7%/70%
Other MHC genes	HLA-B60, *DRB1*0101*	HLA-DR4	HLA-B38, B39, Cw6, DR4	*DRB1*0103*
Non-MHC genes	*CYP2D6, IL-1 genes, (ANKH?)*	n.s.*	*NOD2/CARD15*	*NOD2/CARD15 (IBD1)*
Chromosomal regions implicated in genome scans	Chr.2q, 6q, 10q, 11q, 16q, 19q	n.s.	PSORS1 (chr. 6), PSORS2 (chr.17q)	IBD2, IBD3

*n.s., not studied.

environmental antigens.[33] This is further suggested by the demonstration of CD8[+] T-cell autoreactivity to an HLA-B27-restricted self-epitope correlating with the presence of AS[34] and shared TCR β-chain sequences among different HLA-B27–positive patients with ReA.[35,36] The strongest evidence against this theory is that a specific "arthritogenic peptide" has yet to be demonstrated and that none of the supportive evidence described earlier has yet explained the reduced association of HLA-B*2706 and B*2709 with disease.

2. *HLA-B27 homodimer formation.* Self-association is a unique property of the HLA-B27 molecule. HLA-B27 heavy chains can form homodimers in vitro that depend on disulfide binding through their cysteine-67 residues in the extracellular α_1 domain.[37,38] This occurs as a result of B27 misfolding within the endoplasmic reticulum, and the accumulation of misfolded protein may result in a proinflammatory intracellular stress response. HLA-B27 homodimers are detectable at the cell surface in patients with spondyloarthritis, are capable of peptide binding, and are more abundantly expressed when the antigen-presenting function of the cell is impaired. They are ligands for a number of NK and related cell surface receptors. Populations of synovial and peripheral blood monocytes and B and T lymphocytes from patients with spondyloarthritis and control subjects carry receptors for HLA-B27 homodimers, including KIR3DL1 and KIR3DL2, which are receptors for NK cells, and immunoglobulin-like transcript 4 (ILT4).[39] It is possible that these homodimers may act as a proinflammatory target or receptor for humoral or cell-mediated autoimmune responses. However, the presence of cysteine-67 in the HLA-B27 molecule is not required for the development of arthritis in HLA-B27 transgenic rats. Moreover, it is not yet known whether HLA-B27 homodimer formation is specific for or even correlates with the presence of spondyloarthritis.

3. *Alteration of intracellular invasion/killing.* Intracellular persistence of arthritogenic organisms may contribute to the cellular basis for ReA, but the molecular basis of the bactericidal pathways in synoviocytes has not been fully resolved. HLA-B27–positive U937 cells kill *Salmonella* less efficiently than controls, and show up-regulated production of interleukin-10 and to a lesser extent tumor necrosis factor (TNF)-α. HLA–B27–associated modulation of cytokine response profiles may have importance in the pathogenesis of ReA.[40,41]

4. *HLA-B27 as an autoantigen.* HLA-B27 can be recognized by CD4[+] T cells[42] and can be presented by HLA class II (DR, DQ, and DP) heterodimers to CD4[+] T lymphocytes. HLA-B27–transgenic rats are tolerant of B27 immunization using either B27[+] splenocytes or plasmid DNA and do not develop anti-B27 cytotoxic T lymphocytes. If splenocytes from such immunized animals are exposed to *Chlamydia* in vitro, cytotoxic T lymphocytes are generated that lyse HLA-B27[+] targets but not targets transfected with control HLA-B7, -B14, -B40, or -B44,[43] suggesting that HLA-B27 per se or an altered form thereof may actually drive disease development.

Other major histocompatibility complex genes and susceptibility to ankylosing spondylitis

Studies to date have suggested that HLA-B27 constitutes only part of the overall risk for spondyloarthritis. Less than 5% of HLA-B27–positive individuals in the general population develop a spondyloarthritis.[3] On the other hand, 20% of HLA-B27–positive relatives of AS patients will develop a spondyloarthritis. Family studies have suggested that HLA–B27 contributes only about 37% of the overall genetic risk for spondyloarthritis.[6,7] The entire effect of the MHC, on the other hand, is about 50%.

Other MHC genes also have been implicated in AS in addition to B27. Identifying those genes is particularly complex given the complicated patterns of linkage disequilibrium found within the MHC and the consequent difficulty in identifying true associations with those due to linkage disequilibrium alone. Large systematic studies are now being performed, but there is strong evidence from studies of individual MHC genes to date to support the presence of other non-B27 MHC genetic effects on susceptibility to AS.

HLA-B60, a serologically defined HLA specificity that correlates with HLA-B*4001 on DNA analysis,[44] has been described as augmenting the risk for AS in both HLA-B27-positive and -negative individuals from Europe and Taiwan.[45–48]

Major histocompatibility complex class I associated chain genes

In addition to HLA-B genes, other MHC loci have been suggested as being operative in susceptibility to AS.[49] Several MIC genes and pseudogenes are found in the class I region of the MHC. Two of them, MICA and MICB, located 46.4 and 110 kb, respectively, centromeric from HLA-B, are known to be functional. MICA encodes a polypeptide of 383 amino acids with the same overall organization as an HLA class I molecule, but with only 15% to 36% sequence homology, and is the most polymorphic, with more than 50 alleles described. MIC proteins are considered to be markers of "stress" in the epithelia and act as ligands for cells expressing a common activatory NK receptor (NKG2D). Although several groups have examined MIC polymorphisms in patients with AS, any associations that were seen were better explained by linkage to HLA-B27.[50–53]

Tumor Necrosis Factor-α.

With the striking proinflammatory properties of TNF and the dramatic response of AS to anti-TNF therapy, it is entirely reasonable to implicate the TNF gene complex in pathogenesis. Patients with AS have been shown to have altered cytokine profiles, especially with TNF-α.[54] Numerous studies have examined this, with association of the TNF-308 polymorphism being reported in Scots and Germans.[49,55,56] However this finding has not been universally replicated even in adequately powered studies in other populations.[57,58] Part of the inability to demonstrate an independent association of TNF genes may be due to the linkage disequilibrium of these genes with HLA-B.

HSP70

The physical proximity of the *HSP70* genes to the HLA-B locus makes it difficult to discern whether any

demonstrated association would be better explained by HLA-B27 itself. One study of 150 Mexican patients with AS and other types of spondyloarthritis found an association with *HSP70-1, HSP70-2,* and *HSP70-hom* genotypes in both HLA-B27–positive and HLA-B27–negative individuals.[59] This observation must be confirmed elsewhere.

HLA-DRB1

MHC class II alleles, including the HLA-DRB1*01 and DRB1*04 alleles, have been implicated also in providing additional susceptibility to AS.[60,61] However, linkage to HLA-B27 haplotypes has made it difficult to discern an independent contribution to susceptibility to AS and spondyloarthritis. In addition, HLA-DRB1*08 has been implicated both in susceptibility to uveitis in the setting of AS and to juvenile-onset AS.[62] In patients with the latter, an additional influence of HLA-DPB1*0301 has also been proposed[63] although this has not been evaluated elsewhere.

TAP genes

Despite one early study in AS[64] and another in ReA[65] suggesting an association with *TAP* alleles, a subsequent study showed that the polymorphism of human *TAP* does not affect the translocated repertoire of HLA-B27 ligands and is therefore unlikely to play a decisive role in the development of HLA-B27–associated disease.[66] Hence, that a subsequent analysis in Spanish patients with AS[67] failed to show a role for *TAP* alleles in pathogenesis is not surprising.

LMP2 genes

A few studies have implicated *LMP* genes in subgroups of AS, including *LMP2* genes in patients with juvenile AS in reports from Mexico and Norway[63,68] and in patients with AS and uveitis from Canada[69] as well as *LMP7* alleles in patients from Spain.[70] Until these inconsistent findings are more widely replicated, it is premature to assign a definite role for this locus in AS susceptibility or subsets.

Genome-Wide Screens of Susceptibility Regions to Spondyloarthritis

Although the MHC is probably the primary mediator of genetic susceptibility to AS, it explains less than 50% of the total genetic risk for AS.[6,7,71,72] Genome-wide linkage scans from Britain, France, and North America have implicated numerous non-MHC genomic regions including chromosomes 2q, 3p, 5q, 9q, 10q, 11q, 16q, 17p, and 19q[71–73] (Fig. 3.5). A recent study in AAU susceptibility has identified, in addition to the MHC, regions on chromosome 9p and 1q32.[74] Although only a preliminary genome-wide scan has been conducted

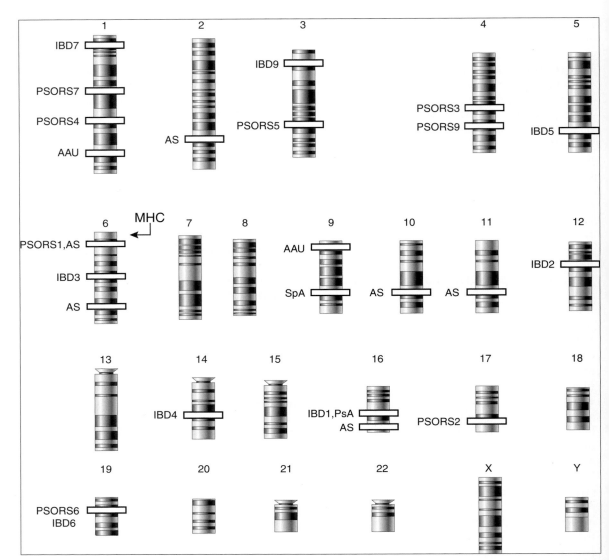

Fig. 3.5 Chromosomal regions implicated in susceptibility to spondyloarthritis and related diseases. Included here are regions on chromosomes 2q, 6p (the MHC), 6q, 10q, 11q, and 16q where linkage to AS occurs; regions on 1q and 9p in acute anterior uveitis (AAU); a region on 9q linked to spondyloarthritis (SpA); nine regions linked to psoriasis susceptibility (PSORS1 through 7 and PSORS9); a locus on 16q linked to psoriatic arthritis (PsA) susceptibility; and eight regions linked to irritable bowel disease (IBD1 through 7 and IBD9). Chromosomal locations of *IBD* and *PSORS* genes are listed at www.ncbi.nlm.nih.gov/entrez/dispomim.cg.

in PsA, genome-wide scans in psoriasis itself have mapped a major susceptibility locus to a 60-kb interval telomeric to HLA-C in the MHC known as PSORS1[75] (Fig. 3.1). PSORS1 is closely linked to the corneodesmosin (*CDSN*) gene, 160-kb telomeric of HLA-C, which functions in corneocyte cohesion and desquamation and whose potential identity as PSORS1 is controversial (Fig. 3.1). Also seen in some scans in families with psoriasis are two other regions on chromosome 17q (PSORS2)[76] and on chromosome 4 (PSORS3).[77] Since the first genome-wide scan for IBD was published in 1996, numerous other scans have identified seven genomic regions for susceptibility to IBD, designated IBD1 to IBD7 and located on chromosomes 1, 5, 6, 12, 14, 16, and 19.[77–79] However, only IBD1, at chromosome 16q12, has been universally replicated.[77] The most consistent region for susceptibility to IBD on genome-wide screens has been found on chromosome 16q (IBD1) at *NOD 2* (otherwise known as *CARD15*) (see later).[79]

Non-Major Histocompatibility Complex Genes

CYP2D6

Few candidate genes have been definitively implicated outside the MHC. The first to be identified was debrisoquine hydroxylase (*CYP2D6*), located on chromosome

22q.[80,81] This gene is involved in the metabolism of xenobiotics, which include certain drugs, metals, and industrial and naturally occurring chemicals. Xenobiotics have been shown to be promoters of inflammation via T cells. Within-family and case-control analyses have reported association of *pm* (poor metabolizer) alleles with AS.[80,81]

Interleukin-1

The interleukin (IL)-1α and IL-1β proteins and their natural antagonist IL-1 receptor antagonist (IL-1RA) are synthesized by a variety of cell types, including activated macrophages, keratinocytes, stimulated B lymphocytes, and fibroblasts, and are potent mediators of inflammation and immunity. There are two structurally distinct forms of IL-1: IL-1α and IL-1β. IL-1RA is a protein that binds to IL-1 receptors and inhibits the binding of IL-1α and IL-1β. It is encoded by the gene *IL1RN*. The genes encoding these proteins form part of a complex of highly homologous genes on chromosome 2q13 termed the *IL-1 gene family complex* (Fig. 3.6).[82]

Studies of IL-1 levels in patients with AS have produced contradictory results, with some showing increased serum levels.[83] However, a genome-wide scan of families from Britain showed suggestive linkage of AS to the region on chromosome 2q13 containing the IL-1 family gene cluster.[71,84] In two studies from Scotland and the Netherlands,[85,86] association of AS was found with a VNTR in intron 2 of *IL1RN*. Furthermore, an association of two synonymous single nucleotide polymorphisms in exon 6 of *IL1RN* and their haplotypes with a large Canadian cohort of AS patients has been recently described[87] although no association with *IL1RN* was seen in a large collection of North American families.[88] A further family and case-control study demonstrated association broadly across the IL-1 gene cluster, with the strongest association being with haplotypes of the *IL-1B* gene, and another member of the IL-1 gene complex lying closed to *IL1RN*, termed *IL-1F10*.[84] Thus, the IL-1 gene complex has emerged as the most significant non-MHC susceptibility locus identified to date, but the primary associated genetic variant(s) remain uncertain.

CARD15

CARD15 (caspase-activating recruitment domain 15), previously known as *NOD2* (nucleotide oligomerization domain 2), located on chromosome 16q12, has been identified as the site of the IBD1 susceptibility region.[79,89] *CARD15* is an important molecule for activation of the NF-κB system in response to bacterial liposaccharide. It is expressed mainly on monocytes, macrophages, and B cells and is thought to be an important component of innate immunity for maintenance of the intestinal barrier. Mutant alleles of *CARD15*

have been associated with susceptibility to Crohn's disease in most ethnic groups. Between 10% and 30% of patients with Crohn's disease are heterozygotes, and 3% to 15% are homozygotes for one of three *CARD15* mutations compared with 8% to 15% and 0% to 1% of control subjects, respectively.[89,90] The presence of *CARD15* mutations explains about 20% of the overall genetic susceptibility to Crohn's disease. Also, in patients with Crohn's disease, *CARD15* mutations are more strongly associated with ileal and right colonic involvement, younger age at onset, and a tendency to develop strictures. Studies of patients with AS and spondyloarthritis from the United Kingdom[91] and France,[92] however, have failed to reveal a role for *CARD15* in pathogenesis. An examination of *CARD15* variants in patients with PsA from Newfoundland demonstrated convincing associations,[93] although no role for them in psoriasis susceptibility per se was seen in another study from Italy.[94]

ANKH

ANKH is a multipass transmembrane protein that exports inorganic pyrophosphate from intracellular to extracellular compartments and in humans is encoded on chromosome 5p.[95] A spontaneous mutation at the mouse *progressive ankylosis* locus causes a generalized, progressive arthritis accompanied by mineral deposition, aberrant new bone formation resulting in ankylosis, and joint destruction. Two novel polymorphic sites, one in the 5′ noncoding region of *ANKH* and the other in the promoter region have been described in humans. Genetic studies in 112 unrelated North American patients with AS and in 124 multiplex families have shown both association and linkage to AS, with an overall relative risk in sibs of 1.9.[95] In another family study from Britain, however, linkage or association with AS could not be confirmed.[96] More recently, it has been shown that two markers in the 3′ end of the *ANKH* gene were significantly associated with AS only in male patients, which may account in part for the gender difference seen in the prevalence of AS.[97]

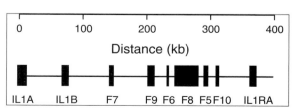

Fig. 3.6 The genomic organization of the IL-1 gene complex at chromosome 2q13. Shown here are locations of *IL1A* and *IL1B* genes, IL-1RA (otherwise known as *IL1RN*), and other members of the IL-1 cytokine family (IL-1F5 to F10), which have been shown to activate the pathway leading to NF-κB.

Clearly, more work is needed to discern whether *ANKH* plays a role in AS susceptibility.

Genes not associated with ankylosing spondylitis
A number of genes have been evaluated in AS susceptibility, and convincing associations have not been seen. Genes that have not shown convincing associations with AS include IL-6, androgen receptor genes, IL-10, transforming growth factor-β (*TGFβ*) genes, and matrix metalloproteinase 3 (*MMP3*).[98–104]

Genes and Severity of Ankylosing Spondylitis

In the past few years, outcome measures have been developed and validated to quantitate disease activity and disease severity, both functionally and radiographically.[105] Not only is susceptibility to AS largely determined by genetic factors but also disease severity in AS has a hereditary component. Classifying severity by disease activity, defined by the Bath Ankylosing Spondylitis Disease Activity Index (BASDAI) and by loss of function, defined by the Bath Ankylosing Spondylitis Functional Index (BASFI), Hamersma et al.[106] demonstrated that these traits are highly heritable. Although MHC genes do not appear to be involved in disease severity, regions on other chromosomes have been implicated, specifically a region on chromosome 18 and disease activity (defined by the BASDAI), age at symptom onset with a region of chromosome 11p, and functional impairment with a region on chromosome 2q.[107] In contrast to the genetic determinants of susceptibility to AS, clinical manifestations of the disease measured by the BASDAI, the BASFI, and age at symptom onset are largely determined by a small number of genes not encoded within the MHC.

INFECTION

A role for triggering infections has been better documented in spondyloarthritis than in most other rheumatic diseases. The most frequent type of ReA in developed countries follows urogenital infections with *C. trachomatis* (endemic ReA).[108] Postdysenteric ReA, more commonly encountered in less technologically advanced countries follows various *Shigella* and *Salmonella* (especially *Salmonella typhimurium* and *enteritidis*), *Campylobacter jejuni* and *fetus* and, in Europe, *Yersinia enterocolitica* infections. Microorganisms implicated in ReA share common biologic features: 1) they can invade mucosal surfaces and replicate intracellularly and 2) they contain lipopolysaccharide in their outer membrane. Of particular note, antigens from *Salmonella*, *Yersinia*, and *Chlamydia* have been found in synovial tissues and fluids of patients with ReA,[104] often many years after the initial infection. Although only bacterial fragments of the enteric pathogens have been found, evidence for viable *C. trachomatis* and perhaps *Chlamydia pneumoniae* have been demonstrated in several studies.[109,110] *Chlamydia* and other organisms also have been reported in the joints of healthy individuals, thus raising questions about the pathogenic significance of these findings.[111] Other data, however, support the likelihood that bacterial persistence plays an important role in ReA, including the finding of specific IgA antibodies and synovial T-cell proliferation to the initiating infectious agent.[112,113] It may also be significant that there are high serum IgA levels in AS, although studies to identify significant IgA antibodies to a variety of organisms have been unrewarding.[114]

The contribution of infection to other types of spondyloarthritis is less clear. In older studies *Klebsiella pneumoniae* was implicated in the pathogenesis of AS,[115] although recent data have not confirmed this finding.[114] An analysis of fecal microflora in patients with AS has suggested instead that *Bacteroides* may play a role.[116] It may also be significant that there are high serum IgA levels in AS, although studies to find significant IgA antibodies to a variety of organisms have been unrewarding (reviewed in reference 1). In fact, it has been proposed that there might be no specific infectious trigger in AS—that it may result from gut flora and may thus be "ubiquitous."[7]

THE GUT AND SPONDYLOARTHRITIS

In studies from Belgium and from Scandinavia, up to 50% of patients with AS have microscopic ileal inflammation seen on ileocolonoscopy.[117,118] Moreover, two-thirds of patients with undifferentiated spondyloarthritis have histologic gut inflammation. This is reviewed elsewhere in this textbook in greater detail. Gut inflammation in AS appears to be immunologically related to that seen in Crohn's disease. These observations have raised speculation that the inciting event in spondyloarthritis may be a breakdown of the gut-blood barrier to intestinal bacteria, although this suggestion has yet to be proven. It has been established that patients with AS and their relatives have increased intestinal permeability compared with healthy control subjects.[119]

CONCLUSION

Great progress has been made in elucidation of the factors involved in the pathogenesis of AS in recent years. It has become clear that HLA-B27, the primary genetic factor identified in AS pathogenesis, functions in a variety of roles including "classical" antigen presentation. How these lead to AS remains to be seen.

That other genes in the MHC contribute to AS suscep-tibility is strongly suspected, although despite the study of a number of candidate genes, this "second" MHC gene has yet to be identified. Genome-wide scans have identified a number of regions that may contain other susceptibility genes for AS, and these are being charac-terized. Most of the extensive studies of non-MHC candidate genes that might function in susceptibility to AS or severity have been inconclusive or unrewarding, although recent data implicating the IL-1 genes has been most promising. Other candidate genes are being examined, especially through international collabora-tions that will address the power concerns.

On the other hand, less recent progress has been made in non-MHC factors. Despite what has been learned in ReA, no infectious trigger has been identi-fied in AS (and in fact there might be no specific trig-ger). The link of gut inflammation to the triggering of AS is strongly suggested by data thus far but has still not been defined—this clearly is an area of promise for further investigation.

REFERENCES

1. Schlosstein L, Terasaki PI, Bluestone R, Pearson CM. High associ-ation of an HL-A antigen, W27, with ankylosing spondylitis. N Engl J Med. 1973;288:704–706.
2. Brewerton DA, Hart FD, Nicholls A, Caffrey M, James DC, Sturrock RD. Ankylosing spondylitis and HL-A 27. Lancet. 1973; 1:904–907.
3. van der Linden SM, Valkenburg HA, de Jongh BM, Cats A. The risk of developing ankylosing spondylitis in HLA-B27 positive individuals. A comparison of relatives of spondylitis patients with the general population. Arthritis Rheum. 1984;27:241–249.
4. Khan MA, Kushner I, Braun WE, Schacter BZ, Steinberg AG. HLA-B7 and ankylosing spondylitis in American blacks. N Engl J Med. 1977;297:513.
5. Jacobs JH, Rose FC. The familial occurrence of ankylosing spondylitis. Br Med J. 1954;4897:1139–1140.
6. Brown MA, Laval SH, Brophy S, Calin A. Recurrence risk model-ling of the genetic susceptibility to ankylosing spondylitis. Ann Rheum Dis. 2000;59:883–886.
7. Brown MA, Kennedy LG, MacGregor AJ, et al. Susceptibility to ankylosing spondylitis in twins: the role of genes, HLA, and the environment. Arthritis Rheum. 1997;40:1823–1828.
8. Porcher R, Said-Nahal R, D'Agostino MA, Miceli-Richard C, Dougados M, Breban M. Two major spondyloarthropathy phenotypes are distinguished by pattern analysis in multiplex families. Arthritis Rheum. 2005;53:263–271.
9. Ott J. Analysis of Human Genetic Linkage. Baltimore, Md: Johns Hopkins University Press; 1991.
10. Kelley J, Walter L, Trowsdale J. Comparative genomics of major histocompatibility complexes. Immunogenetics. 2005; 56:683–695.
11. Borrego F, Masilamani M, Kabat J, Sanni TB, Coligan JE. The cell biology of the human natural killer cell CD94/NKG2A inhibitory receptor. Mol Immunol. 2005;42:485–488.
12. Clements CS, Kjer-Nielsen L, Kostenko L, et al. Crystal structure of HLA-G: a nonclassical MHC class I molecule expressed at the fetal-maternal interface. Proc Natl Acad Sci USA. 2005;102:3360–3365.
13. Lee N, Geraghty DE. HLA-F surface expression on B cell and monocyte cell lines is partially independent from tapasin and completely independent from TAP. J Immunol. 2003;171: 5264–5271.
14. Reveille JD. Genetic studies in the rheumatic diseases: The present status and implications for the future. J Rheumatol. 2005;72:10–13.
15. Brocke P, Garbi N, Momburg F, Hammerling GJ. HLA-DM, HLA-DO and tapasin: functional similarities and differences. Curr Opin Immunol. 2002;14:22–29.
16. Deshaies F, Brunet A, Diallo DA, Denzin LK, Samaan A, Thibodeau J. A point mutation in the groove of HLA-DO allows egress from the endoplasmic reticulum independent of HLA-DM. Proc Natl Acad Sci USA. 2005;102:6443–6448.
17. Paulsson KM. Evolutionary and functional perspectives of the major histocompatibility complex class I antigen-processing machinery. Cell Mol Life Sci. 2004;61:2446–2460.
18. Matsuzaka Y, Makino S, Nakajima K, et al. New polymorphic microsatellite markers in the human MHC class III region. Tissue Antigens. 2001;57:397–404.
19. Allcock RJ, Baluchova K, Cheong KY, Price P. Haplotypic single nucleotide polymorphisms in the central MHC gene IKBL, a potential regulator of NF-κB function. Immunogenetics. 2001;52:289–293.
20. Wei J, Hemmings GP. TNXB locus may be a candidate gene predis-posing to schizophrenia. Am J Med Genet B Neuropsychiatr Genet. 2004;125:43–49.
21. Lindor NM, Bristow J. Tenascin-X deficiency in autosomal reces-sive Ehlers-Danlos syndrome. Am J Med Genet A. 2005;135:75–80.
22. Tazi-Ahnini R, Cork MJ, Wengraf D, et al. NOTCH4, a non-HLA gene in the MHC is strongly associated with the most severe form of alopecia areata. Hum Genet. 2003;112:400–403.
23. Schmidt AM, Stern DM. Receptor for AGE (RAGE) is a gene within the major histocompatibility class III region: implications for host response mechanisms in homeostasis and chronic disease. Front Biosci. 2001;6:D1151–D1160.
24. Reveille JD, Ball EJ, Khan, MA. HLA-B27 and genetic predisposing factors in spondyloarthropathies. Curr Opin Rheumatol, 2001;13:265–272.
25. Brown MA, Wordsworth BP, Reveille JD. Genetics of ankylosing spondylitis. Clin Exp Rheumatol. 2002;20(6 suppl 28):S43–S49.
26. Mody GM, Parke FA, Reveille JD. Articular manifestations of human immunodeficiency virus infection. Best Pract Res Clin Rheumatol. 2003;17:265–287.
27. Martin TM, Smith JR, Rosenbaum JT. Anterior uveitis: current concepts of pathogenesis and interactions with spondy-loarthopathies. Curr Opin Rheumatol. 2002;14:337–341.
28. Steiner NK, Gans C, Baldassarre L, et al. Twenty-five novel HLA-B alleles. Tissue Antigens. 2003;62:263–266.
29. Ramos M, Lopez de Castro JA. HLA-B27 and the pathogenesis of spondyloarthritis. Tissue Antigens. 2002;60:191–205.
30. Boyle LH, Gaston JS. Breaking the rules: the unconventional recognition of HLA-B27 by CD4+ T lymphocytes as an insight into the pathogenesis of the spondyloarthropathies. Rheumatology (Oxford) 2003;42:404–412.
31. Boyle LH, Goodall JC, Opat SS, Gaston JS. The recognition of HLA-B27 by human CD4+ T lymphocytes. J Immunol. 2001; 167:2619–2624.
32. Kuon W, Holzhutter HG, Appel H, et al. Identification of HLA-B27-restricted peptides from the Chlamydia trachomatis proteome with possible relevance to HLA-B27-associated diseases. J Immunol. 2001;167:4738–4746.
33. Montserrat V, Marti M, Lopez de Castro JA. Allospecific T cell epitope sharing reveals extensive conservation of the antigenic features of peptide ligands among HLA-B27 subtypes differentially associated with spondyloarthritis. J Immunol. 2003; 170: 5778–5785.
34. Fiorillo MT, Maragno M, Butler R, Dupris ML, Sorrentino R. CD8+ T-cell autoreactivity to an HLA-B27-restricted self-epitope corre-lates with ankylosing spondylitis. J Clin Invest. 2000;106:47–53.

35. Dulphy N, Peyrat MA, Tieng V, et al. Common intra-articular T cell expansions in patients with reactive arthritis: identical β-chain junctional sequences and cytotoxicity toward HLA-B27. J Immunol. 1999;162:3830–3839.

36. May E, Dulphy N, Frauendorf E, et al. Conserved TCR β chain usage in reactive arthritis; evidence for selection by a putative HLA-B27-associated autoantigen. Tissue Antigens. 2002;60: 299–308.

37. Dangoria NS, DeLay ML, Kingsbury DJ, et al. HLA-B27 misfolding is associated with aberrant intermolecular disulfide bond formation (dimerization) in the endoplasmic reticulum. J Biol Chem. 2002;277:23459–23468.

38. Bird LA, Peh CA, Kollnberger S, Elliott T, McMichael AJ, Bowness P. Lymphoblastoid cells express HLA-B27 homodimers both intracellularly and at the cell surface following endosomal recycling. Eur J Immunol. 2003;33:748–759.

39. Kollnberger S, Bird L, Sun MY, et al. Cell-surface expression and immune receptor recognition of HLA-B27 homodimers. Arthritis Rheum. 2002;46:2972–2982.

40. Ekman P, Saarinen M, He Q, et al. HLA-B27-transfected (Salmonella permissive) and HLA-A2-transfected (Salmonella nonpermissive) human monocytic U937 cells differ in their production of cytokines. Infect Immun. 2002;70:1609–1614.

41. Inman RD, Payne U. Determinants of synoviocyte clearance of arthritogenic bacteria. J Rheumatol. 2003;30:1291–1297.

42. Popov I, Dela Cruz CS, Barber BH, Chiu B, Inman RD. Breakdown of CTL tolerance to self HLA-B*2705 induced by exposure to Chlamydia trachomatis. J Immunol. 2002;169:4033–4038.

43. Ekman P, Kirveskari J, Granfors K. Modification of disease outcome in Salmonella-infected patients by HLA-B27. Arthritis Rheum. 2000;43:1527–1534.

44. Pimtanothai N, Rizzuto GA, Slack R, et al. Diversity of alleles encoding HLA-B40: relative frequencies in United States populations and description of five novel alleles. Hum Immunol. 2000;61:808–815.

45. Robinson WP, van der Linden SM, Khan MA, et al. HLA-Bw60 increases susceptibility to ankylosing spondylitis in HLA-B27+ patients. Arthritis Rheum. 1989;32:1135–1141.

46. Rubin LA, Amos CI, Wade JA, et al. Investigating the genetic basis for ankylosing spondylitis. Linkage studies with the major histocompatibility complex region. Arthritis Rheum. 1994; 37:212–220.

47. Brown MA, Pile KD, Kennedy LG, Calin A, Darke C, Bell J, Wordsworth BP, Cornelis F. HLA class I associations of ankylosing spondylitis in the white population in the United Kingdom. Ann Rheum Dis. 1996;55:268–270.

48. Wei JC, Tsai WC, Lin HS, Tsai CY, Chou CT. HLA-B60 and B61 are strongly associated with ankylosing spondylitis in HLA-B27-negative Taiwan Chinese patients. Rheumatology (Oxford). 2004;43:839–842.

49. Milicic A, Lindheimer F, Laval S, et al. Interethnic studies of TNF polymorphisms confirm the likely presence of a second MHC susceptibility locus in ankylosing spondylitis. Genes Immun. 2000;1:418–422.

50. Singal DP, Li J, Zhang G. Microsatellite polymorphism of the MICA gene and susceptibility to rheumatoid arthritis. Clin Exp Rheumatol. 2001;19:451–452.

51. Ricci-Vitiani L, Vacca A, Potolicchio I, et al. MICA gene triplet repeat polymorphism in patients with HLA-B27 positive and negative ankylosing spondylitis from Sardinia. J Rheumatol. 2000;27:2193–2197.

52. Yabuki K, Ota M, Goto K, et al. Triplet repeat polymorphism in the MICA gene in HLA-B27 positive and negative Caucasian patients with ankylosing spondylitis. Hum Immunol. 1999;60:83–86.

53. Martinez-Borra J, Gonzalez S, Lopez-Vazquez A, et al. HLA-B27 alone rather than B27-related class I haplotypes contributes to ankylosing spondylitis susceptibility. Hum Immunol. 2000; 61:131–139.

54. Rudwaleit M, Siegert S, Yin Z, et al. Low T cell production of TNFα and IFNγ in ankylosing spondylitis: its relation to HLA-B27 and influence of the TNF-308 gene polymorphism. Ann Rheum Dis. 2001;60:36–42.

55. McGarry F, Walker R, Sturrock R, Field M. The −308.1 polymorphism in the promoter region of the tumor necrosis factor gene is associated with ankylosing spondylitis independent of HLA-B27. J Rheumatol. 1999;26:1110–1116.

56. Hohler T, Schaper T, Schneider PM, Meyer zum Buschenfelde KH, Marker-Hermann E. Association of different tumor necrosis factor α promoter allele frequencies with ankylosing spondylitis in HLA-B27 positive individuals. Arthritis Rheum. 1998;41: 1489–1492.

57. Verjans GM, Brinkman BM, Van Doornik CE, Kijlstra A, Verweij CL. Polymorphism of tumour necrosis factor-α (TNF-α) at position −308 in relation to ankylosing spondylitis. Clin Exp Immunol. 1994; 97:45–47.

58. Gonzalez S, Torre-Alonso JC, Martinez-Borra J, et al. TNF-238A promoter polymorphism contributes to susceptibility to ankylosing spondylitis in HLA-B27 negative patients. J Rheumatol. 2001;28:1288–1293.

59. Vargas-Alarcon G, Londono JD, Hernandez-Pacheco G, et al. Heat shock protein 70 gene polymorphisms in Mexican patients with spondyloarthropathies. Ann Rheum Dis. 2002;61:48–51.

60. Brown MA, Kennedy LG, Darke C, et al. The effect of HLA-DR genes on susceptibility to and severity of ankylosing spondylitis. Arthritis Rheum. 1998;41:460–465.

61. Said-Nahal R, Miceli-Richard C, Gautreau C, et al. The role of HLA genes in familial spondyloarthropathy: a comprehensive study of 70 multiplex families. Ann Rheum Dis. 2002;61:201–206.

62. Monowarul-Islam SM, Numaga J, Fujino Y, et al. HLA-DR8 and acute anterior uveitis in ankylosing spondylitis. Arthritis Rheum. 1995;38:547–550.

63. Ploski R, Flato B, Vinje O, Maksymowych W, Forre O, Thorsby E. Association to HLA-DRB1*08, HLA-DPB1*0301 and homozygosity for an HLA-linked proteasome gene in juvenile ankylosing spondylitis. Hum Immunol 1995;44:88–96.

64. Burney RO, Pile KD, Gibson K, et al. Analysis of the MHC class II encoded components of the HLA class I antigen processing pathway in ankylosing spondylitis. Ann Rheum Dis. 1994;53: 58–60.

65. Barron KS, Reveille JD, Carrington M, Mann DL, Robinson MA. Susceptibility to Reiter's syndrome is associated with alleles of TAP genes. Arthritis Rheum. 1995;38:684–689.

66. Kuipers JG, Raybourne RB, Williams KM, Zeidler H, Yu DT. Specificities of human TAP alleles for HLA-B27 binding peptides. Arthritis Rheum. 1996;39:1892–1895.

67. Fraile A, Collado MD, Mataran L, Martin J, Nieto A. TAP1 and TAP2 polymorphism in Spanish patients with ankylosing spondylitis. Exp Clin Immunogenet. 2000;17:199–204.

68. Vargas-Alarcon G, Gamboa R, Zuniga J, et al. Association study of LMP gene polymorphisms in Mexican patients with spondyloarthritis. Hum Immunol. 2004;65:1437–1442.

69. Maksymowych WP, Adlam N, Lind D, Russell AS. Polymorphism of the LMP2 gene and disease phenotype in ankylosing spondylitis: no association with disease severity. Clin Rheumatol. 1997;16:461–465.

70. Fraile A, Nieto A, Vinasco J, Beraun Y, Martin J, Mataran L. Association of large molecular weight proteasome 7 gene polymorphism with ankylosing spondylitis. Arthritis Rheum. 1998; 41:560–562.

71. Laval SH, Timms A, Edwards S, et al. Whole-genome screening in ankylosing spondylitis: evidence of non-MHC genetic-susceptibility loci. Am J Hum Genet. 2001;68:918–926.

72. Zhang G, Luo J, Bruckel J, et al. Genetic studies in familial ankylosing spondylitis susceptibility. Arthritis Rheum. 2004; 50:2246–2254.

73. Miceli-Richard C, Zouali H, Said-Nahal R, et al. Significant linkage to spondyloarthropathy on 9q31-34. Hum. Mol Genet. 2004;13:1641–1648.

74. Martin TM, Zhang G, Luo J, et al. A locus on chromosome 9p predisposes to a specific disease manifestation, acute anterior uveitis, in ankylosing spondylitis, a genetically complex, multisystem, inflammatory disease. Arthritis Rheum. 2005;52:269–274.

75. Nair RP, Stuart P, Henseler T, et al. Localization of psoriasis-susceptibility locus PSORS1 to a 60-kb interval telomeric to HLA-C. Am J Hum Genet. 2000;66:1833–1844.

76. Tomfohrde J, Silverman A, Barnes R, et al. Gene for familial psoriasis susceptibility mapped to the distal end of human chromosome 17q. Science. 1994;264:1141–1145.

77. Becker KG, Simon RM, Bailey-Wilson JE, et al. Clustering of non-major histocompatibility complex susceptibility candidate loci in human autoimmune diseases. Proc Natl Acad Sci USA. 1998;95:9979–9984.

78. Hugot J-P, Laurent-Puig P, Gower-Rousseau C, et al. Mapping of a susceptibility locus for Crohn's disease on chromosome 16. Nature. 1996;379:821–823.

79. Bonen DK, Cho JH. The genetics of inflammatory bowel disease. Gastroenterology. 2003;124:521–536.

80. Beyeler C, Armstrong M, Bird HA, Idle JR, Daly AK. Relationship between genotype for the cytochrome P450 CYP2D6 and susceptibility to ankylosing spondylitis and rheumatoid arthritis. Ann Rheum Dis. 1996;55:66–68.

81. Brown MA, Edwards S, Hoyle E, et al. Polymorphisms of the CYP2D6 gene increase susceptibility to ankylosing spondylitis. Hum Mol Genet. 2000;9:1563–1566.

82. Nicklin MJH, Weith A, Duff GW. A physical map of the region encompassing the human interleukin-1-α, interleukin-1-β, and interleukin-1 receptor antagonist genes. Genomics. 1994; 19:382–384.

83. Vazquez-Del MM, Garcia-Gonzalez A, Munoz-Valle JF, et al. Interleukin 1β(IL-1β), IL-10, tumor necrosis factor-α, and cellular proliferation index in peripheral blood mononuclear cells in patients with ankylosing spondylitis. J Rheumatol. 2002;29: 522–526.

84. Timms AE, Crane AM, Sims AM, et al. The interleukin 1 gene cluster contains a major susceptibility locus for ankylosing spondylitis. Am J Hum Genet. 2004;75:587–595.

85. McGarry F, Neilly J, Anderson N, Sturrock R, Field M. A polymorphism within the interleukin 1 receptor antagonist (IL-1Ra) gene is associated with ankylosing spondylitis. Rheumatology (Oxford). 2001;40:1359–1364.

86. van der Paardt M, Crusius JB, Garcia-Gonzalez MA, et al. Interleukin-1β and interleukin-1 receptor antagonist gene polymorphisms in ankylosing spondylitis. Rheumatology (Oxford). 2002;41:1419–1423.

87. Maksymowych WP, Reeve J, Reveille JD, et al. High throughput single nucleotide polymorphism (SNP) analysis of the interleukin-1 receptor antagonist (IL-1 RN) locus in patients with ankylosing spondylitis (AS) by MALDI-TOF mass spectroscopy. Arthritis Rheum. 2003;48:2011–2018.

88. Jin L, Weisman MA, Zhang G, et al. Lack of linkage of IL1RN genotypes with ankylosing spondylitis susceptibility. Arthritis Rheum. 2004;50:3047–3048.

89. Hugot JP, Chamaillard M, Zouali H, et al. Association of NOD2 leucine-rich repeat variants with susceptibility to Crohn's disease. Nature. 2001;411:599–603.

90. Ogura Y, Bonen DK, Inohara N, et al. A frameshift mutation on NOD2 associated with susceptibility to Crohn's disease. Nature. 2001;411:537–539.

91. Crane AM, Bradbury L, van Heel DA, et al. Role of NOD2 variants in spondylarthritis. Arthritis Rheum. 2002;46:1629–1633.

92. Miceli-Richard C, Zouali H, Lesage S. CARD15/NOD2 analyses in spondyloarthropathy. Arthritis Rheum. 2002;46:1405–1406.

93. Rahman P, Bartlett S, Siannis F, et al. CARD15: a pleiotropic autoimmune gene that confers susceptibility to psoriatic arthritis. Am J Hum Genet. 2003;73:677–681.

94. Borgiani P, Vallo L, D'Apice MR, et al. Exclusion of CARD15/NOD2 as a candidate susceptibility gene to psoriasis in the Italian population. Eur J Dermatol. 2002;12:540–542.

95. Tsui FW, Tsui HW, Cheng EY, et al. Novel genetic markers in the 5'-flanking region of ANKH are associated with ankylosing spondylitis. Arthritis Rheum. 2003;48:791–797.

96. Timms AE, Zhang Y, Bradbury L, Wordsworth BP, Brown MA. Investigation of the role of ANKH in ankylosing spondylitis. Arthritis Rheum. 2003;48:2898–2902.

97. Tsui HW, Inman RD, Paterson AD, Reveille JD, Tsui FWL. ANKH variants associated with ankylosing spondylitis: Gender differences. Arthritis Res Ther. 2005;7:513–525.

98. Mori K, Ushiyama T, Inoue K, Hukuda S. Polymorphic CAG repeats of the androgen receptor gene in Japanese male patients with ankylosing spondylitis. Rheumatology (Oxford). 2000;39:530–532.

99. Collado-Escobar MD, Nieto A, Mataran L, Raya E, Martin J. Interleukin 6 gene promoter polymorphism is not associated with ankylosing spondylitis. J Rheumatol. 2000;27:1461–1463.

100. Goedecke V, Crane AM, Jaakkola E, et al. Interleukin 10 polymorphisms in ankylosing spondylitis. Genes Immun. 2003;4: 74–76.

101. Jaakkola E, Crane AM, Laiho K, et al. The effect of transforming growth factor β1 gene polymorphisms in ankylosing spondylitis. Rheumatology (Oxford). 2004;43:32–38.

102. Howe HS, Cheung PL, Kong KO, et al. Transforming growth factor β-1 and gene polymorphisms in oriental ankylosing spondylitis. Rheumatology (Oxford). 2005;44:51–54.

103. van der Paardt M, Crusius JB, Garcia-Gonzalez MA, Dijkmans BA, Pena AS, van der Horst-Bruinsma IE. Susceptibility to ankylosing spondylitis: no evidence for the involvement of transforming growth factor β 1 (TGFB1) gene polymorphisms. Ann Rheum Dis. 2005;64:616–619.

104. Jin L, Weisman M, Zhang G, et al. Lack of association of matrix metalloproteinase 3 (MMP3) genotypes with ankylosing spondylitis susceptibility and severity. Rheumatology (Oxford). 2005;44:55–60.

105. van der Heijde D, Bellamy N, Cbalin A, et al. Preliminary core sets for endpoints in ankylosing spondylitis. Assessments in Ankylosing Spondylitis Working Group. J Rheumatol. 1997; 24:2225–2229.

106. Hamersma J, Cardon LR, Bradbury L, et al. Is disease severity in ankylosing spondylitis genetically determined? Arthritis Rheum. 2001;44:1396–1400.

107. Brown MA, Brophy S, Bradbury L, et al. Identification of major loci controlling clinical manifestations of ankylosing spondylitis. Arthritis Rheum. 2003;48:2234–2239.

108. van der Linden SJ, van der Heijde D. Spondylarthopathies. Ankylosing spondylitis. In: Ruddy S, Harris ED, Sledge CB, eds. Kelley's Textbook of Rheumatology. 6th ed. Philadelphia, Pa: Saunders;2000:1039–1053.

109. Nikkari S, Rantakokko K, Ekman P, et al. Salmonella-triggered reactive arthritis: use of polymerase chain reaction, immunocytochemical staining, and gas chromatography-mass spectrometry in the detection of bacterial components from synovial fluid. Arthritis Rheum. 1999;42:84–89.

110. Gerard HC, Branigan PJ, Schumacher HR Jr, Hudson AP. Synovial Chlamydia trachomatis in patients with reactive arthritis/Reiter's syndrome are viable but show aberrant gene expression. J Rheumatol. 1998;25:734–742.

111. Schumacher HR Jr, Arayssi T, Crane M, et al. Chlamydia trachomatis nucleic acids can be found in the synovium of some asymptomatic subjects. Arthritis Rheum. 1999;42: 1281–1284.

112. Arnett FC. Seronegative spondyloarthropathies. In: Dale Dc, Federman DD, eds. Scientific American Medicine, 2003 edition (www.samed.com). New York, NY: Web MD; 2003:1304–1315.

113. Cowling P, Ebringer R, Ebringer A. Association of inflammation with raised serum IgA in ankylosing spondylitis. Ann Rheum Dis. 1980;39:545–549.

114. Stone MA, Payne U, Schentag C, Rahman P, Pacheco-Tena C, Inman RD. Comparative immune responses to candidate arthritogenic bacteria do not confirm a dominant role for Klebsiella pneumoniae in the pathogenesis of familial ankylosing spondylitis. Rheumatology (Oxford). 2003;43:148–155.

115. Ebringer RW, Cawdell DR, Cowling P, Ebringer A. Sequential studies in ankylosing spondylitis. Association of Klebsiella pneumoniae with active disease. Ann Rheum Dis. 1978;37: 146–151.

116. Stebbings S, Munro K, Simon MA, et al. Comparison of the faecal microflora of patients with ankylosing spondylitis and controls using molecular methods of analysis. Rheumatology (Oxford). 2002;41:1395–1401.

117. Mielants H, Veys EM, Goemaere S, Goethals K, Cuvelier C, De Vos M. Gut inflammation in the spondyloarthropathies: clinical, radiologic, biologic and genetic features in relation to the type of histology. A prospective study. J Rheumatol. 1991;18: 1542–1551.

118. Leirisalo-Repo M, Turunen U, Stenman S, Helenius P, Seppala K. High frequency of silent inflammatory bowel disease in spondylarthropathy. Arthritis Rheum. 1994;37:23–31.

119. Martinez-Gonzalez O, Cantero-Hinojosa J, Paule-Sastre P, Gomez-Magan JC, Salvatierra-Rios D. Intestinal permeability in patients with ankylosing spondylitis and their healthy relatives. Br J Rheumatol. 1994;33:644–647.

4 Infection and Spondyloarthritis

Robert D. Inman and Millicent A. Stone

INTRODUCTION

The seronegative spondyloarthropathies (SpAs) refer to a group of diseases that share several common features: 1) a strong association with HLA-B27; 2) asymmetric oligoarthritis; 3) axial involvement, particularly of the sacroiliac joints; 4) enthesitis; and 5) characteristic extraarticular features including acute anterior uveitis. The role of infection as a triggering factor is implicated with varying degrees of certainty among the subcategories: probable in reactive arthritis (ReA), possible in ankylosing spondylitis (AS), and unresolved in psoriatic arthritis and enteropathic arthritis. The very definition of ReA—a sterile synovitis after an extraarticular infection—clearly implicates infection in its inclusion criteria. SpAs, and ReA in particular, continue to occupy the conceptual ground somewhere between septic arthritis and the autoimmune rheumatic diseases such as rheumatoid arthritis (RA).

There have been attempts to bring more order into the nomenclature of the SpAs.[1–4] The etiologic classification has the most intrinsic appeal and has fueled the search for definitive links between particular pathogens and ReA. Many of these studies represent "guilt by association," in that the demonstration of a particular immune response profile by serology or cellular responses comes to define the identity of the causative pathogen even when there is no direct demonstration of the organism or its antigens in synovial tissues or fluid. However, the predictive power of a diagnostic test critically depends on the prevalence of positive results in the healthy population at large.[5] What constitutes the appropriate control group for these studies has not been consistently defined or applied, as will be discussed later in the controversial relationship of *Klebsiella* to AS. The mechanistic approach to classification of the SpAs awaits a better understanding of the molecular and cellular mechanisms underlying the chronic inflammation, but advances in clinical and experimental ReA hold the promise for this in the near future. Recent studies in ReA and undifferentiated oligoarthritis indicate that about 50% of such cases can be attributed to a specific pathogen by a combination of culture and serologic analysis, the predominant organisms being *Salmonella*, *Yersinia*, and *Chlamydia*.[6] Species-specific analysis of serological responses to pathogens may further enhance this detection rate.[7]

APPROACHES TO DETECTING MICROBES IN JOINTS

The most direct causal proof for microbes in ReA derives from demonstrations of microbial antigens in the joint. The case for persisting intraarticular pathogens is strongest for *Chlamydia*, and several investigators have demonstrated *Chlamydia* DNA or RNA by polymerase chain reaction (PCR) in joints of patients with *Chlamydia*-induced ReA. In an experimental model, it has been shown that synoviocyte-packaged *Chlamydia* can induce a chronic aseptic arthritis and that the synoviocyte can serve as an important reservoir of microbial antigens within the joint tissues long after the organism can be cultured from the joint.[8] There is some evidence that these persisting organisms in the joints are metabolically altered and may have entered a quiescent phase that renders them more resistant to antibiotic treatment. This has been shown for *Chlamydia pneumoniae*,[9] which, in terms of viability and metabolic activity, has been shown to have characteristics comparable to those of *Chlamydia trachomatis*. There is, however, a lower prevalence of *C. pneumoniae* DNA compared with *C. trachomatis* DNA in synovial tissues,[10] but the significance of such findings for the pathogenesis of joint disease remains an ongoing discussion.[11] *Chlamydia* nucleic acids have been found in the synovium of some asymptomatic patients.[12] Conversely, bacterial DNA or RNA from a wide spectrum of bacteria, including species not previously associated with ReA, have been demonstrated in patients with chronic arthritis in reports from Latin America,[13,14] England,[15] and the United States.[16] In some patients in these studies DNA from a number of different strains of bacteria is found in the same joint. Thus, although the application of PCR results has heightened the sensitivity of this quest, it has raised important questions about the specificity of the results. In addition to PCR analysis, gas chromatography-mass spectrometry (GC-MS) has been applied to search for bacterial components in joint tissues.[17] Once again, enhanced sensitivity has complicated the analysis of specificity.[18] These different approaches to microbe hunting in the joints are summarized in Table 4.1.

BITS OF BUGS IN THE JOINT: THE CHALLENGE OF PROVING CAUSALITY

The quest for infectious triggers in rheumatic diseases is not confined to SpA, and there are instructive lessons from studies in chronic arthritis in general. RA is considered an autoimmune disease, but the notion that the process may be triggered by an infectious agent has been a long-standing theory in the pathogenesis of RA. After several decades of searching for such causative agents in the joints, the direct evidence is still elusive. Recently, Chen et al.[17] provided new insights in this area by searching with GC-MS for muramic acid, a component derived from bacterial cell walls, in the joint tissues of patients with RA. For ReA, infectious agents triggering the joint inflammation have been well established.[19,20] One of the strongest links is the demonstration by PCR of chlamydial DNA in joints of patients with post-*Chlamydia* ReA.[21,22] However, after a prolonged search for bacterial DNA in joints in RA, whether an organism or its antigenic fragments persist locally in these joints remains unresolved. It may still be argued that the causative agent is present at such a low concentration that it cannot be detected with current microbiologic techniques. To date, many methods have been used in hunting for microbes in joints in RA as well as in joints in ReA, AS, and osteoarthritis (OA) (Table 4.1). Chen et al.[17] screened for bacteria in joint tissues of patients with RA using a sensitive pan-bacteria PCR that can detect DNA of almost any bacterial species. However, no bacterial DNA was found in their study. Despite the absence of bacterial DNA, they probed for evidence of the bacterial cell wall, which represents the major constituent of bacteria. The skeleton of the bacterial cell wall consists mainly of polysaccharide, peptidoglycan, and cell wall–associated proteins. Peptidoglycan is the major constituent of the gram-positive bacterial cell wall, whereas lipopolysaccharide (LPS) is the dominant component of the gram-negative bacterial cell wall. Chen et al. selected muramic acid, a component of the peptidoglycan moiety of the bacterial cell wall. Muramic acid is unique to bacteria and is not present in the mammalian proteome, making it an ideal chemical marker for detecting bacteria.[31] Muramic acid was detected by using a GC-MS with a

TABLE 4.1 DETECTION OF MICROBES IN JOINT TISSUES BY DIFFERENT METHODS*

Method	RA	ReA	AS	OA	Septic Arthritis
Culture	–	–	–	–	+
EM	–	+[†]	ND	ND	+
IF/IHC	–	+[‡]	ND	ND	+
PCR	+[§]/–[¶]	+[†]	+[¶]/–[**]	+[†]	+
GC-MS	+[¶]	+[††]	ND	+[¶]	+

*Culture, electron microscopy (EM), immunofluorescence (IF) and immunohistochemistry (IHC) are used for detecting intact organisms or their antigenic fragments, PCR for their nucleic acids, and GC-MS for their cell wall components. ND, not done.
[†]*Chlamydia* only.[22-24]
[‡]*Chlamydia, Salmonella,* and *Yersinia*[25-28]
[§]Pan-bacterial PCR[29,30]
[¶]Mass spectrometry.[17]
[¶]In patients with juvenile AS patients.[29]
[**]Nested PCR.[30]
[††]Detection of muramic acid.[24]

chemical ionization method sensitive enough to detect even picogram amounts (2 pg/injected amount). GC-MS has previously been used successfully to detect muramic acid in joints of patients with septic arthritis.[32,33] These investigators were able to demonstrate the presence of muramic acid in the joints of some patients with RA, suggesting that bacterial cell wall components, rather than bacterial DNA, persist in the joints in chronic RA (duration longer than 5 years). Their findings are in line with earlier reports that bacterial cell wall components were present in joints in RA by immunohistochemical analysis, using an antibody against bacterial cell wall peptidoglycan.[27] However, the important observation from this study is that the presence of bacterial cell wall components is not specific for RA, because they were also found in joint tissues of patients with OA.

The question of how these bacterial cell wall components might play a biological role if they persist in the joints for prolonged periods has remained open. Are they pathogenic? Several studies have suggested that bacterial cell wall components have multiple immunologic activities that may contribute to joint inflammation. 1) The recently discovered receptors of the first line of host defense—the Toll-like receptors (TLR)—recognize a range of microbes and their products. For example, TLR2 recognizes bacterial peptidoglycan.[34] 2) Bacterial peptidoglycan is capable of stimulating synovial macrophages to express the costimulatory molecules CD80 and CD86 and to produce proinflammatory cytokines such as tumor necrosis factor (TNF)-α and interleukin (IL)-6.[35] 3) Certain bacterial cell walls are able to induce experimental arthritis in rats with histopathologic features resembling RA.[36,37] 4) Small fragments of the arthritogenic bacterial peptidoglycan such as muramyl peptides possess potent proinflammatory capacity.[38] All these lines of evidence suggest that the bacterial cell wall components are potential arthritogenic agents. If they appear in the joints under certain circumstances and persist chronically, the stage may be set in this microenvironment of inflammation and injury for a breakdown in immune tolerance to local self-antigens, thereby initiating an autoimmune response that leads to self-perpetuating inflammation and ultimately bone and cartilage destruction.

Conversely, the stimulatory potential of TLR ligands such as LPS or peptidoglycan is relatively short-lived, raising questions about their potential as *chronic* stimuli. After an initial challenge with LPS, dendritic cells or macrophages enter into a programmed hyporesponsive stage in which the TLR4 signaling pathway has been shown to be down-regulated.[39,40] This hyporesponsiveness has also been analyzed for TLR2 ligands such as mycobacterial lipopeptides and lipoteichoic acid, and cross-hyporesponsiveness induction between TLR2 and TLR4 has been proposed.[40,41] Therefore, chronic persistence of bacterial components in the joints does not necessarily mean a chronic inflammatory stimulus in the joint. This fact may explain the discordance between inflammation and the presence of muramic acid in the synovial tissues of OA. The potential of muramic acid as a proinflammatory factor in RA synovitis is unsolved. Nevertheless, genetic polymorphisms in the molecules involved in the recognition and signaling pathways for bacterial components might explain different individual susceptibilities. This question has been addressed for TLR2 mutations and gram-positive (staphylococcal) infection[42] as well as for TLR4 polymorphisms and gram-negative infections.[43,44]

These recent data demonstrate the presence of stable bacterial degradation products, rather than whole bacteria, not only in the joints of patients with RA but also in joints of patients with OA. This finding raises important issues about the clinical significance of these events for the pathogenesis of inflammatory joint disease generally and has an interesting parallel in the PCR analysis of ReA joint tissues, in which chlamydial nucleic acids have been found not only in patients with ReA but also in joints of patients with OA as well.[23,45] Conversely, this study illustrates the fact that targeting the bacterial cell wall components by current techniques may be an alternative way to hunt microbes in the joints. Several methods have been used to detect the bacterial cell wall components in the joints of experimental cell wall–induced arthritis. These methods detecting unique bacterial cell wall components can be considered as a valuable approach to study the role of microbes and their products in chronic joint diseases. With these more sophisticated techniques a more definitive statement on the microbial contribution to the pathogenesis of inflammatory joint disease may be forthcoming.

MICROBE-HOST INTERACTIONS: A DYNAMIC STRUGGLE

There is great diversity in the clinical and immunologic sequelae to infection, and there is improved understanding of the biochemical events that reflect the host-microbe interaction at the cellular level. The attachment and invasion of bacteria represent an interplay between invasion-related proteins of the bacteria and surface receptors on host target cells. Analysis of these events has refined the concept of virulence of an organism from one that is a fixed property of a microorganism to a dynamic concept that reflects both bacterial and host factors. Similarly, the B-cell and T-cell immune responses to viral and bacterial infections are shedding new light on antigenic recognition, cell signaling pathways in activation, and immunologic memory. Thus, the pathways from antecedent infection to subsequent arthritis are gradually becoming better defined. Local persistence of the intact pathogen may prove elusive to define at first, as was the case for *Borrelia burgdorferi* in Lyme disease-associated arthritis. Local persistence of bacterial antigens is exemplified by post-*Yersinia* ReA and perhaps in the broader range of the SpAs. Deposition of circulating immune complexes, as occurs in bacterial endocarditis, may result in a chronic synovitis that remains culture negative. Generation of arthritogenic toxins may occur as a sequela to infection with *Clostridium difficile* or in the course of toxic shock syndrome. Antecedent infection may initiate an autoimmune attack on articular structures if the foreign antigens exhibit immunologic cross-reactivity with normal host tissues. Such molecular mimicry is reflected in the relationship between the M protein of group A *Streptococcus* and cardiac myosin, and in this regard the molecular mimicry aspects of acute rheumatic fever has significantly influenced theories of microbial pathogenesis.

Yet even molecular mimicry, a cornerstone of this line of investigation, has come under rigorous scrutiny.[46] The central notion of that theory is that if microbial antigens share elements recognized as antigenic by the immune system, then the stage is set for an activation of otherwise quiescent autoreactive T cells and B cells. However, it is evident that sequence homology between self-proteins and microbial proteins may be a relatively common event in biology and that there is a degree of degeneracy in the binding of peptides to both major histocompatibility complex (MHC) molecules on antigen-presenting cells (APCs) and to T-cell receptors on responding T cells. Thus, rigorous proof of molecular mimicry in the pathogenesis of human arthritis and autoimmunity has proved elusive, but infection may provide the stimulus for breaking tolerance to self-antigens through several nonspecific mechanisms unrelated to mimicry. Tissue damage and local necrosis of cells may uncover cryptic epitopes of self-antigens. Reactivation of resting autoreactive T cells may occur in this manner.[47] Inappropriate activation may occur owing to up-regulation of MHC molecules and costimulatory molecules on APCs. Alternatively, nonspecific T-cell activation can occur as the result of the elaboration of bacterial proteins known as superantigens.

MECHANISMS OF INFECTION AND ARTHRITIS

How most organisms gain access to the joints is unresolved, but leukocytes that have internalized these pathogens may display altered migratory patterns that would accentuate homing to the joints.[48] Several studies support the notion of the presence of a viable organism, at least transiently, in the early stages of the synovitis. It is speculated that this may reflect defective killing of the organism, either by failure to internalize the pathogen or to effectively initiate intracellular killing. There has been interest in particular in the *Chlamydia* heat shock proteins, notably hsp60, and recent studies have identified differential expression of three *C. trachomatis* hsp60-encoding genes that may differ in active versus persistent infections.[49] The cellular response to *Chlamydia* infection has been studied by microarray techniques, and 18 genes appeared to be selectively up-regulated after infection with *C. trachomatis.*[50] In a more recent examination a detailed expression profile for 14 genes induced by *C. trachomatis* and *C. pneumoniae* was shown.[50] Of interest, the genes were induced by *Salmonella typhimurium,* but this approach may shed light on common arthritogenic factors playing a role in ReA. In this study inactivated bacteria induced no specific gene expression, suggesting that innate immunity may play a role in these events. Profiling *Chlamydia* infection of U937 monocytic cells[51] and human lung epithelial cells[52] has provided a profile of induced gene expression and, in particular, has indicated which cytokines are induced by this microbial challenge.

Infection of synoviocytes with *Chlamydia* induces IL-6 production[53] and HLA class I expression.[54] The latter appears to be mediated by induction of interferon (IFN)-β, which in turn stimulates synthesis of ISFG3γ, a transcription factor participating in the regulation of the human leukocyte antigen (HLA) class I genes. Synoviocytes may represent not only a reservoir of proinflammatory bacterial antigens but also may

themselves mediate the disease process. RANKL (receptor activator of NF-κB ligand) expression was undetectable in resting synoviocytes but was dose dependently up-regulated in synoviocytes after *Salmonella* infection.[55] Osteoprotegerin was constitutively expressed by synoviocytes and was not up-regulated by infection. Infected synovioctyes induced the formation of multinucleated tartrate-resistant acid phosphatase–positive cells and formation of bone resorption pits in co-cultures of bone marrow–derived osteoclast precursors. Arthritogenic bacteria may thus induce erosive changes in bone via synoviocyte intermediaries, providing a link between infection and osteoclastogenesis. This may relate to the phenomenon of culture-negative erosive sacroiliitis that can occur as a sequela of ReA.

Salmonella infection inhibits cell surface expression of MHC class II, and this event involves the *sifA* gene locus and thus may represent a mechanism whereby this organism interferes with the development of an adaptive immune response.[56] Significant systemic effects induced by exposure to microbial factors may set the stage for the subsequent development of arthritis by several means. *Yersinia enterocolitica* O:3 isolated from patients with ReA was shown to induce polyclonal activation of B cells and autoantibody production in vivo.[57] Oligodeoxynucleotides, containing unmethylated CpG motifs characteristic of bacterial DNA, were shown to significantly increase susceptibility to arthritis in mice.[58] The host susceptibility to arthritis in this scenario was mediated by CD11c+ cells, which were the dominant source of TNF-α.

With the identification of TLR, the role of innate immunity in arthritis has come under closer scrutiny, because TLRs may mediate not only the initial host response to a pathogenic challenge but may also play key role in the development of adaptive immunity by up-regulation of key costimulatory molecules.[34] Recent studies have addressed the role of TLR-2 and TLR-4 in both RA and collagen-induced arthritis.[59,60] With respect to SpA, the relationship between TLR-4 polymorphisms and AS and no significant relationship was found.[61] In experimental *Chlamydia*-induced arthritis, TLR-4 and neutrophil Rac 1/2 have been shown to define the severity and chronicity of joint inflammation and injury,[62] and it will be important to extend such analyses into the clinical setting.

B27 IMPACT ON HOST–PATHOGEN INTERACTIONS

This host–pathogen interaction has proved to be a fertile ground for exploring noncanonical roles for HLA-27, the latter being raised in part because of the sustained difficulties in applying conventional structure and function to a mechanistic hypothesis of how B27 contributes to disease. By using transfected U937 cell lines, it has been observed that B27-positive cells kill *Salmonella* less efficiently than control cells[63] and that LPS stimulation of these transfected cells suggests that HLA-B27 enhances nuclear factor-κB activation and TNF-α secretion.[64] This phenomenon of more permissive intracellular replication of *Salmonella* may depend on the unique characteristics of the B pocket on HLA-B27, in particular the glutamic acid residue at position 45.[65] In contrast, some investigators have found that HLA-B27 expression does not alter infection nor replication of *C. trachomatis* in cell lines.[66] An alternative approach to studying transfected cell lines has been to analyze host-microbial interactions in the context of synoviocytes harvested from HLA-B27+ synoviocytes.[67] By using this approach, it was observed that HLA-B27 did not appear to play a direct role in internalization of *S. typhimurium,* nor in the kinetics of intracellular killing of this organism. In some patients there was a paradoxical response to IFN-γ, which may provide a clue to aberrant handling of pathogens in the joint, but this is unresolved at present. A biochemical approach has been to examine endogenously labeled B27-bound peptides by mass spectrometry.[68] With this approach, there was no evidence for significant changes in endogenous peptide repertoire by B*2704 after infection of the target cells with *S. typhimurium.* Although this does not exclude a role for altered cytotoxic T-lymphocyte (CTL) recognition of infected B27+ target cells, the sensitivity of mass spectrometry suggests that harvesting "arthritogenic peptides" using such an approach will be a difficult undertaking, if at all possible.

HOST HUMORAL RESPONSES

Evidence implicating microbes in SpAs has depended largely and indirectly on the humoral or cellular immune response of the host. Serologic studies continue to contribute to this body of evidence. For *Chlamydia,* the high prevalence of antichlamydial antibodies in the normal population[69] has led investigators to seek an antibody profile with sufficient sensitivity and specificity to be of diagnostic value. It has been proposed that immunoglobulin (Ig) G and IgA antibodies against major outer membrane protein—derived peptides and pgp3 may be useful in the diagnosis of *Chlamydia*-induced ReA.[70] Conversely, ReA may reflect a failure of host response to the infection. The male predominance of ReA may be related to a deficient humoral immune response to

Chlamydia, secondarily leading to systemic dissemination of the organism.[71]

HOST CELLULAR RESPONSES

Analysis of the cellular immune response has continued to shed light both on potential triggering pathogens as well as on effector mechanisms. Isolation of T-cell clones from synovial fluid (SF) of patients with post-*Yersinia* ReA identified the triggering antigens to be proteins secreted by the organism, including a phosphatase, YopH, and determined that the clones used a limited set of T-cell receptor variable region gene segments.[72] By using a similar approach for post-*Chlamydia* ReA, it has been observed that two antigens were immunodominant: the 57-kD heat shock protein and the 18-kD histone-like protein Hc1.[73] Mapping the epitope in Hc1 using synthetic peptides identified a peptide containing a sequence motif compatible with binding to HLA-DR1, the restricting element for the T-cell clones. There has been an extensive body of evidence to support the notion of local generation of SF T cells specific for the triggering bacterium. In one study the corresponding T-cell reactivity in peripheral blood was addressed.[74] In 24 of 87 patients with a bacteria-specific T-cell proliferative response in SF, there was a corresponding peripheral blood response to the same bacterium. The longitudinal profile of SF T-cell reactivity was studied in 28 patients with ReA.[75] At different time points the same bacterium was always recognized in arthritis triggered by *Chlamydia, Shigella,* and *B. burgdorferi,* with a significant degree of variation in the magnitude of the proliferative response. Only the *Yersinia*-specific responses changed specificity, suggesting that the proliferative response to *Yersinia* is nonspecific in some patients. An analysis of the specificity of CD4+ T-cell clones for *Yersinia* peptides was reported.[76] With overlapping synthetic peptides from hsp60 of *Yersinia,* the specificity of the clones identified a core epitope that was presented in an MHC promiscuous manner, and this epitope was almost identical with the B27-restricted epitope of *Yersinia* hsp60. Analysis of CR4+ T-cell responses to *C. trachomatis* revealed that in patients with ReA there were abundant blood and SF T cells specific for the 60-kD cysteine-rich outer membrane protein of *Chlamydia* and that this epitope was presented by HLA-DRB1*0401.[77] Expression libraries have also been used to provide a more comprehensive analysis of chlamydial antigenic recognition by CD4+ T cells, and flow cytometry may be a method to quantitate the number of antigen-specific T cells against the triggering pathogen in ReA.[78]

KLEBSIELLA PNEUMONIAE AND ANKYLOSING SPONDYLITIS: A CONTROVERSIAL RELATIONSHIP

Conceptual Issues Relating to the Role for *K. pneumoniae* in Ankylosing Spondylitis

Several studies in the literature have suggested a role for *K. pneumoniae* in the pathogenesis of AS. Earlier observations date to the studies of Ebringer et al.,[79,80] who demonstrated increased fecal carriage of *K. pneumoniae* in active disease. However, other investigators have been unable to confirm a difference in fecal colonization with *K. pneumoniae* between case-patients and control subjects.[81] Subsequently there have been several theories set forth to explain a possible etiopathogenetic link between *K. pneumoniae* and AS. The theory of molecular mimicry postulated antigenic cross-reactivity of microbial and host determinants. It was demonstrated, for example, by Schwimmbeck et al.[82] that there was a degree of sequence homology between HLA-B27 and the nitrogenase enzyme of *K. pneumoniae*.[82] Molecular mimicry, however, although a common biochemical reality, has been difficult to prove as a pathogenic mechanism.[46] A second theory proposed that *K. pneumoniae* antigens were capable of specifically modifying HLA-B27 or a hypothetical HLA-B27-associated receptor and that tissue damage is caused by the cytolytic activity of a circulating antibody to the infecting organism.[83] These investigators then provided evidence that CTLs can recognize certain bacterial antigens in association with HLA-B27 and suggested that this interaction may contribute directly to an immune-mediated inflammation during the initial stages of the disease.[83] Again, these events have proved difficult to rigorously prove as pathogenic mechanisms.[84,85] Finally, the arthritogenic peptide model has been proposed as an explanation of how HLA B27 may mediate disease. It suggests that AS is mediated by CTLs with specificity for a peptide of exogenous or endogenous origin. The latter might result from articular tissue, which, when presented by HLA-B27, triggers autoimmunity in the joints. This model of disease may explain the pathogenic role of microbial triggers in ReA because the candidate organisms are commonly intracellular pathogens (e.g., *Chlamydia trachomatis*) and thereby would be presented by an MHC class I molecule such as HLA-B27. However, this raises an issue for the AS-*Klebsiella* theory. *K. pneumoniae* is an extracellular organism that would normally be expected to be presented by MHC class II molecules. Despite these conceptual problems the AS-*Klebsiella* hypothesis has persisted for several years and warrants a thorough discussion because it highlights the complexities surrounding microbial triggers in SpAs generally.

Prior Studies on the Role of *K. pneumoniae* in the Pathogenesis of Ankylosing Spondylitis

There have been numerous reports implicating *K. pneumoniae* in AS that have been based primarily on detection of a distinctive humoral immune response to this organism.[86–91] Some of these studies have shown polyclonal serum antibody responses to *K. pneumoniae*.[91] Enzyme-linked immunoabsorbent assay (ELISA) analyses by Sahly et al.[90] indicated that there was an increase in serum IgG against several strains of *K. pneumoniae* in patients with AS in contrast to control subjects. Maki-Ikola et al.[92] reported that active AS was associated with increased IgG, IgM, and IgA against *Klebsiella* LPS and that there was a decline in antibody titer after treatment with sulfasalazine. However, there remains significant controversy in the literature over the specificity of antibodies against *K. pneumoniae*. In a recent study no evidence was found for AS-specific serologic responses to multiple serotypes of *K. pneumoniae* in a cohort of 187 patients with AS compared with 195 control subjects.[93] Furthermore, attempts to identify *Klebsiella* DNA by PCR in sacroiliac biopsy specimens of patients with AS have not been successful.[94] No clinical improvement in the disease activity has been demonstrated with antibiotic therapy,[95] which further weakens the argument for the role of at least an *active* infection in AS. Finally, there has been no evidence to date that *K. pneumoniae* demonstrates any joint tropism. All of these factors raise important questions about the role of *K. pneumoniae* as an important microbial trigger in AS, but the controversy persists as investigators continue to report elevation of serum antibodies to *K. pneumoniae* in this disease. There are several reasons that might contribute to the discrepancies in the literature and the lack of reproducibility of results. First, in most studies addressing microbial pathogenesis in AS only serum antibody profiles have been used to implicate potential pathogens. There are far fewer studies in which T-cell responses to candidate organisms in AS have been evaluated, yet this may represent a more complete approach to detecting an immune fingerprint of a recent or remote infection in an individual with AS. Second, the prevalence of the test pathogen in the control population has generally not been adequately addressed. Finally, there have been a variety of antigenic preparations used in these studies, not always accompanied by microbial control antigens.

Family Studies Evaluating the Role of *K. pneumoniae* in Ankylosing Spondylitis

Recently, we conducted a case-control study to compare the immune profile of patients with AS in

25 multiplex AS families with unaffected family members and normal healthy control subjects to resolve whether there was evidence of a predominant immune response to *K. pneumoniae* in AS.[96] Twenty-five families with two or more individuals affected with AS and 34 normal age-, sex-, and ethnically matched control subjects were enrolled in the study. All affected ($n = 57$) and unaffected ($n = 39$) family members had a detailed clinical evaluation. Peripheral blood was drawn to measure T-lymphocyte proliferation and IgG and IgA (by ELISA analysis) immune response to *K. pneumoniae*, *S. typhimurium*, *Y. enterocolitica*, and *C. trachomatis*. Immune responses to each of the four candidate organisms were compared in affected and unaffected individuals and normal healthy control subjects. With respect to cell proliferation to microbial antigens, there were no differences in the response profiles between affected and unaffected individuals. In profiling antibody responses to the microbial antigens there are no differences between affected or unaffected family members for each of the candidate organisms Figure 4.1 provides a representative result from the study, depicting the IgA anti-*Klebsiella* profile among affected and unaffected family members and healthy control subjects. This result highlights the importance of careful selection of environmental controls such as unaffected family members, which we used in this study. In addition, this observation may shed some light on the elevated serum anti-*Klebsiella* antibodies reported in previous studies in which affected individuals were compared with normal healthy control subjects as opposed to family members. Thus, although we confirmed the results of prior investigations that there appears to be a heightened serum antibody pattern against *K. pneumoniae*, we found no specificity for AS. This finding speaks against a pathogenic role for this organism in AS. Finally, we were unable to demonstrate any associations

between clinical characteristics and immune responses. Because one of the unique aspects of this study was the familial case-control design, we addressed whether there was any clustering of specific antimicrobial immune response within families, but we saw none.

Relatively few researchers have addressed T-cell responses to *Klebsiella* antigens in the literature to date. Dominguez-Lopez et al.[97] evaluated T-cell responses in a small cohort of 13 patients with AS. With peripheral blood mononuclear cells (PBMCs), cellular proliferation to a GroEL-like protein (hsp60) of *K. pneumoniae* was demonstrated in 7 of 13 patients. However, numbers were small in this study, and the antigen preparation used was different from that used in our study. Furthermore, the key control group was patients with RA, whereas in our study the unaffected family members served as the control group. Interestingly, these same authors also showed that HLA-B27–positive individuals recognized not only the GroEL-like HSP protein from *K. pneumoniae* but also GroEL-like proteins from other organisms such as *Mycobacterium*.[87] This finding suggests that the humoral immune response they detected in AS may be related to HSP from a range of microbes, but without specificity for *K. pneumoniae*. In one prior study addressing cellular immune responses in familial AS, Hohler et al.[98] reported that there were no differences in T-cell responses between affected and unaffected twins in a study of 11 monozygotic twins. Affected twins, however, had a decrease in the calculated frequency of *K. pneumoniae*–responsive T cells in peripheral blood lymphocytes compared with healthy HLA-B27+ subjects. It was speculated that this quantitative reduction in specific T cells might reflect a defective host defense against *Klebsiella*. In this study, various antigen preparations of *K. pneumoniae* (K21 and K43) were used for ELISA antibody studies, and there were no differences between affected and unaffected subjects for K21, but there was a lower response to K43 in affected subjects. In our study we used K43 as the antigen preparation because it has been the antigen used most consistently in prior studies implicating *K. pneumoniae* in the pathogenesis of AS.[88] Hermann et al.[99] also reported a quantitative reduction in *K. pneumoniae*-responsive T cells in the peripheral blood lymphocytes of patients with AS compared with healthy control subjects. Furthermore, those authors reported that PBMC responses to *K. pneumoniae* may be depressed in comparison with concurrent synovial fluid mononuclear cell (SFMC) responses. We analyzed paired samples of PBMCs and SFMCs from four patients with AS, but found there was no significant difference in the pattern of PBMC and SFMC responses to *K. pneumoniae* in these patients. In conclusion, in our study we tried to address the shortcomings of study design of some prior approaches to this question. Examining the immune

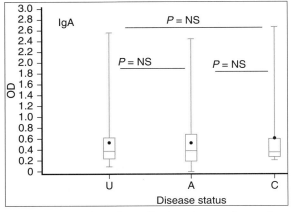

Fig. 4.1 IgA anti-*Klebsiella* profiles in patients and control subjects.

response to *K. pneumoniae* in affected versus unaffected individuals in familial AS, we found no evidence supporting a causal role for *K. pneumoniae* in AS.

CYTOKINES

Analysis of T-cell subsets with respect to cytokine profiles is a further method for studying the link between infection and ReA. Exposure to different pathogens can stimulate at least two patterns of cytokine production by CD4$^+$T cells (Th1 and Th2). It has been long held that Th1 cells mediate a protective role against intracellular pathogens. Thus, it would seem appropriate that these cells would be central in clinical complications of such infections. In a study of 11 patients with ReA, it was observed that stimulation of SFMCs resulted in secretion of low amounts of IFN-γ and TNF-α but high amounts of IL-10.[100] IL-10 was responsible for suppression of IFN-γ and TNF-α as judged by the effect of adding IL-10 or anti-IL-10 to the cells. The suppression of Th1-like cytokines is probably mediated through suppression of IL-12 synthesis. In the synovial tissues of these patients, a higher number of cells were positive for the Th2 cytokine IL-4, compared with the number of IFN-γ-secreting cells. This IL-10/IL-12 balance, resulting in a predominance of Th2 cytokines, may contribute to the persistence of bacteria in the joint. In comparison with RA, SF levels of TNF-α in ReA are lower, despite comparable levels of IL-2 receptor, again implicating a relative deficiency of protective, antimicrobial cytokines in the local environment.[101] SF cytokines have been studied in patients with *Chlamydia*-induced arthritis, and it was found that B27$^+$ patients had lower SF IFN-γ levels and also had a more chronic disease course.[102] This finding suggests that diminished IFN-γ generation might account for the persistence of the arthritis. The source of these cytokines may not only be the infiltrating immunoreactive mononuclear cells, but also the resident synoviocytes. When human synoviocytes are infected with *C. trachomatis* in vitro, there is generation of IL-6, transforming growth factor-β, and granulocyte-macrophage colony-stimulating factor.[103] The cells respond to IFN-γ with secretion of TNF-α, so this represents another contributory population of cells in the joint, in addition to B cells and T cells. Whether these cytokine profiles are primarily genetically defined is an important unanswered question.[104,105] The non-B27 genes that are contributing to disease susceptibility in patients with SpA have not been characterized adequately for a definitive answer. Enhanced production of TNF-α and IFN-γ is observed in chronic ReA compared with either acute ReA or RA.[106] The TNF dependence of chronic inflammation in the spine draws indirect support from the dramatic changes that follow the institution of anti-TNF therapies in these patients. Yet cytokine in the setting of infection can be helpful or harmful, depending on the time under observation. In studies of murine experimental *Yersinia*-induced arthritis, it has been observed that TNF-α is deleterious for the host in the acute phase of the infection, because there is a TNF-mediated apoptosis of CD4$^+$ cells.[107] However, in the chronic phase of the disease TNF-α is helpful for host defense, because TNF-mediated production of nitric oxide plays a critical role in clearance of the pathogen.[108] It is recognized that reactivation of tuberculosis can occur after the institution of anti-TNF therapy in patients with SpA, but experience to date has not unmasked quiescent arthritogenic pathogens in the treated patients in this population. Clearly vigilance is warranted as long-term experience with these agents grows.

B27 EFFECT ON HOST IMMUNE RESPONSES

The strong association of HLA-B27 with SpAs has indirectly implicated microbial antigen-specific, MHC class I–restricted CD8$^+$ CTLs as playing a role in the pathogenesis of these diseases. It is important to note in this context that CD8$^+$ T cells in SF may express natural killer (NK) cell receptors.[109] Such cells reflect a high degree of heterogeneity in the expression of NK cell receptors, which may modulate their cytotoxicity and contribute to disease pathogenesis as a result. The fact that certain subtypes of HLA-B27 are more strongly associated with SpAs than others has implicated T-cell specificities in a more precise fashion.[110,111] The HLA-B*2709 subtype, although differing by a single amino acid (His116 → Asp116), from the strongly AS-associated subtype B27*2705, is not found in patients with AS. It has been shown that CD8$^+$ T cells can distinguish these two B27 subtypes when presenting the same epitope derived from Epstein-Barr virus low molecular weight proteosome (LMP)-2, suggesting that the subtypes may differ in presenting an arthritogenic peptide derived from microbial sources.[112] A recent approach using peptide binding has addressed what might differentiate HLA-B*2704 (associated with SpAs) from HLA-B*2706 (not associated with SpAs). The main structural feature of peptides differentially bound to B*2704 was the presence of COOH-terminal Tyr or Arg together with a strong preference for aliphatic/aromatic P3 residues. This provides a distinctive profile of B*2704 and B*2706 binding that correlates with their differential association with SpAs. An analysis of the specificity of T-cell clones demonstrated that target cells pulsed with *Yersinia* 60-kD heat shock protein, but not with other *Yersinia* proteins, were successfully lysed by the CTLs and that this killing was restricted by B27.[113] It was also observed that a single nonamer, 321 to 329, derived from *Yersinia* hsp60 was the dominant epitope in this recognition event. In another approach to this interaction, it was shown that T cells themselves can be infected with *Yersinia* and that infected CTLs have a reduced lytic capacity against syngeneic and allogeneic infected target cells, implicating a breakdown in immune surveillance that could occur by this mechanism during the course of gram-negative bacterial infection.[114] By using a computer-generated algorithm that incorporated HLA-B27 binding motifs and proteosome-generated motifs, an approach to identifying immunodominant peptides from *C. trachomatis* has been undertaken.[115] Nine peptides so identified proved to be stimulatory for CD8+ T cells, and many of these same peptides were recognized by CD8+ T cells derived from patients with ReA. Peptide binding to these T cells was also demonstrated by tetramer staining. This approach may prove to be valuable for identifying key peptides from arthritogenic pathogens. In a recent study HLA-B27 tetramers were successfully used to identify low-frequency antigen-specific T cells in *Chlamydia*-induced ReA.[116] Such cells could be expanded ex vivo, suggesting a functional capability that may contribute to the arthritis.

Whether microbial peptides share functional homology with self-proteins, such as B27 itself, has remained unresolved. There is some supportive evidence for this notion of molecular mimicry in SpA,[117,118] but the theory leaves important questions unanswered. For example, the target-organ specificity of AS remains unexplained, as well as the apparent frequency of homologous sequences even among bacteria not commonly thought to be arthritogenic on clinical grounds. An immuno-dominant epitope from the *S. typhimurium* GroEL molecule was recognized by CD8+ cytotoxic T lymphocytes after natural infection in mice,[119] and these CTLs cross-reacted with peptides derived from mouse hsp60. This cross-reaction provided a model that might link bacterial immunity with autoimmunity, although several aspects of this relationship remain unexplained.[120] A dodecamer derived from the intracytoplasmic tail of HLA-B27 was found to be a natural ligand for disease-associated subtypes (B*2702, B*2704, and B*2705) but for non-disease–associated subtypes (B*2706 and B*2709). This peptide showed striking homology to a region of the DNA primase from *C. trachomatis*, indicating that some mimicry exists between B27-derived and chlamydial peptides that might relate to cross-reactivity of immune responses against microbial and endogenous antigens.[121] In a study of CTL recognition of B27, it was observed in an animal model that a prior expansion of an immune response against HLA-B27 results in a reduced threshold for generating a primary antichlamydial CTL response.[122] A subsequent study applied this system in

B27-transgenic animals.[123] Such animals are tolerant of immunization with B27 DNA, but if splenocytes from these animals are exposed to *Chlamydia* in vitro, then autoreactive CTLs with specificity for B27 are generated. The autoreactive epitope of HLA-B27 involves Lys70 in a critical way. This involvement indicates a dynamic interrelationship between the pathogen and host B27 that may have important implications for the pathogenesis of ReA. These interactions might result in a break in self-tolerance or perhaps impaired clearance of the organism on the basis of impaired recognition of the organism as nonself.

EPIDEMIOLOGIC STUDIES

Studies on the epidemiology of ReA have shed new light on the frequency of this complication of enteric infections. A prospective study of the annual incidence of inflammatory joint disease in Sweden showed that the annual incidence of ReA (28 per 100,000) exceeded that of RA (24 per 100,000), emphasizing the importance of ReA in the overall burden of rheumatic diseases.[123a] In that same study population it was determined that 45% of patients with new-onset arthritis had had a prior infection and that *Campylobacter* was the dominant organism in this cohort.[124] Studies on both sporadic[125] and outbreak[126] *S. typhimurium* infections have further substantiated the role of *Salmonella* in triggering ReA. The frequency of this event has generally been in the range of 10%,[127] but in a recent study of 91 individuals exposed to food-borne *Salmonella enteritidis* 17 developed ReA, indicating that this event may occur more often than previously thought.[128] In a population-based study, it was determined that ReA after *Campylobacter* infections is common, with an annual incidence of 4.3 per 100,000.[129] These incidence figures are no doubt strongly influenced by the population under study. The frequency of ReA after an outbreak of *Campylobacter jejuni* was 2.6%, and the clinical course was benign.[130] Conversely, ReA after an outbreak of *Yersinia pseudotuberculosis* O:3 was more common (15%), and the clinical course was more severe.[131] ReA appears to be more prevalent in Alaskan Eskimo populations[132] whereas the incidence of ReA after a *Salmonella* outbreak appears to be lower in children than in adults.[133]

One mechanism that may indirectly implicate microbial antigens of gut origin is the coexistence of inflammation in the gastrointestinal (GI) tract and the joint. This relationship relates both to postdysenteric ReA as well as to the arthritis associated with inflammatory bowel disease. It appears that inflammatory lesions in the gut occur in 68% of patients with SpAs, including patients with classic AS and no history of GI symptomatology.[134–136] There is a correlation between the resolution of GI and joint inflammation, and this relationship may reflect altered bowel permeability and repeated microbial antigenemia as a mechanism, but formal proof is needed. The range of pathogens may be broader than those classically linked to SpAs (*Yersinia, Salmonella, Shigella,* and *Chlamydia*), but often these organisms are not associated with the common clinical features summarized earlier. More sophisticated techniques such as PCR may broaden the definition of the arthritogenic pathogens even further. Poststreptococcal ReA continues to attract the attention of investigators,[137] and *Streptococcus* is the most common arthritogenic bacteria beyond the gram-negative pathogens listed. Poststreptococcal arthritis in children is a potential predecessor of rheumatic heart disease, although the relationship to acute rheumatic fever is not clearly defined.[138] A recent report of six adult patients with poststreptococcal ReA highlighted the imprint contribution of this entity in the differential diagnosis of acute polyarthritis.[139] Another discriminating feature between poststreptococcal ReA and the more common forms is its association with HLA-DR alleles (DRB1*01) rather than with HLA-B27, suggesting that the cellular basis for the inflammation in the two syndromes may differ fundamentally.[140] Other microbial triggers that have been implicated in association with arthritis recently have included bacille Calmette-Guérin,[141,142] hepatitis B virus vaccination,[143] Lyme disease vaccination,[144] enterotoxigenic *Escherichia coli,*[145] and a broad range of parasites.[146]

Researchers have attempted to define the relative contributions of different pathogens to the general picture of ReA. However, the lack of universally agreed-upon classification criteria continue to pose problems for population studies of incidence and prevalence. In an urban sexually transmitted disease clinic, it was observed that 4.1% of patients with genital infection or inflammation had objective ReA, and chlamydial or nongonococcal sexually transmitted disease syndromes accounted for 88% of these cases.[147] SpA represents an interplay of environmental and genetic factors, and recent population studies have begun to unravel new aspects of this dynamic interaction. In a study of twins with AS, it was concluded that genetic factors accounted for 97% of the determining influence, suggesting that an environmental trigger for the disease is likely to be ubiquitous and may contribute little to the population variance.[148] When one includes the broader spectrum of the SpAs and the interplay between infection and genetics, the picture may be very different. In a large study addressing the prevalence of SpA in HLA-B27–positive and HLA-B27–negative blood donors, there was a prevalence of 13.6% among B27-positive individuals and 0.7% in the B27-negative population.[149] The relative risk of developing SpA in B27-positive subjects

was calculated as 20.7. Taking into account the frequency of B27 in the population studied, it was concluded that the SpAs have a prevalence of 1.9%, making this group of arthropathies among the most common rheumatic diseases. With respect to environmental triggers, other genetically defined modulators of immune response, particularly those affecting host innate immunity, are attractive candidates for non-MHC genes that may contribute to disease susceptibility. Mannose-binding lectin was examined but did not differentiate ReA patients from control subjects.[150] Conversely, enhanced gene expression of host defense scavenger receptors was demonstrated both in patients with ReA and in patients with RA.[151] This continues to be an area of active investigation.

CLINICAL COURSE, ANTIBIOTIC TRIALS

Clinical studies have provided a more complete picture of the manifestations and the clinical course of ReA. Thomson et al.[152] reported on a large cohort of patients with post-*Salmonella* ReA at a 5-year follow-up interval after the initial infection. In 9 of the 27 patients the arthritis resolved within 4 months of onset. Eighteen patients continued to have symptoms 5 years after onset, and in 4 of these patients the symptoms were severe enough to force a change of work. At the 5-year point, 37% had objective changes in the joints. The important long-term sequelae have kept the question of antibiotic therapy as an important area for study. In a 3-month, double-blind, randomized, placebo-controlled study no benefit was found for ciprofloxacin treatment in patients with ReA and undifferentiated oligoarthritis.[153] In subgroup analysis ciprofloxacin was better than a placebo in *Chlamydia*-induced ReA but not in *Salmonella*- or *Yersinia*-induced ReA. This general impression was borne out in a report that lymecycline decreased the duration of acute arthritis in *Chlamydia*-induced ReA but not in other ReA.[154] Of 17 patients followed for 10 years in this study, 1 patient had AS, 3 had radiographic sacroiliitis, and 3 had radiographic changes in peripheral joints, but long-term lymecycline treatment did not change the natural history of the disease. A 3-month trial of doxycycline for chronic SpA was no better than a placebo for pain or functional status, but few patients had a causative organism identified.[155]

In a group of patients with undifferentiated SpA it was reported that a combination of doxycycline and rifampin was superior to doxycycline alone, although no placebo was included in the study design.[156] In a 4- to 7-year follow-up of an earlier ReA trial, it was noted that chronic arthritis developed in 41% of patients initially treated with placebo in contrast to 8% of patients initially treated with ciprofloxacin, suggesting that the long-term prognosis might be favorably influenced by antibiotic treatment.[157] At present, the consensus that *Chlamydia*-induced ReA alone may be responsive to antibiotic treatment raises the interesting question that the pathogenesis of acute and chronic ReA induced by this organism may be very different from that induced by the enteric pathogens, but the critical differences at the cellular level have not been defined. Recently the results of a 3-month, placebo-controlled trial of azithromycin in ReA was reported.[158] With 152 patients who were analyzed for response, it was concluded that azithromycin, given orally for 13 weeks, was ineffective in ReA.

The role of infectious triggers in rheumatic diseases in general has been a long-standing pursuit for many investigators, and the potential of antimicrobial therapies to modify disease course has been a corollary of this search.[159] It should be recalled that the initial reports of *Helicobacter pylori* recovered from the gastric tissues of patients with peptic ulcer disease were met with great skepticism.[160] Eradicating this organism is now considered optimal therapy for this disease[161]—perhaps a word of caution for the critics and a word of encouragement for the microbe hunters in the joints.

REFERENCES

1. Inman RD. Classification criteria for reactive arthritis. J Rheumatol. 1999;26:1219–1221.
2. Pacheo-Tena C, Burgos-Vargas R, Vazquez-Mellado J, et al. A proposal for the classification of patients to enter clinical and experimental studies on reactive arthritis. J Rheumatol. 1999;26:1338–1347.
3. Sieper J, Braun J. Problems and advances in the diagnosis of reactive arthritis. J Rheumatol. 1999;26:1124–1222.
4. Braun J, Kingsley G, van der Heijde D, Sieper J. On the difficulties of establishing a consensus on the definition and diagnostic criteria for reactive arthritis. J Rheum. 2000;27:185–192.
5. Sieper J, Rudwaleit M, Braun J, van der Heigde D. Diagnosing reactive arthritis: role of clinical setting in the value of serologic and microbiologic assays. Arthritis Rheum. 2002;46:319–327.
6. Fendler C, Laitko S, Sorensen H, et al. Frequency of triggering bacteria in patients with reactive arthritis and undifferentiated oligoarthritis and the relative importance of the tests used for diagnosis. Ann Rheum Dis. 2001;60:337–343.
7. Nikkari S, Puolakkainen M, Narvanen A, AAkre O, Toivanen P, Leirisalo-Repo M. Use of a peptide based enzyme immunoassay in diagnosis of *Chlamydia trachomatis* triggered reactive arthritis. J Rheumatol. 2001;28:2487–2493.
8. Inman RD, Chiu B. Synoviocyte-packaged *Chlamydia trachomatis* induces a chronic aseptic arthritis. J Clin Invest. 1998;102:1776–1782.
9. Gerard HC, Schumacher HR, El-Gabalawy H, Goldbach-Mansky R, Hudson AP. *Chlamydia pneumoniae* present in the human synovium are viable and metabolically active. Microb Pathog. 2000;29:17–24.
10. Schumacher HR Jr, Gerard HC, Arayssi TK, et al. Lower prevalence of *Chlamdydia pneumoniae* DNA compared with *Chlamydia trachomatis* DNA in synovial tissue of arthritis patients. Arthritis Rheum. 1999;42:1889–1893.
11. Sigal LH. Synovial fluid polymerase chain reaction detection of pathogens—what does it really mean? Arthritis Rheum. 2001;44:2463–2485.
12. Schumacher HR Jr, Arayssi T, Crane M, et al. *Chlamydia trachomatis* nucleic acids can be found in the synovium of some asymptomatic subjects. Arthritis Rheum. 1999;42:1281–1284.
13. Cuchacovich R, Japa S, Huang WQ, et al. Detection of bacterial DNA in Latin American patients with reactive arthritis by polymerase chain reaction and sequencing analysis. J Rheumatol. 2002;29:1426–1429.
14. Pacheco-Tena P, De La Barrerra A, Lopez-Vidal Y, et al. Bacterial DNA in synovial fluid cells of patients with juvenile onset spondyloarthopathies. Rheumatology (Oxford). 2001;40:920–927.
15. Cox CJ, Kempsell KE, Gaston JS. Investigation of infectious agents associated with arthritis by reverse transcription PCR of bacterial rRNA. Arthritis Res Ther. 2003;5:R1–R8.
16. Gerard HC, Wang Z, Wang GF, et al. Chromosomal DNA from a variety of bacterial species is present in synovial tissue from patients with various forms of arthritis. Arthritis Rheum. 2001; 44:1689–1697.
17. Chen T, Rimpilainen M, Luukkainen R, et al. Bacterial components in the synovial tissue of patients with advanced rheumatoid arthritis or osteoarthritis: analysis with gas chromatography-mass spectrometry and pan-bacterial polymerase chain reaction. Arthritis Rheum. 2003;49:328–334.
18. Zhang X, Pacheco-Tena C, Inman RD. Microbe hunting in the joints. Arthritis Rheum. 2003;49:479–482.
19. Toivanen A, Toivanen P. Reactive arthritis. Curr Opin Rheumatol. 2000;12:300–305.
20. Hyrich KL, Inman RD. Infectious agents in chronic rheumatic diseases. Curr Opin Rheumatol. 2001;13:300–304.
21. Bas S, Griffais R, Kvien TK, Glennas A, Melby K, Vischer TL. Amplification of plasmid and chromosome Chlamydia DNA in synovial fluid of patients with reactive arthritis and undifferentiated seronegative oligoarthropathies. Arthritis Rheum. 1995; 38:1005–1013.
22. Branigan PJ, Gerard HC, Hudson AP, Schumacher HR Jr, Panbdo J. Comparison of synovial tissue and synovial fluid as the source of nucleic acids for detection of *Chlamydia trachomatis* by polymerase chain reaction. Arthritis Rheum. 1996;39:1740–1746.
23. Olmez N, Wang GF, Li Y, Zhang H, Schumacher HR. Chlamydial nucleic acids in synovium in osteoarthritis: what are the implications? J Rheumatol. 2001;28:1874–1880.
24. Schumacher HR Jr, Magge S, Cherian PV, et al. Light and electron microscopic studies on the synovial membrane in Reiter's syndrome. Immunocytochemical identification of chlamydial antigen in patients with early disease. Arthritis Rheum. 1988; 31:937–946.
25. Nikkari S, Rantakokko K, Ekman P, et al. *Salmonella*-triggered reactive arthritis: use of polymerase chain reaction, immunocytochemical staining, and gas chromatography-mass spectrometry in the detection of bacterial components from synovial fluid. Arthritis Rheum. 1999;42:84–89.
26. Granfors K, Jalkanen S, von Essen R, et al. *Yersinia* antigens in synovial-fluid cells from patients with reactive arthritis. N Engl J Med. 1989;320:216–221.
27. van der Heijden IM, Wilbrink B, et al. Presence of bacterial DNA and bacterial peptidoglycans in joints of patients with rheumatoid arthritis and other arthritides. Arthritis Rheum. 2000;43: 593–598.
28. Gerard HC, Wang Z, Wang GF, et al. Chromosomal DNA from a variety of bacterial species is present in synovial tissue from patients with various forms of arthritis. Arthritis Rheum. 2001;44:1689–1697.
29. Pacheco-Tena C, Alvarado De La Barrera C, et al. Bacterial DNA in synovial fluid cells of patients with juvenile onset spondyloarthropathies. Rheumatology (Oxford). 2001;40:920–927.
30. Braun J, Tuszewski M, Ehlers S, et al. Nested polymerase chain reaction strategy simultaneously targeting DNA sequences of multiple bacterial species in inflammatory joint diseases.

II. Examination of sacroiliac and knee joint biopsies of patients with spondyloarthropathies and other arthritides. J Rheumatol. 1997;24:1101–1105.

31. Gilbart J, Fox A, Whiton RS, Morgan SL. Rhamnose and muramic acid: chemical markers for bacterial cell walls in mammalian tissues. J Microbiol Methods. 1986;5:272–282.

32. Christensson B, Gilbart J, Fox A, Morgan SL. Mass spectrometric quantitation of muramic acid, a bacterial cell wall component, in septic synovial fluids. Arthritis Rheum. 1989;32:1268–1272.

33. Lehtonen L, Kortekangas P, Oksman P, Eerola E, Aro H, Toivanen A. Synovial fluid muramic acid in acute inflammatory arthritis. Br J Rheumatol. 1994;33:1127–1130.

34. Pacheco-Tena C, Zhang X, Stone M, Burgos-Vargas R, Inman RD. Innate immunity in host-microbial interactions: Beyond B27 in the spondyloarthropathies. Curr Opin Rheumatol. 2002;14:373–382.

35. Schrijver IA, Melief M-J, Tak PP, Hazenberg MP, Laman JD. Antigen-presenting cells containing bacterial peptidoglycan in synovial tissues of rheumatoid arthritis patients coexpress costimulatory molecules and cytokines. Arthritis Rheum. 2000;43:2160–2168.

36. Simelyte E, Rimpiläinen M, Lehtonen L, Zhang X, Toivanen P. Bacterial cell wall-induced arthritis: chemical composition and tissue distribution of four Lactobacillus strains. Infect Immun. 2000;68:3535–3540.

37. Zhang X, Rimpiläinen M, Simelyte E, Toivanen P. Characterization of Eubacterium cell wall: peptidoglycan structure determines arthritogenicity. Ann Rheum Dis. 2001;60:269–274.

38. Zhang X, Rimpilainen M, Simelyte E, Toivanen P. Enzyme degradation and proinflammatory activity in arthritogenic and nonarthritogenic Eubacterium aerofaciens cell walls. Infect Immun. 2001;69:7277–7284.

39. Sato S, Takeuchi O, Fujita T, Tomizawa H, Takeda K, Akira S. A variety of microbial components induce tolerance to lipopolysaccharide by differentially affecting MyD88-dependent and -independent pathways. Int Immunol. 2002;14:783–791.

40. Jacinto R, Hartung T, McCall C, Li L. Lipopolysaccharide- and lipoteichoic acid-induced tolerance and cross-tolerance: distinct alterations in IL-1 receptor-associated kinase. J Immunol. 2002;168:6136–6141.

41. Medvedev AE, Henneke P, Schromm A, et al. Induction of tolerance to lipopolysaccharide and mycobacterial components in Chinese hamster ovary/CD14 cells is not affected by overexpression of Toll-like receptors 2 or 4. J Immunol. 2001;167:2257–2267.

42. Lorenz E, Mira JP, Cornish KL, Arbour NC, Schwartz DA. A novel polymorphism in the toll-like receptor 2 gene and its potential association with staphylococcal infection. Infect Immun. 2000;68:6398–6401.

43. Arbour NC, Lorenz E, Schutte BC, et al. TLR4 mutations are associated with endotoxin hyporesponsiveness in humans. Nat Genet. 2000;25:187–191.

44. Agnese DM, Calvano JE, Hahm SJ, et al. Human Toll-like receptor 4 mutations but not CD14 polymorphisms are associated with an increased risk of gram-negative infections. J Infect Dis. 2002;186:1522–1525.

45. Schumacher HR Jr, Gerard HC, Arayssi TK, et al. Lower prevalence of Chlamydia pneumoniae DNA compared with Chlamydia trachomatis DNA in synovial tissue of arthritis patients. Arthritis Rheum. 1999;42:1889–1893.

46. Albert LJ, Inman RD. Molecular mimicry and autoimmunity. N Engl J Med. 1999; 341:2068–2074.

47. Horwitz MS, Bradley LM, Halberston J, Krahl T, Lee J, Sarvetnick N. Diabetes induced by Coxsackie virus: initiation by bystander damage and not by molecular mimicry. Nat Med. 1998;4:781–785.

48. Wuorela M, Tohka S, Granfors K, Jalkanen S. Monocytes that have ingested Yersinia enterocolitica serotype O:3 acquire capacity to bind to nonstimulated vascular endothelial cells via P-selectin. Infect Immun. 1999;67:726–732.

49. Gerard HC, Whittum-Hudson JA, Schumacher HR, Hudson AP. Differential expression of three Chlamydia trachomatis hsp60-encoding genes in active vs. persistent infections. Microb Pathog. 2004;36:35–39

50. Hess S, Rheinheimer C, Tidow F, et al. The reprogrammed host: Chlamydia trachomatis-induced upregulation of glycoprotein 130 cytokines, transcription factors and antiapoptotic genes. Arthritis Rheum. 2001;44:2392–2401.

51. Virok D, Loboda A, Kari L, et al. Infection of U937 monocytic cells with Chlamydia pneumoniae induces extensive changes in host cell gene expression. J Infect Dis. 2003;188:1310–1321.

52. Yang J, Hooper WC, Phillips DJ, Tondella ML, Talkington DF. Induction of proinflammatory cytokines in human lung epithelial cells during Chalmydia pneumoniae infection. Infect Immun. 2003;71:614–620.

53. Hanada H, Ikeda-Dantsuji Y, Naito M, Nagayama A. Infection of human fibroblast-like synovial cells with Chlamydia trachomatis results in persistent infection and IL-6 production. Microb Pathog. 2003;34:57–63.

54. Rodel JM, Vogelsang H, Prager K, Hartmann M, Schmidt KH, Straube E. Role of IFN-stimulated gene factor 3γ and β-interferon in HLA class I enhancement in synovial fibroblasts upon infection with Chlamydia trachomatis. Infect Immun. 2002;70:6140–6146.

55. Xiang Z, Aubin JE, Kim TH, Payne U, Chiu B, Inman RD. Synovial fibroblasts infected with Salmonella enterica serovar Typhimurium mediate osteoclast differentiation and activation. Infect Immun. 2004;72:7183–7189.

56. Mitchell EK, Mastroeni P, Kelly AP, Trowsdale J. Inhibition of cell surface MHC class II expression by Salmonella. Eur J Immunol. 2004;34:2559–2567.

57. Silva EE, Ramos OP, Bauab TM, Falcao DP, de Medeiros BM. Yersinia enterocolitica 0:3 isolated from patients with or without reactive arthritis induces polyclonal activation of B cells and autoantibody production in vivo. Autoimmunity. 2003;36:261–268.

58. Zeuner RA, Verthelyi D, Gursel M, Ishii KJ, Klinman DM. Influence of stimulatory and suppressive DNA motifs on host susceptibility to inflammatory arthritis. Arthritis Rheum. 2003;48:1701–1707.

59. Radstake TR, Roelofs MF, Jenniskens YM, et al. Expression of Toll-like receptors 2 and 4 in rheumatoid synovial tissue and regulation by proinflammatory cytokines IL-12 and IL-18 via γ interferon. Arthritis Rheum. 2004;50:3856–3865.

60. Lee EK, Kang SM, Pail DJ, Kim JM, Youn J. Essential roles of TLR-4 signaling in arthritis induced by type II collagen antibody and LPS. Int Immunol. 2005;17:325–333.

61. van der Paardt M, Crusius JB, de Koning MH, et al. No evidence for involvement of the TLR-4 A896G and CD-14-C260T polymorphism in susceptibility to ankylosing spondylitis. Ann Rheum Dis. 2005;64:235–238.

62. Zhang X, Glogauer M, Zhu F, Kim TH, Chiu B, Inman RD. Effective pathogen clearance in Chlamydia-induced arthritis is dependent on neutrophil Rac1/2 and TLR4. Arthritis Rheum. 2005;52:1297–1304.

63. Ekman P, Saarinen M, He Q, et al. HLA-B27-transfected and HLA-A2-transfected human monocytic U937 cells differ in their production of cytokines. Infect Immun. 2002;70:1609–1614.

64. Pentinnen MA, Holmberg CI, Sistonen LM, Granfors K: HLA-B27 modulates NFκB activation in human monocytic cells exposed to lipopolysaccharide. Arthritis Rheum. 2002;46:2172–2180.

65. Pentinnen MA, Heiskanen KM, Mohaptra R, et al. Enhanced intracellular replication of Salmonella enteritidis in HLA-B27-expressing human monocytic cells. Arthritis Rheum. 2004;50: 2225–2263.

66. Young JL, Smith L, Matyszak MK, Gaston JS. HLA-B27 expression does not modulate intracellular Chlamydia trachomatis infection of cell lines. Infect Immun. 2001;69:6670–6675.

67. Payne U, Inman RD. Determinants of synovocyte clearance of arthritogenic bacteria. J Rheumatol. 2003;30:1291–1297.

68. Ringrose JH, Meiring HD, Spiejer D, et al. Major histocompatibility complex class I peptide presentation and Salmonella enterica serovar typhimurium infection assessed via a stable isotope tagging of the B27-presented peptide repertoire. Infect Immun. 2004;72:5097–5105.

69. Erlacher L, Wintersberger W, Menschik M, et al. Reactive arthritis: urogenital swab culture is the only useful diagnostic method for detection of the arthritogenic infection in extra-articularly asymptomatic patients with undifferentiated oligoarthritis. Br J Rheumatol. 1995;34:838–842.

70. Bas S, Genevay S, Schenkel MC, Vischer TL. Importance of species-specific antigens in the serodiagnosis of Chlamydia trachomatis reactive arthritis. Rheumatology (Oxford). 2002;41:1017–1020.

71. Bas S, Scieux C, Vischer TL. Male sex predominance in Chlamydia trachomatis sexually acquired reactive arthritis: are women more protected by anti-Chlamydia antibodies? Ann Rheum Dis. 2001;60:605–611.

72. Lahesmaa R, Soderberg C, Bliska J, et al. Pathogen antigen- and superantigen-reactive synovial fluid T cells in reactive arthritis. J Infect Dis. 1995;172:1290–1297.

73. Gaston JS, Deane KH, Jecock RM, Pearce JH. Identification of 2 Chlamydia trachomatis antigens recognized by synovial fluid T cells from patients with Chlamydia-induced reactive arthritis. J Rheumatol. 1996;23:130–136.

74. Fendler C, Braun J, Eggens U, et al. Bacteria-specific lymphocyte proliferation in peripheral blood in reactive arthritis and related diseases. Br J Rheumatol. 1998;37:520–524.

75. Fendler C, Wu P, Eggens U, et al. Longitudinal investigation of bacterium-specific synovial lymphocyte proliferation in reactive arthritis and Lyme arthritis. Br J Rheumatol. 1998;37:784–788.

76. Mertz AK, Wu P, Stuniolo T, et al. Multispecific CD4+ T cell response to a single 12-mer epitope of the immunodominant heat shock protein 69 of Yersinia enterocolitica in Yersinia-triggered reactive arthritis. J Immunol. 2000;164;1529–1537.

77. Goodall JC, Beacock-Sharp H, Deane KH, Gaston JS. Recognition of the 60 kD cysteine-rich outer membrane protein OMP2 by CD4+ T cells from humans infected with Chlamydia trachomatis. Clin Exp Immunol. 2001;136:488–493.

78. Thiel A, Wu P, Lauster R, Braun J, Radbruch A, Sieper J. Analysis of the antigen-specific T cell response in reactive arthritis by flow cytometry. Arthritis Rheum. 2000;43:2834–2842.

79. Ebringer A. The relationship between Klebsiella infection and ankylosing spondylitis. Baillieres Clin Rheumatol. 1989;3:321–338.

80. Ebringer R. Acute anterior uveitis and faecal carriage of gram-negative bacteria. Br J Rheumatol. 1988;27(suppl 2):42–45.

81. Stebbings S, Munro K, Simon MA, et al. Comparison of the faecal microflora of patients with ankylosing spondylitis and controls using molecular methods of analysis. Rheumatology (Oxford). 2002;41:1395–1401.

82. Schwimmbeck PL, Yu DT, Oldstone MB. Autoantibodies to HLA B27 in the sera of HLA B27 patients with ankylosing spondylitis and Reiter's syndrome. Molecular mimicry with Klebsiella pneumoniae as potential mechanism of autoimmune disease. J Exp Med. 1987;166:173–181.

83. Sullivan JS, Prendergast JK, Geczy AF, Edmonds JP, McGuigan LE, Edwards CM. Cross-reacting bacterial determinants in ankylosing spondylitis. Am J Med. 1988; 85:54–55.

84. Czitrom AA, Pototschnik R, Edwards S, Gladman DD, Falk JA. Analysis of HLA B27 in ankylosing spondylitis with human alloreactive cytolytic T lymphocyte clones: failure to detect disease-related T cell epitopes. Exp Clin Immunogenet. 1986;3: 129–137.

85. van KE, Huber-Bruning O, Vandenbroucke JP, Willers JM. No conclusive evidence of an epidemiological relation between Klebsiella and ankylosing spondylitis. J Rheumatol. 1991;18:384–388.

86. Ahmadi K, Wilson C, Tiwana H, Binder A, Ebringer A. Antibodies to Klebsiella pneumoniae lipopolysaccharide in patients with ankylosing spondylitis. Br J Rheumatol. 1998;37:1330–1333.

87. Cancino-Diaz ME, Perez-Salazar JE, Dominguez-Lopez L, et al. Antibody response to Klebsiella pneumoniae 60 kDa protein in familial and sporadic ankylosing spondylitis: role of HLA-B27 and characterization as a GroEL-like protein. J Rheumatol. 1998; 25:1756–1764.

88. Cooper R, Fraser SM, Sturrock RD, Gemmell CG. Raised titres of anti-Klebsiella IgA in ankylosing spondylitis, rheumatoid arthritis, and inflammatory bowel disease. Br Med J (Clin Res Ed). 1988;296:1432–1434.

89. Maki-Ikola O, Leirisalo-Repo M, Turunen U, Granfors K. Association of gut inflammation with increased serum IgA class Klebsiella antibody concentrations in patients with axial ankylosing spondylitis (AS): implication for different aetiopathogenetic mechanisms for axial and peripheral AS? Ann Rheum Dis. 1997;56:180–183.

90. Sahly H, Podschun R, Ullmann U. Increased antibody responses to Klebsiella serotypes K26, K36, and K50 in patients with ankylosing spondylitis. Rheumatology (Oxford). 1999;38:481–482.

91. Tiwana H, Walmsley RS, Wilson C, et al. Characterization of the humoral immune response to Klebsiella species in inflammatory bowel disease and ankylosing spondylitis. Br J Rheumatol. 1998;37:525–531.

92. Maki-Ikola O, Nissila M, Lehtinen K, et al. Antibodies to Klebsiella pneumoniae, Escherichia coli and Proteus mirabilis in the sera of patients with axial and peripheral form of ankylosing spondylitis. Br J Rheumatol. 1995;34:413–417.

93. Toivanen P, Hansen DS, Mestre F, et al. Somatic serogroups, capsular types, and species of fecal Klebsiella in patients with ankylosing spondylitis. J Clin Microbiol. 1999;37:2808–2812.

94. Braun J, Tuszewski M, Ehlers S, et al. Nested polymerase chain reaction strategy simultaneously targeting DNA sequences of multiple bacterial species in inflammatory joint diseases. II. Examination of sacroiliac and knee joint biopsies of patients with spondyloarthropathies and other arthritides. J Rheumatol. 1997;24:1101–1105.

95. Smieja M, MacPherson DW, Kean W, et al. Randomised, blinded, placebo controlled trial of doxycycline for chronic seronegative arthritis. Ann Rheum Dis. 2001;60:1088–1094.

96. Stone MA, Payne U, Schentag C, Rahman R, Pacheco-Tena C, Inman RD. Comparative immune responses to candidate arthritogenic bacteria do not confirm a role for Klebsiella pneumoniae in the pathogenesis of familial ankylosing spondylitis. Rheumatology (Oxford). 2004;43:148–155.

97. Dominguez-Lopez ML, Cancino-Diaz ME, Jimenez-Zamudio L, et al. Cellular immune response to Klebsiella pneumoniae antigens in patients with HLA-B27+ ankylosing spondylitis. J Rheumatol. 2000;27:1453–1460.

98. Hohler T, Hug R, Schneider PM, et al. Ankylosing spondylitis in monozygotic twins: studies on immunological parameters. Ann Rheum Dis. 1999;58:435–440.

99. Hermann E, Sucke B, Droste U, Meyer zum Buschenfelde KH. Klebsiella pneumoniae-reactive T cells in blood and synovial fluid of patients with ankylosing spondylitis. Comparison with HLA-B27+ healthy control subjects in a limiting dilution study and determination of the specificity of synovial fluid T cell clones. Arthritis Rheum. 1995;38:1277–1282.

100. Yin Z, Braun J, Neure L, et al. Crucial role of interleukin-10/interleukin-12 balance in the regulation of the type 2 T helper cytokine response in reactive arthritis. Arthritis Rheum. 1997; 40:1788–1797.

101. Steiner G, Studnicka-Benke A, Witzmann G, et al. Soluble receptors for tumor necrosis factor and interleukin-2 in serum and synovial fluid of patients with rheumatoid arthritis, reactive arthritis, and osteoarthritis. J Rheumatol. 1985;22:406–412.

102. Bas S, Kvien TK, Buchs N, Fulpius T, Gabay C. Lower level of synovial fluid IFN-γ in HLA-B27-positive than in HLA-B27-negative patients with Chlamydia trachomatis reactive arthritis. Rheumatology (Oxford). 2003;42:461–467.

103. Rodel J, Straube E, Lungerhausen W, Hartmann M, Groh A. Secretion of cytokines by human synoviocytes during in vitro infection with Chlamydia trachomatis. J Rheumatol. 1998;24: 2161–2168.

104. Stone MA, Inman RD. The genetics of cytokines in ankylosing spondylitis. J Rheumatol. 2001;28:1288–1293.

105. Repo H, Anttonen K, Kilpinen SK, et al. CD14 and TNF-α promoter polymorphisms in patients with acute arthritis. Special reference to development of chronic spondyloarthropathy. Scand J Rheumatol. 2002;31:355–361.

106. Butrimiene I, Jarmalaite S, Ranceva J, Venalis A, Jasiuleviciute L, Zvirbliene A. Different cytokine profiles in patients with chronic and acute arthritis. Rheumatology (Oxford). 2004;43:1300–1304.

107. Zhao YX, Lajoie G, Zhang H, Chiu B, Payne U, Inman RD. Tumor necrosis factor p55-receptor-deficient mice respond to acute Yersinia enterocolitica infection with less apoptosis and more effective host resistance. Infect Immun. 2000;68:1243–1251.

108. Zhao YX, Zhang H, Chiu B, Payne U, Inman RD. Tumor necrosis factor receptor p55 controls the severity of arthritis in experimental Yersinia enterocolitica infection. Arthritis Rheum. 1999;42:1662–1672.

109. Dulphy N, Rabian C, Douay C, et al. Functional modulation of expanded CD8+ synovial fluid T cells—NK cell receptor expression in HLA-B27-associated reactive arthritis. Int Immunol. 2002;14:471–479.

110. Ren EC, Koh WH, Sim D, Boey ML, Wee GB, Chan SH. Possible protective role of HLA-B*2706 for ankylosing spondylitis. Tissue Antigens. 1997;49:67–69.

111. D'Amato M, Fiorillo MT, Carcassi C, et al. Relevance of residue 116 of HLA-B27 in determining susceptibility to ankylosing spondylitis. Eur J Immunol. 1995;25:3199–3201.

112. Fiorillo MT, Greco G, Maragno M, et al. The naturally occurring polymorphism Asp116 → His116, differentiating the ankylosing spondylitis-associated HLA-B*2705 from the non-associated HLA-B*2709 subtype, influences peptide-specific CD8 T cell recognition. Eur J Immunol. 1998;28:2508–2516.

113. Ugrinovic S, Mertz A, Wu P, Braun J, Sieper J. A single nonamer from the Yersinia 60-kDa heat shock protein is the target of HLA-B27-restricted CTL response in Yersinia-induced arthritis. J Immunol. 1997;159:5715–5723.

114. Ackermann B, Staege MS, Reske-Kunz AB, et al. Enterobacteria-infected T cells as antigen-presenting cells for cytotoxic CD8 T cells: a contribution to the self-limitation of cellular immune reactions in reactive arthritis? J Infect Dis. 1997;175: 1121–1127.

115. Kuon W, Holzhutter HG, Appel H, et al. Identification of HLA-B27-restricted peptides from the Chlamydia trachomatis proteome with possible relevance to HLA-B27-associated diseases. J Immunol. 2001;167:4738–4746.

116. Appel H, Kuon W, Kuhne, et al. Use of HLA-B27 tetramers to identify low-frequency antigen-specific T cells in Chlamydia-triggered reactive arthritis. Arthritis Res Ther. 2004;6:R521–R534.

117. Lopez-Larrea C, Gonzalez S, Martinez-Borra J. The role of HLA-B27 polymorphism and molecular mimicry in spondyloarthropathy. Mol Med Today. 1998;4:540–549.

118. Williams RC, Tsuchiya N, Husby G. Molecular mimicry, ankylosing spondylitis and reactive arthritis. Scand J Rheumatol. 1992;21:105–108.

119. Lo WF, Woods AS, DeCloux A, Cotter RJ, Metcalf ES, Soloski MJ. Molecular mimicry mediated by MHC class Ib molecules after infection with gram-negative pathogens. Nat Med. 2000;6: 215–218.

120. Albert LJ, Inman RD. Gram-negative pathogens and molecular mimicry: is there a case for mistaken identity? Trends Microbiol. 2000;8:446–447.

121. Ramos M, Alvarez I, Sesma L, Logean A, Rognan D, Lopez de Castro JA. Molecular mimicry of HLA-B27-derived peptide ligand of arthritis-linked subtypes with chlamydial proteins. J Biol Chem. 2002:277:37573–37581.

122. Popov I, Dela Cruz CS, Barber BH, Chiu B, Inman RD. The effect of an anti-B27 immune response on CTL recognition of Chlamydia. J Immunol. 2001;167:3375–3382.

123. Popov I, Dela Cruz CS, Barber BH, Chiu B, Inman RD. Breakdown of CTL D, tolerance to self HLA-B*2705 induced by exposure to Chlamydia trachomatis. J Immunol. 2002;169: 4033–4038.

123a. Soderlin MK, Borjesson O, Kautiainen H, et al. Annual incidence of inflammatory joint diseases in a population-based study in southern Sweden. Ann Rheum Dis. 2002;61:911–915.

124. Soderlin MK, Kautiainen H, Puolakkainen M, et al. Infections preceding early arthritis in southern Sweden: a prospective population-based study. J Rheumatol. 2003;30:459–464.

125. Buxton JA, Fyfe M, Berger S, Cox MB, Northcott KA, Multiprovinicial Salmonella typhimurium Case-Control Study Group. Reactive arthritis and other sequelae following sporadic Salmonella typhimurium infection in British Columbia, Canada—a case control study. J Rheumatol. 2002;29:2154–2158.

126. Hannu T, Mattila L, Siitonen A, Leirisalo-Repo M. Reactive arthritis following an outbreak of Salmonella typhimurium phage type 193 infection. Ann Rheum Dis. 2002;61:264–266.

127. Hannu T, Mattila L, Siitonen A, Leirisalo-Repo M. Reactive arthritis following an outbreak of Salmonella typhimurium phage type 193 infection. Ann Rheum Dis. 2002;61:264–266.

128. Locht H, Molbak K, Krogfelt KA. High frequency of reactive arthritis symptoms after an outbreak of Salmonella enteritidis. J Rheumatol. 2002;29:767–771.

129. Hannu T, Mattila L, Rautelin H, et al. Campylobacter-triggered reactive arthritis: a population-based study. Rheumatology (Oxford). 2002;41:312–318.

130. Hannu T, Kauppi M, Tuomala M, Laaksonen I, Klemets P, Kuusi M. Reactive arthritis following an outbreak of Campylobacter jejuni infection, J Rheumatol. 2004;31:528–530.

131. Hannu T, Mattila L, Nuorti JP, et al. Reactive arthritis after an outbreak of Yersinia pseudotuberculosis serotype 0:3 infection. Ann Rheum Dis. 2003;62:866–869.

132. Boyer GS, Templin DW, Bowler A, et al. Spondyloarthropathy in the community: clinical syndromes and disease manifestations in Alaskan Eskimo populations. J Rheumatol. 1999;26: 1537–1544.

133. Rudwaleit M, Richter S, Braun J, Sieper J. Low incidence of reactive arthritis in children following a salmonella outbreak. Ann Rheum Dis. 2001;60:1055–1057.

134. Mielants H, Veys EM, Cuvelier C, et al. The evolution of spondyloarthropathies in relation to gut histology. III. Relation between gut and joint. J Rheumatol. 1995;22:2279–2284.

135. Mielants H, Veys EM, Cuvelier C, et al. The evolution of spondyloarthropathies in relation to gut histology. II. Histological aspects. J Rheumatol. 1995;22:2273–2278.

136. Mielants H, Veys EM, De Vos M, et al. The evolution of spondyloarthropathies in relation to gut histology. I. Clinical aspects. J Rheumatol. 1995;22:2266–2272.

137. Birdi N, Hosking M, Clulow MK, Duffy CM, Allen U, Petty RE. Acute rheumatic fever and poststreptococcal reactive arthritis: diagnostic and treatment practices of pediatric subspecialists. J Rheumatol. 2001;28:1681–1688.

138. Moon RY, Greene MG, Rehe GT, Katona IM. Poststreptococcal reactive arthritis in children: a potential predecessor of rheumatic heart disease. J Rheumatol. 1995;22:529–532.

139. Aviles RJ, Ramakrishna G, Mohr DN, Michet CJ. Poststreptococcal reactive arthritis in adults: a case series. Mayo Clin Proc. 2000; 75:144–147.

140. Shulman ST, Ayoub EM. Poststreptococcal reactive arthritis. Curr Opin Rheumatol. 2002;14:562–565.

141. Schwartzenberg JM, Smith DD, Lindsley HB. BCG-associated arthropathy mimicking undifferentiated spondyloarthropathy. J Rheumatol. 1999;26:933–935.

142. Mas AJ, Romera M, Valverde-Garcia JM. Articular manifestations after the administration of intravesical BCG. Joint Bone Spine. 2002;69:92–93.

143. Maillefert JF, Sibilia J, Toussirot E, et al. Rheumatic disorders developed after hepatitis B vaccination. Rheumatology (Oxford). 1999;38:978–983.

144. Rose CD, Fawcett PT, Gibney KM. Arthritis following recombinant outlet surface protein A vaccination for Lyme disease. J Rheumatol. 2001;28:2555–2557.

145. Locht H, Krogfelt KA. Comparison of rheumatological and gastrointestinal symptoms after infection with Campylobacter jejuni/coli and enterotoxigenic Escherichia coli. Ann Rheum Dis. 2002:61:448–452.

146. Peng SL. Rheumatic manifestations of parasitic diseases. Semin Arthritis Rheum. 2002;31:228–247.

147. Rich E, Hook EW 3rd, Alarcon GS, et al. Reactive arthritis in patients attending an urban sexually transmitted diseases clinic. Arthritis Rheum. 1996;39:1172–1177.

148. Brown MA, Kennedy LG, MacGregor AJ, et al. Susceptibility to ankylosing spondylitis in twins—the role of genes, HLA, and environment. Arthritis Rheum. 1997;40:1823–1828.

149. Braun J, Bollow M, Remlinger G, et al. Prevalence of spondyloarthropathies in HLA-B27 positive and negative blood donors. Arthritis Rheum. 1998;41:58–67.

150. Locht H, Christiansen M. Laursen I: Reactive arthritis and serum levels of mannose binding lectin-lack of association. Clin Exp Immunol. 2003;131:169–173.

151. Seta N, Granfors K, Sahly H, et al. Expression of host defense scavenger receptors in spondyloarthropathy. Arthritis Rheum. 2001;44:931–939.

152. Thomson GT, DeRubeis DA, Hodge MA, Rajanayagam C, Inman RD. Post-salmonella reactive arthritis: late sequelae in a point source cohort. Am J Med. 1995;38:618–627.

153. Sieper J, Fendler C, Laitko S, et al. No benefit of long-term ciprofloxacin treatment in patients with reactive arthritis and undifferentiated oligoarthritis: a three-month, multicenter, double-blind, randomized, placebo-controlled study. Arthritis Rheum 1999;42:1386–1396.

154. Laasila K, Lassonen L, Leirisalo-Repo M. Antibiotic treatment and long term prognosis of reactive arthritis. Ann Rheum Dis. 2003;62:655–658.

155. Smieja M, MacPherson DW, Kean W, et al. Randomised, blinded, placebo-controlled trial of doxycycline in chronic seronegative arthritis. Ann Rheum Dis. 2001;60:1088–1094.

156. Carter JD, Valeriano J, Vasey FB. Doxycycline versus doxycycline and rifampin in undifferentiated spondyloarthropathy, with special reference to *Chlamydia*-induced arthritis. A prospective, randomized 9-month comparison. J Rheumatol. 2004;31: 1973–1980.

157. Yli-Kerttula T, Luukkainen R, Yli-Kettula U, et al. Effect of a three-month course of ciprofloxacin on the late prognosis of reactive arthritis. Ann Rheum Dis. 2003;62:880–884.

158. Kvien TK, Gaston JSH, Bardin T, et al. Three month treatment of reactive arthritis with azithromycin: a EULAR double-blind, placebo-controlled study. Ann Rheum Dis. 2004;63: 1113–1119.

159. Inman, RD, Perl A. Infectious agents in chronic rheumatic diseases. In Koopman WJ, Moreland LW, eds. Arthritis and Allied Conditions. Philadelphia, Pa: Lippincott Williams & Wilkins; 2005:647–677.

160. Przyklenk B, Bauernfeind A, Bornschein W, Emminger G, Heilmann K, Schweighart S. The role of *Campylobacter* (*Helicobacter*) *pylori* in disorders of the gastrointestinal tract. Infection. 1990;18:3–7.

161. Tulassay Z, Kryszewski A, Dite P, et al. One week of treatment with esomeprazole-based triple therapy eradicates *Helicobacter pylori* and heals patients with duodenal ulcer disease. Eur J Gastroenterol Hepatol. 2001;13:1457–1465.

5

Reactive Spondyloarthritis: Epidemiology, Clinical Features, and Treatment

Marjatta Leirisalo-Repo and Joachim Sieper

EPIDEMIOLOGY AND CLASSIFICATION

The term *reactive spondyloarthritis* has not been used before but we are using it in the context of this book to discuss both arthritis and sacroiliitis/spondylitis as associated with previous infection and the potential etiologic role of infection in spondyloarthritis. We first discuss acute rheumatic manifestations after previous bacterial infections, including arthritis, enthesitis, and sacroiliitis/spondylitis, then chronic courses of reactive arthritis (ReA), and finally the potential role of these infections in the long-term development of ankylosing spondylitis (AS).

Spondyloarthritis is the covering diagnosis for a group of joint diseases with several features in common.[1] Patients have mono- or oligoarthritis with or without inflammatory back symptoms. Extraarticular inflammatory symptoms also characterize the diseases. The diagnostic subgroups in the spondyloarthritis family include ReA/Reiter's disease, AS, arthritis associated with inflammatory bowel disease (IBD), psoriatic arthritis (PsA), and some forms of juvenile onset arthritis. These diseases have a strong association with a genetic marker, HLA-B27. In addition, rheumatoid factor is absent (thus, the condition was previously referred to as *seronegative spondyloarthritis*), there is a tendency for family aggregation, and extraarticular symptoms often occur (Table 5.1). *Undifferentiated arthritis* is a term used when patients do not exhibit the typical features of spondyloarthritis; some of these patients most probably have a condition belonging to the spondyloarthritis family that does not yet fulfill diagnostic/classification criteria.

Spondyloarthritides are nowadays regarded as a common cause for musculoskeletal symptoms, but the true incidence is hard to calculate, because numbers depend on the background genetic susceptibility in the population (HLA-B27) as well as possible triggering factors such as infections. A recent population study from Finland found the annual incidence of spondyloarthritis (excluding AS, undifferentiated arthritis, and PsA) to be 13 per 100,000.[2]

REACTIVE ARTHRITIS AS A SEQUEL OF INFECTION

The prevalence of infections capable of triggering ReA in different populations is unknown. Based on the presence of antibodies in healthy populations, infection as the cause of acute joint symptoms has been suggested to play a role in 9% to 18% of patients with inflammatory joint disease of less than 6 months' duration.[3,4] There have been only a few population-based studies on the annual incidence of ReA, mostly from Scandinavia. The total incidence has been estimated to be 10 to 30 per 100,000[2,5-7] (Table 5.2). *Campylobacter* has recently been recognized as one of the most important infections causing gastroenteritis in countries in the Western world, such as in Finland,[8] where the annual incidence of ReA due to *Campylobacter* infection is 4.3 per 100,000.[9] This is a much higher figure than that for a recent analysis of *Shigella*-induced ReA (1.3 per 100,000).[10]

CLINICAL FEATURES IN ACUTE REACTIVE ARTHRITIS

The arthritis is usually followed by gastrointestinal (enteroarthritis) or urogenital (uroarthritis) infections. Enteritis can be caused by gram-negative bacteria such as *Yersinia* (especially *Yersinia enterocolitica* and less commonly *Yersinia pseudotuberculosis*), *Salmonella*, *Shigella*, and *Campylobacter*. A few reports also link joint symptoms with *Clostridium difficile*. Genital infections caused by *Chlamydia trachomatis* are the most common triggering infections, whereas *Chlamydia pneumoniae* has also been implicated as the triggering infection in about 10% of patients with ReA.[11,12] In about 60% of patients, evidence of previous infection can be detected either by serology or by

and validated in patients with acute ReA or reactive spondyloarthritis.

TREATMENT OF ACUTE JOINT INFLAMMATION

General measures include the use of local cold treatment and avoidance of overuse of weight-bearing joints, if inflamed. For knee synovitis, atrophy of the vastus medialis of the quadriceps muscle usually develops rapidly and should be prevented by muscle exercise.

Nonsteroidal anti-inflammatory drugs are a cornerstone in the treatment of spondyloarthritis. In acute ReA, the patients need active treatment for joint inflammation. Local corticosteroid injections can be applied and are usually also of benefit in patients with mono- or oligoarticular disease. Enthesopathy also responds to local corticosteroid injections. Systemic use of corticosteroids is indicated rarely when the patient is bedridden due to severe polyarthritis or if atrioventricular conduction disturbances are present.

TREATMENT OF THE TRIGGERING INFECTION IN ACUTE REACTIVE ARTHRITIS

Often the microbes causing infection cannot be isolated at the time the patient presents with arthritis. Urethral samples are positive in about half of the patients with *C. trachomatis* infection.[63,64] In enteroarthritis, results of stool cultures are usually negative by the time the patient presents with arthritis.[16,17] Thus, the important question is whether antibiotic therapy is of benefit both for the infection and arthritis.

In patients with *C. trachomatis* or gonococcal infections, irrespective of whether complicating arthritis is present, it is important to give conventional antibiotic therapy for both the patient and the partner to eradicate the infection and to prevent late complications. Treatment of *C. trachomatis* for 10 to 14 days does not influence the course of ongoing arthritis. For enteric infections, there is no need for antibiotic treatment, unless the patient has septic symptoms. Also, there is no evidence that a routine 2-week course of therapy with antibiotics modifies the ongoing ReA.[65] However, if the antimicrobial therapy has been started for the infection before arthritis is present, it may prevent the development of ReA.[66,67]

ANTIMICROBIAL CHEMOTHERAPY FOR TREATMENT OF REACTIVE ARTHRITIS

As discussed previously, there is evidence that antigenic material persists in the joints of a patient with ReA. Because most of the triggering bacteria are intracellular, a prolonged course of chemotherapy would probably be needed to eradicate the (possible) viable bacteria. There have been few controlled and open studies to address this question (Table 5.4).

A 3-month placebo-controlled, prospective study on patients with acute ReA showed a positive effect on the duration of acute arthritis in patients with *C. trachomatis*-triggered arthritis when they were treated with lymecycline (a tetracycline derivative) compared with those treated with placebo.[68] Such a difference in favor of chemotherapy was not observed in patients with enteroarthritis.

With the exception of the above-mentioned study, there is no evidence favoring prolonged (a duration of 3 months has been the most common time in the studies) use of antibiotics (ciprofloxacin has been usually used) on the duration of arthritis.[69-71] A recent European League against Rheumatism (EULAR)-supported placebo-controlled multicenter study on patients with acute mono- or oligoarthritis with clinical picture of ReA, who were treated for 3 months with azithromycin, did not show any evidence in favoring the active drug[72] (see Table 5.4).

NATURAL HISTORY

The duration of acute ReA varies among reports. In Finnish studies, the average duration of arthritis was

TABLE 5.4 RANDOMIZED, DOUBLE-BLIND, PLACEBO-CONTROLLED STUDIES ON THE EFFECT OF ANTIMICROBIAL CHEMOTHERAPY ON ReA				
Ref.	Etiology	Duration of Therapy (mo)	Treatment	Result
68	a) Chlamydia	3	Lymecycline	Lymecycline effective
	b) Enteric infections	3	Lymecycline	No difference
69	*Yersinia*	3	Ciprofloxacin	No difference
70	Various triggers	3	Ciprofloxacin	No difference
71	Various triggers	3	Ciprofloxacin	No difference
72	Clinical suspicion of reactive arthritis	3	Azithromycin	No difference

3 to 5 months, and about 15% of patients developed chronic sequels or chronic spondyloarthritis.[16] In some other studies, chronicity has been reported in a vast majority of patients with Reiter's disease,[73] a form of severe arthritis usually triggered by *C. trachomatis* infection. A prolonged (>1 year) extension of the acute arthritis has been described in about 4% of patients with *Yersinia*-induced arthritis, in 19% of patients with *Salmonella*-induced arthritis, in 19% of patients with *Shigella*-induced arthritis, and in 17% of patients with *Chlamydia*-induced arthritis.[13,16,74–76] Enthesopathy tends to persist even after the joint inflammation has disappeared and laboratory markers of inflammation have returned to normal.[77]

CHRONIC REACTIVE ARTHRITIS

During the next few years after the acute episode, mild joint pain or enthesopathy is common in patients with previous ReA. Also, one third of the patients have occasional attacks of low-back pain.[16,73,74] In 14% of patients with previous postenteric ReA, signs and symptoms of chronic SpA have been described.[78] During the next 10 to 20 years, recurrent attacks of acute ReA seldom occur in patients with previous *Yersinia*-associated arthritis but occur more often in patients with previous *Salmonella*- or *Shigella*-associated arthritis (Table 5.5). Depending on the triggering infection and on the follow-up time, chronic arthritis is observed in 2% to 18%,[75,76] sacroiliitis in 14% to 49%,[77] and AS in 12% to 26%[75,79] (see Table 5.5). It is still uncertain to what extent ReA contributes to the development of sacroiliitis or AS or whether sacroiliac changes would have been proceeding in a subject with a genetic tendency for spondyloarthritis even in the absence of intervening ReA. Also, a minority of the patients manifest sacroiliitis on a radiologic study during the first known attack of arthritis.[16,74,75]

ROLE OF INFECTION IN THE DEVELOPMENT OF CHRONIC SPONDYLOARTHRITIS

Factors determining the progression of acute ReA to chronic SpA are incompletely known, but persistent or recurrent urogenital infection or chronic inflammatory focus in the gut could be good candidates. In addition to evidence of the presence of *Yersinia*[80] and *Salmonella*[81] antigens in synovial fluid cells or in synovial tissue[82] of patients with ReA, *Yersinia* structures have been shown to persist in submucosa of the gut,[83] and in lymph nodes of patients with prolonged or chronic *Yersinia*-associated arthritis.[84,85] *C. trachomatis* might also persist for prolonged period in the infected host. There is evidence for the presence of whole *Chlamydia* organisms in the synovial fluid in patients with seronegative arthritis with persisting synovitis for months or even for 2 years.[86–88]

Thus, infection plays a definite role in the etiology of acute ReA. Also in some other forms of spondyloarthritis, infection is suggested to contribute to the clinical activity or to the exacerbation of the disease. In addition to infection, the presence of HLA-B27 is also an important factor in the development of severe SpA or AS.

ANTIBIOTIC TREATMENT WITH RESPECT TO THE OUTCOME OF REACTIVE ARTHRITIS

The question of antibiotic therapy during acute ReA on the outcome of patients in the long run is an interesting. This question was addressed in two recent studies, in which patients participating in placebo-controlled studies were analyzed with respect to the development of chronic SpA. The first was based on the study by Lauhio et al.,[68] which originally included 40 patients with very early ReA who were randomly assigned to lymecycline or placebo groups. The follow-up study was performed on 17 of the patients, all HLA-B27 positive

TABLE 5.5 OUTCOME OF REA AFTER 10 TO 20 YEARS WITH RESPECT TO TRIGGERING INFECTION				
	Yersinia	*Salmonella*	*Shigella*	*C. trachomatis*
Recovered (%)	45	40	20	30
Occasional or chronic joint pain (%)	20	20	NA	68
Recurrent arthritis (%)	6	22	18	38
Chronic arthritis (%)	2	16	18	16
Ankylosing spondylitis (%)	15	12	14	26
Radiologic sacroiliitis (%)	20	14	32	49

Data collected from refs. 16, 73–76, and 79. NA, not available.

(9 originally in the lymecycline and 8 in the placebo group). There was not even a trend for a higher risk for chronic rheumatic diseases in the placebo group.[69] Similarly, Yli-Kerttula et al.[90] published a follow-up study on 53 patients who had previously participated in a placebo-controlled study with ciprofloxacin.[71] According to these results, patients originally in the placebo group developed various chronic joint diseases significantly more often and also had more often sacroiliitis on magnetic resonance imaging (MRI) examination (Table 5.6). This finding suggests that effective treatment of bacterial infections with antibiotics can prevent the occurrence of AS or related conditions. However, these data also suggest that persistent infection has to be accompanied by HLA-B27 positivity. The results of the two studies are contradictory. The reasons for that might be the small number of patients in the study of Laasila et al.,[89] use of a different set of study protocols, different follow-up times, and of course, different antibiotics used. In the first study,[89] all patients, irrespective of clinical symptoms or findings, underwent radiologic examination of the lumbar spine and sacroiliac joints at the follow-up, whereas in the study of Yli-Kerttula et al.,[90] only those patients with suspicion of inflammatory lesions had x-ray and MRI studies. Of course, the patient groups are small, and the results must be confirmed in a study with a follow-up of a larger cohort.

Recently, Carter et al.[91] reported a beneficial effect of a combination treatment with doxycycline and rifampicin, used for 9 months on patients with chronic spondyloarthritis (10-year duration of disease) induced by *Chlamydia* infection, compared with doxycycline as a single treatment. The results are promising but should be confirmed in a larger number of patients.

At the moment, there is no hard evidence favoring the use of antibiotics in the treatment of ReA. On the basis of the available evidence, we recommend that 1) all patients with acute *C. trachomatis* infection should have the routine treatment (e.g., azithromycin 2 g as single therapy, with partners treated as well) and 2) all patients with acute ReA associated with *C. trachomatis* infection could probably receive a prolonged course of antibiotics. The impact of antibiotic therapy during acute arthritis on the long-term outcome is unsolved at the moment and should be analyzed by performance of follow-up studies on patients participating in some of the previous large placebo-controlled studies.

BACTERIA AND ANKYLOSING SPONDYLITIS

Of all the possible autoimmune diseases, probably the best evidence that bacterial infections are a crucial trigger is available for AS. Between a few days and 6 weeks after a preceding bacterial infection of the gut with enterobacteria or the urogenital tract with *C. trachomatis*, ReA occurs in 1% to 4% of these patients, with 30% to 70% of them being positive for HLA-B27. Even more interesting in the context of a discussion on infection and autoimmunity, 20% to 40% of these patients develop, if they are positive for HLA-B27, the full clinical picture of AS 10 to 20 years after the initial infection.[92]

In a discussion on infection and autoimmunity AS is also of special interest because, on one hand, a chronic immune response against self-antigens is assumed to be crucial for the immunopathologic changes and, on the other hand, bacteria seem to be necessary to trigger the disease.[93] AS is a chronic inflammatory disease that affects primarily the spine and the sacroiliac joints, but extraspinal structures such as peripheral joints, the enthesis (insertion of tendons/ligaments at bone), the eye (uveitis), and the aorta can also be involved. Histologic studies[94-96] and MRI investigations[95] suggest that the primary site of inflammation is the cartilage-bone interphase. Mononuclear cell infiltrates are mainly found in cartilage and subchondral bone. In early and active sacroiliitis T cells and macrophages are dominant in these infiltrates, underlining the relevance of a specific cellular immune response.[96]

There is increasing evidence for the role of gut in the maintenance of joint symptoms in patients with chronic spondyloarthropathies even without the history of preceding enteritis[97,98] analogously to the patients with IBD, in whom an increased load of gram-negative pathogens via an inflamed and leaking gut mucosa is probably contributing to the development of peripheral and axial arthritis.[99] *Klebsiella* has been proposed to be involved in spondyloarthropathies[100] and with AS, especially in association with peripheral arthritis.[101]

From 10% to 20% of patients with IBD can develop a peripheral arthritis at some time during the course of their disease, and AS has been reported in between 5% and 10% of patients with IBD. Patients with IBD who are also positive for HLA-B27 have an especially high risk of developing AS. In one large study including 231 patients with Crohn's disease, 54% of HLA-B27–positive patients developed AS, whereas the disease could be diagnosed in only 2.6% of HLA-B27–negative patients.[102] Thus, at least half of the HLA-B27–positive patients with IBD will develop AS, which cannot be differentiated from primary AS. Although IBD cannot be seen as a bacterial infection, stimulation of the immune system by local gut bacteria because of lesions in the gut mucosa probably serves a similar purpose.

Although a preceding infection or IBD is evident only in less than 10% of patients with AS, infections with ReA-associated bacteria and gut lesions in patients with IBD are often subclinical.[93] The question of whether asymptomatic or uncomplicated infection would lead to the development of AS has not been properly answered yet. There are some reports that

TABLE 5.6 OUTCOME OF PATIENTS WITH PREVIOUS REA AFTER TREATMENT WITH ANTIBIOTICS OR PLACEBO FOR 3 MONTHS DURING THE ACUTE PHASE

Characteristics	Study by Laasila et al., 2003[89]			Study by Yli-Kerttula et al., 2003[90]		
	Lymecycline (n = 9)	Placebo (n = 8)	Total (n = 17)	Ciprofloxacin (n = 26)	Placebo (n = 27)	Total (n = 53)
Mean age at acute phase, years	36	32	34	36	37	34.5
Male patients, number (%)	4 (44)	7 (87)	14 (82)	NA	NA	30 (57)
Triggering infection				NA	NA	
Enteritis, n (%)	7 (78)	2 (25)	9 (53)			85
Urogenital, n (%)	1 (11)	4 (50)	5 (29)			15
Not known, n (%)	1 (11)	0 (0)	1 (6)			0
HLA-B27 positive, n (%)	9 (100)	8 (100)	17 (100)	20 (77)	25 (93)	45 (85)
Follow-up time, mean or range, years	10.3	10.5	10.4	NA	NA	4–7
Follow-up						
IBP	4 (44)	3 (38)	7 (41)	0 (0)	4 (15)	4 (8)
Patients with tender joints, n (%)	3 (33)	3 (38)	6 (35)	NA	NA	NA
Patients with swollen joints, n (%)	1 (11)	2 (25)	3 (18)	1 (4)	2 (7)	3 (6)
Chronic arthritis, n (%)	0	0 (0)	0	2 (8)	1 (4)	3 (6)
Recurrent reactive arthritis, n (%)	2 (22)	0 (0)	2 (12)	NA	NA	NA
Recurrent iritis, n (%)	1 (11)	2 (25)	3 (12)	0	3 (11)	3 (6)
Lumbosacral X-ray: inflammatory, n (%)	3 (33)	1 (13)	4 (24)	0/4 (0)	2/7 (29)	2/11

IBP, inflammatory low back pain; NA, not available.

would argue in favor the hypothesis. Interestingly, 2 of 94 patients who had an acute uncomplicated gut infection due to a *Y. enterocolitica* outbreak had AS when examined 13 years later, and both were HLA-B27–positive.[103] Also, patients with pelvic inflammatory disease due to *C. trachomatis* can develop sacroiliitis, with intermittent or persistent low back pain; HLA-B27–positive patients have a higher frequency of symptomatic sacroiliitis.[104] Also, Lehtinen[105] reported a higher frequency of positive results for *Chlamydia* antibodies in patients with AS of long duration (33%) compared with patients with rheumatoid arthritis (8%) or control subjects (18%). The presence of *Chlamydia* antibodies was associated with a history of acute anterior uveitis whereas active *Chlamydia* infection was as common in patients with AS as in matched control subjects.[105] This indicates that an infection might be able to trigger the pathogenic mechanisms that later manifest as "primary AS." Thus, probably in most, if not all, patients with AS, a bacterial trigger is essential in the pathogenesis of the disease. These patients are normally positive for HLA-B27.

In established AS or chronic spondyloarthritis, a flare of the disease is not usually suspected to be related to an infection. However, it is interesting that Martínez et al.[107] described a relationship between the disease activity and a history of recent infection, especially an enteric infection in patients with spondyloarthritides, and in particular those with AS and undifferentiated spondyloarthritis. Furthermore, Lange et al.[108] reported *Chlamydia*-induced urethral syndrome in 15 of 32 female patients with AS; the infected patients had a higher incidence of enthesopathy, involvement of the spinal column, and higher sedimentation rates and C-reactive protein levels than the rest of the patients.

The crucial question is whether the assumed autoimmune disease runs an independent course after the initial bacterial trigger or whether a chronic interaction of the immune system with bacteria is necessary to result in a chronic immune response against self-antigens. As reviewed recently,[109,110] bacteria seem to persist for prolonged periods and trigger immune responses in patients with acute ReA. A cytokine imbalance with a relative lack of T-helper 1 type cytokines may play a role during acute infection, indicating poor elimination and permitting the survival of the microbes. With a prolonged or chronic course of ReA and the development of spondyloarthritis, the interaction between microbial antigens and HLA-B27 seems to be important. The arthritogenic peptide hypothesis is one of the most popular to explain the association, and HLA-B27-restricted peptides from *Chlamydia* and *Yersinia* have been identified; the peptides are stimulatory for CD8+ T cells derived from patients with ReA. In addition to aberration in the T-cell immune response, defective innate immunity has been suggested to be playing a role in the first-line defense and clearing of the infection.[111]

Factors leading to chronic ReA and the development of spondyloarthritis are even less well understood. Recurrent infection might be important to the development of chronic spondyloarthritis. This suggestion is supported by animal studies. HLA-B27 transgenic rats are tolerant of HLA-B27 immunization. However, when exposed to *Chlamydia* in vitro, splenocytes of the animals induce cytotoxic T lymphocytes that lyse HLA-B27-positive target cells.[112] Synovial fibroblasts, when infected with arthritogenic *Salmonella* induce the up-regulation of RANKL (receptor activator of nuclear factor-κB ligand) expression and enhance osteoclast precursor maturation to osteoclast-like cells.[113] These results were discussed with respect to the development of chronic peripheral arthritis and even sacroiliitis, known to occur in a proportion of patients with previous ReA. Thus, infection can break down tolerance in this experimental setting.

There are no good studies on the effect of the healing of gut lesions in Crohn's disease on symptoms and progression of AS. In an uncontrolled study, chronic gut lesions observed at ileocolonoscopy in patients without a history of IBD, inflammatory axial pain, evidence of inflammation in laboratory tests (a high erythrocyte sedimentation rate and high C-reactive protein levels) and the presence of HLA-B27 also predicted the chronicity of SpA and the development of AS within 2 to 9 years, whereas the presence of HLA-Bw62 was associated with undifferentiated SpA and predicted remission.[98]

Urogenital infections may also contribute in chronic SpA. Prostatitis has been shown to support the ongoing joint/axial inflammation in uroarthritis and in AS.[114] In the 1940s and 1950s arthritis (not yet called *reactive arthritis*) associated with urogenital infections, usually prostatitis was seen with development of AS in Sweden in a higher percentage than 20 to 30 years later,[114] when investigated by the same authors. In the earlier period about one third of their patients with AS had a previous urogenital ReA whereas in the later period AS was diagnosed in only 1 of 62 patients (1.6%) with urogenital ReA after a follow-up of 6 years. As pointed out by these authors, consequent and long-term antibiotic treatment for prostatitis in the later period was the main difference in the management of these patients, suggesting that persistent infection played an important role for the development of AS in patients with urogenital infections. In 1983, Schiefer et al.[115] reported a high frequency (38%) of urogenital tract infections in male patients with AS, usually due to *C. trachomatis* and *Ureaplasma urealyticum*. Although they did not report any association between activity of arthritis and infection, the high frequency of infections confirms the previous association between prostatitis and AS and suggests a more aggressive search for microbes in patients with active AS.

Environmental factors (most probably infections) have also been suggested to play a role in the severity and age of onset of AS. AS and related diseases were more severe in lower social classes with poorer hygiene practices when investigated in North Africa.[116] In this study that included 518 patients, hip involvement was used as the most important severity marker for AS. The risk of hip involvement estimated after 10 years of disease duration was 39%, in contrast to 14% to 17% found in European studies. Bad prognostic factors were age younger that 24 years at onset and a combination of "lower social class" and "'no refrigerator at home," suggesting that infections and/or repeated infections are important for a more severe course of the disease. In another study from the same group hip involvement was reported in 48% of patients with AS in Morocco compared with 16% in France.[117] That this difference is probably due to environmental rather than to genetic factors is suggested by reports from Bernard Amor who found in his large rheumatology outpatient clinic in Paris, France, that the first generation of immigrants from North Africa to France had more severe AS compared with the second generation (Amor B, unpublished observations).

Furthermore, in countries such as Mexico[118] and China[119] AS starts at an earlier age and has a more severe course[118,119] compared with AS in Western Europe. For these countries, repeated bacterial infections of the gastrointestinal tract starting at a young age are common, again especially in the lower social classes. Single and several combinations of bacterial DNA in synovial fluid cells of Mexican patients with juvenile-onset and adult-onset spondyloarthritis have been described by the Mexican group, again emphasizing the environmental load of microbes in propagation of the chronic disease.[120] Although most of the data presented here are not based on controlled prospective studies, they all indicate that persistent or repeated infection, most probably of the gut, is a very important contributor not only for the pathogenesis but also for severity of AS.

IMAGING

Radiographs of the affected joints in patients with acute ReA with or without other features of spondyloarthritis are usually normal and do not aid in the diagnostic process. Ultrasound examination of the entheseal insertions has proved to be a sensitive and accurate method to show enthesopathy, periosteal reaction, and tendinosis and is superior to the clinical examination.[77,121,122] Radiologic examination of the lumbar spine and sacroiliac joints in a patient with ReA, even in the presence of inflammatory low-back pain, is usually normal, thus demonstrating the low sensitivity of plain radiographs in the detection of sacroiliitis. About 10% to 15% of patients with acute ReA have, however, evidence of mild radiologic sacroiliitis[16,75] and this can be interpreted as a sign of previous sacroiliac inflammation or early AS.

Scintigraphy can show joint inflammation and is useful for demonstrating enthesitis. It has also been used as a more sensitive method than plain radiography for the demonstration of sacroiliac inflammation,[123] but it is often too sensitive and of low specificity. Recently, MRI has been applied in the diagnosis of active sacroiliac or spinal inflammation in patients with AS and has been used also in spondyloarthritis. The imaging is very sensitive and can show erosive signs in sacroiliac joints with bone marrow edema, a feature interpreted as inflammation; bone marrow edema can be seen in thoracic and lumbar vertebrae, indicating inflammation. Superior to plain radiographs, MRI scans of these inflammatory lesions are visualizing the typical anatomic lesion in spondyloarthritis, i.e., enthesitis, which can be seen in sacroiliac joints and in interspinal and supraspinal ligaments of the spine.[124] At present this area is developing very fast, but no guidelines on how to use and interpret the new imaging techniques in the diagnostic work-up of a patient with ReA or reactive spondyloarthritis exist.

REFERENCES

1. Dougados M, van der Linden S, Juhlin R, et al. The European Spondylarthropathy Study Group preliminary criteria for the classification of spondylarthropathy. Arthritis Rheum. 1991; 34:1218–1227.
2. Savolainen E, Kaipiainen-Seppanen O, Kroger L, Luosujarvi R. Total incidence and distribution of inflammatory joint diseases in a defined population: results from the Kuopio 2000 arthritis survey. J Rheumatol. 2003;30:2460–2468.
3. Granfors K, Isomaki H, von Essen R, Maatela J, Kalliomaki JL, Toivanen A. *Yersinia* antibodies in inflammatory joint diseases. Clin Exp Rheumatol. 1983;1:215–218.
4. Maki-Ikola O, Viljanen MK, Tiitinen S, Toivanen P, Granfors K. Antibodies to arthritis-associated microbes in inflammatory joint diseases. Rheumatol Int. 1991;10:231–234.
5. Isomaki H, Raunio J, von Essen R, Hameenkorpi R. Incidence of inflammatory rheumatic diseases in Finland. Scand J Rheumatol. 1978;7:188–192.
6. Kvien TK, Glennas A, Melby K, et al. Reactive arthritis: incidence, triggering agents and clinical presentation. J Rheumatol. 1994;21:115–122.
7. Soderlin MK, Borjesson O, Kautiainen H, Skogh T, Leirisalo-Repo M. Annual incidence of inflammatory joint diseases in a

population based study in southern Sweden. Ann Rheum Dis. 2002;61:911–915.

8. Rautelin H, Hanninen ML. Campylobacters: the most common bacterial enteropathogens in the Nordic countries. Ann Med. 2000;32:440–445.

9. Hannu T, Mattila L, Rautelin H, et al. Campylobacter-triggered reactive arthritis: a population-based study. Rheumatology (Oxford). 2002;41:312–318.

10. Hannu T, Mattila L, Siitonen A, Leirisalo-Repo M. Reactive arthritis attributable to Shigella infection: a clinical and epidemiological nationwide study. Ann Rheum Dis. 2005;64:594–598.

11. Braun J, Laitko S, Treharne J, et al. Chlamydia pneumoniae—a new causative agent of reactive arthritis and undifferentiated oligoarthritis. Ann Rheum Dis. 1994;53:100–105.

12. Hannu T, Puolakkainen M, Leirisalo-Repo M. Chlamydia pneumoniae as a triggering infection in reactive arthritis. Rheumatology (Oxford). 1999;38:411–414.

13. Keat A. Reiter's syndrome and reactive arthritis in perspective. N Engl J Med. 1983;309:1606–1615.

14. Laasila K, Leirisalo-Repo M. Recurrent reactive arthritis associated with urinary tract infection by Escherichia coli. J Rheumatol. 1999;26:2277–2279.

15. Locht H, Krogfelt KA. Comparison of rheumatological and gastrointestinal symptoms after infection with Campylobacter jejuni/coli and enterotoxigenic Escherichia coli. Ann Rheum Dis. 2002;61:448–452.

16. Leirisalo M, Skylv G, Kousa M, et al. Followup study on patients with Reiter's disease and reactive arthritis, with special reference to HLA-B27. Arthritis Rheum. 1982;25:249–259.

17. Hannu TJ, Leirisalo-Repo M. Clinical picture of reactive salmonella arthritis. J Rheumatol. 1988;15:1668–1671.

18. Mattila L, Leirisalo-Repo M, Koskimies S, Granfors K, Siitonen A. Reactive arthritis following an outbreak of Salmonella infection in Finland. Br J Rheumatol. 1994;33:1136–1141.

19. Mattila L, Leirisalo-Repo M, Pelkonen P, Koskimies S, Granfors K, Siitonen A. Reactive arthritis following an outbreak of Salmonella bovismorbificans infection. J Infect. 1998;36:289–295.

20. Rudwaleit M, Richter S, Braun J, Sieper J. Low incidence of reactive arthritis in children following a salmonella outbreak. Ann Rheum Dis. 2001;60:1055–1057.

21. Maki-Ikola O, Granfors K. Salmonella-triggered reactive arthritis. Lancet. 1992;339:1096–1098.

22. Maki-Ikola O. Reactive arthritis after unusual Salmonella infections. Lancet. 1990;336:1387.

23. Thomson GT, Rajanayagam C, Chiu B, Thorne C, Falk J, Inman RD. Interplay of microbe and major histocompatibility complex: a family study. J Rheumatol. 1991;18:1756–1759.

24. Thomson GT, Chiu B, De Rubeis D, Falk J, Inman RD. Immunoepidemiology of post-Salmonella reactive arthritis in a cohort of women. Clin Immunol Immunopathol. 1992;64:227–232.

25. Locht H, Kihlstrom E, Lindstrom FD. Reactive arthritis after Salmonella among medical doctors—study of an outbreak. J Rheumatol. 1993;20:845–848.

26. Shrivastava A, Thistlethwaite D. Erythema nodosum and arthritis with Salmonella enteritidis enteritis. Br J Dermatol. 1993;128:704.

27. Huppertz HI, Sandhage K. Reactive arthritis due to Salmonella enteritidis complicated by carditis. Acta Paediatr. 1994;83:1230–1231.

28. Samuel MP, Zwillich SH, Thomson GT, et al. Fast food arthritis—a clinico-pathologic study of post-Salmonella reactive arthritis. J Rheumatol. 1995;22:1947–1952.

29. Thomson GT, DeRubeis DA, Hodge MA, Rajanayagam C, Inman RD. Post-Salmonella reactive arthritis: late clinical sequelae in a point source cohort. Am J Med. 1995;98:13–21.

30. Aragon A, Duran Perez-Navarro A. Familial Salmonella-triggered reactive arthritis. Br J Rheumatol. 1996;35:908–909.

31. Fischel JD, Lipton J. Acute anterior uveitis in juvenile Reiter's syndrome. Clin Rheumatol. 1996;15:83–85.

32. Kanakoudi-Tsakalidou F, Pardalos G, Pratsidou-Gertsi P, Kansouzidou-Kanakoudi A, Tsangaropoulou-Stinga H. Persistent or severe course of reactive arthritis following Salmonella enteritidis infection. A prospective study of 9 cases. Scand J Rheumatol. 1998;27:431–434.

33. Kirveskari J, He Q, Holmstrom T, et al. Modulation of peripheral blood mononuclear cell activation status during Salmonella-triggered reactive arthritis. Arthritis Rheum. 1999;42:2045–2054.

34. Kirveskari J, He Q, Leirisalo-Repo M, et al. Enterobacterial infection modulates major histocompatibility complex class I expression on mononuclear cells. Immunology. 1999;97:420–428.

35. McColl GJ, Diviney MB, Holdsworth RF, et al. HLA-B27 expression and reactive arthritis susceptibility in two patient cohorts infected with Salmonella typhimurium. Aust NZ J Med. 2000;30:28–32.

36. Ekman P, Kirveskari J, Granfors K. Modification of disease outcome in Salmonella-infected patients by HLA-B27. Arthritis Rheum. 2000;43:1527–1534.

37. Paronen I. Reiter's disease. A study of 344 cases observed in Finland. Acta Med Scand. 1948;131(suppl 212):1–113.

38. Berden JH, Muytjens HL, Van de Putte LB. Reactive arthritis associated with Campylobacter jejuni enteritis. Br Med J. 1979;1:380–381.

39. Bekassay AN, Enell H, Schalen C. Severe polyarthritis following Campylobacter enteritis in a 12-year-old boy. Acta Paediatr Scand. 1980;69:269–271.

40. Kosunen TU, Kauranen O, Martio J, et al. Reactive arthritis after Campylobacter jejuni enteritis in patients with HLA-B27. Lancet. 1980;1:1312–1313.

41. Leung FY, Littlejohn GO, Bombardier C. Reiter's syndrome after Campylobacter jejuni enteritis. Arthritis Rheum. 1980;23:948–950.

42. Saari KM, Kauranen O. Ocular inflammation in Reiter's syndrome associated with Campylobacter jejuni enteritis. Am J Ophthalmol. 1980;90:572–573.

43. Van de Putte LB, Berden JH, Boerbooms MT, et al. Reactive arthritis after Campylobacter jejuni enteritis. J Rheumatol. 1980;7:531–535.

44. Kosunen TU, Ponka A, Kauranen O, et al. Arthritis associated with Campylobacter jejuni enteritis. Scand J Rheumatol. 1981;10:77–80.

45. Ponka A, Martio J, Kosunen TU. Reiter's syndrome in association with enteritis due to Campylobacter fetus ssp. jejuni. Ann Rheum Dis. 1981;40:414–415.

46. Schaad UB. Reactive arthritis associated with Campylobacter enteritis. Pediatr Infect Dis. 1982;1:328–332.

47. Short CD, Klouda PT, Smith L. Campylobacter jejuni enteritis and reactive arthritis. Ann Rheum Dis. 1982;41:287–288.

48. Albert J, Spaeth PJ, Ott H, Buetler R. Symmetrical reactive oligoarthritis after Campylobacter jejuni enteritis—case report and study of the synovial complement. Z Rheumatol. 1983;42:104–106.

49. Bengtsson A, Ahlstrand C, Lindstrom FD, Kihlstrom E. Bacteriological findings in 25 patients with Reiter's syndrome (reactive arthritis). Scand J Rheumatol. 1983;12:157–160.

50. Eastmond CJ. Gram-negative bacteria and B27 disease. Br J Rheumatol. 1983;22:67–74.

51. Eastmond CJ, Rennie JA, Reid TM. An outbreak of Campylobacter enteritis—a rheumatological followup survey. J Rheumatol. 1983;10:107–108.

52. Johnsen K, Ostensen M, Melbye AC, Melby K. HLA-B27-negative arthritis related to Campylobacter jejuni enteritis in three children and two adults. Acta Med Scand. 1983;214:165–168.

53. Ebright JR, Ryan LM. Acute erosive reactive arthritis associated with Campylobacter jejuni-induced colitis. Am J Med. 1984;76:321–323.

54. Pipalia DH, Plumber ST, Vora S, Mehta A, Vora IM, Naik SR. Campylobacter jejuni infection with acute self limiting colitis and polyarthritis. Indian J Gastroenterol. 1988;7:47–48.

55. Bremell T, Bjelle A, Svedhem A. Rheumatic symptoms following an outbreak of campylobacter enteritis: a five year follow up. Ann Rheum Dis. 1991;50:934–938.

56. Policastro AM. Index of suspicion. Case 3. Campylobacter gastroenteritis with joint pain. Pediatr Rev. 1994;15:117–119.

57. Goudswaard J, Sabbe L, Te WW. Reactive arthritis as a complication of Campylobacter lari enteritis. J Infect. 1995;31:171.

58. Hannu T, Kauppi M, Tuomala M, Laaksonen I, Klemets P, Kuusi M. Reactive arthritis following an outbreak of Campylobacter jejuni infection. J Rheumatol. 2004;31:528–530.

59. Thomson GT, Alfa M, Orr K, Thomson BR, Olson N. Secretory immune response and clinical sequelae of Salmonella infection in a point source cohort. J Rheumatol. 1994;21:132–137.

60. Heikkila S, Viitanen JV, Kautianen H, Kauppi M. Evaluation of the Finnish versions of the functional indices BASFI and DFI in spondylarthropathy. Clin Rheumatol. 2000;19:464–469.

61. Heikkila S, Ronni S, Kautiainen HJ, Kauppi MJ. Functional impairment in spondyloarthropathy and fibromyalgia. J Rheumatol. 2002;29:1415–1419.

62. Maksymowych WP, Lambert R, Jhangri GS, et al. Clinical and radiological amelioration of refractory peripheral spondyloarthritis by pulse intravenous pamidronate therapy. J Rheumatol. 2001;28:144–155.

63. Kousa M, Saikku P, Richmond S, Lassus A. Frequent association of chlamydial infection with Reiter's syndrome. Sex Transm Dis. 1978;5:57–61.

64. Keat AC, Thomas BJ, Taylor-Robinson D, Pegrum GD, Maini RN, Scott JT. Evidence of Chlamydia trachomatis infection in sexually acquired reactive arthritis. Ann Rheum Dis. 1980;39:431–437.

65. Leirisalo-Repo M. Are antibiotics of any use in reactive arthritis? APMIS. 1993;101:575–581.

66. Bardin T, Enel C, Cornelis F, et al. Antibiotic treatment of venereal disease and Reiter's syndrome in a Greenland population. Arthritis Rheum. 1992;35:190–194.

67. Hannu T, Mattila L, Siitonen A, Leirisalo-Repo M. Reactive arthritis following an outbreak of Salmonella typhimurium phage type 193 infection. Ann Rheum Dis. 2002;61:264–266.

68. Lauhio A, Leirisalo-Repo M, Lahdevirta J, Saikku P, Repo H. Double-blind, placebo-controlled study of three-month treatment with lymecycline in reactive arthritis, with special reference to Chlamydia arthritis. Arthritis Rheum. 1991;34:6–14.

69. Toivanen A, Yli-Kerttula T, Luukkainen R, Merilahti-Palo R, Granfors K, Seppala J. Effect of antimicrobial treatment on chronic reactive arthritis. Clin Exp Rheumatol. 1993;11:301–307.

70. Sieper J, Fendler C, Laitko S, et al. No benefit of long-term ciprofloxacin treatment in patients with reactive arthritis and undifferentiated oligoarthritis: a three-month, multicenter, double-blind, randomized, placebo-controlled study. Arthritis Rheum. 1999;42:1386–1396.

71. Yli-Kerttula T, Luukkainen R, Yli-Kerttula U, et al. Effect of a three month course of ciprofloxacin on the outcome of reactive arthritis. Ann Rheum Dis. 2000;59:565–570.

72. Kvien TK, Gaston JS, Bardin T, et al. Three month treatment of reactive arthritis with azithromycin: a EULAR double blind, placebo controlled study. Ann Rheum Dis. 2004;63:1113–1119.

73. Fox R, Calin A, Gerber RC, Gibson D. The chronicity of symptoms and disability in Reiter's syndrome. An analysis of 131 consecutive patients. Ann Intern Med. 1979;91:190–193.

74. Good AE. Reiter's syndrome: long-term follow-up in relation to development of ankylosing spondylitis. Ann Rheum Dis. 1979;38(suppl 1):suppl 39–45.

75. Leirisalo-Repo M, Helenius P, Hannu T, et al. Long-term prognosis of reactive salmonella arthritis. Ann Rheum Dis. 1997;56:516–520.

76. Leirisalo-Repo M, Suoranta H. Ten-year follow-up study of patients with Yersinia arthritis. Arthritis Rheum. 1988;31:533–537.

77. Lehtinen A, Leirisalo-Repo M, Taavitsainen M. Persistence of enthesopathic changes in patients with spondylarthropathy during a 6-month follow-up. Clin Exp Rheumatol. 1995;13:733–736.

78. Kruger K, Schattenkirchner M. Reactive arthritis—clinical aspects and course. Wien Klin Wochenschr. 1983;95:884–889.

79. Sairanen E, Paronen I, Mahonen H. Reiter's syndrome: a follow-up study. Acta Med Scand. 1969;185:57–63.

80. Granfors K, Jalkanen S, von Essen R, et al. Yersinia antigens in synovial-fluid cells from patients with reactive arthritis. N Engl J Med. 1989;320:216–221.

81. Granfors K, Jalkanen S, Lindberg AA, et al. Salmonella lipopolysaccharide in synovial cells from patients with reactive arthritis. Lancet. 1990;335:685–688.

82. Hammer M, Zeidler H, Klimsa S, Heesemann J. Yersinia enterocolitica in the synovial membrane of patients with Yersinia-induced arthritis. Arthritis Rheum. 1990;33:1795–1800.

83. Hoogkamp-Korstanje JA. Antibiotics in Yersinia enterocolitica infections. J Antimicrob Chemother. 1987;20:123–131.

84. Hoogkamp-Korstanje JA, de Koning J, Heesemann J. Persistence of Yersinia enterocolitica in man. Infection. 1988;16:81–85.

85. Hoogkamp-Korstanje JA, de Koning J, Heesemann J, Festen JJ, Houtman PM, van Oyen PL. Influence of antibiotics on IgA and IgG response and persistence of Yersinia enterocolitica in patients with Yersinia-associated spondylarthropathy. Infection. 1992;20:53–57.

86. Bas S, Griffais R, Kvien TK, Glennas A, Melby K, Vischer TL. Amplification of plasmid and chromosome Chlamydia DNA in synovial fluid of patients with reactive arthritis and undifferentiated seronegative oligoarthropathies. Arthritis Rheum. 1995;38:1005–1013.

87. Sieper J, Braun J, Brandt J, et al. Pathogenetic role of Chlamydia, Yersinia and Borrelia in undifferentiated oligoarthritis. J Rheumatol. 1992;19:1236–1242.

88. Gerard HC, Branigan PJ, Schumacher HR Jr, Hudson AP. Synovial Chlamydia trachomatis in patients with reactive arthritis/Reiter's syndrome are viable but show aberrant gene expression. J Rheumatol. 1998;25:734–742.

89. Laasila K, Laasonen L, Leirisalo-Repo M. Antibiotic treatment and long term prognosis of reactive arthritis. Ann Rheum Dis. 2003;62:655–658.

90. Yli-Kerttula T, Luukkainen R, Yli-Kerttula U, et al. Effect of a three month course of ciprofloxacin on the late prognosis of reactive arthritis. Ann Rheum Dis. 2003;62:880–884.

91. Carter JD, Valeriano J, Vasey FB. Antimicrobial treatment for Chlamydia induced reactive arthritis. Ann Rheum Dis. 2005;64:512–513.

92. Leirisalo-Repo M. Prognosis, course of disease, and treatment of the spondyloarthropathies. Rheum Dis Clin North Am. 1998;24:737–51, viii.

93. Sieper J, Braun J. Pathogenesis of spondylarthropathies. Persistent bacterial antigen, autoimmunity, or both? Arthritis Rheum. 1995;38:1547–1554.

94. Braun J, Bollow M, Neure L, et al. Use of immunohistologic and in situ hybridization techniques in the examination of sacroiliac joint biopsy specimens from patients with ankylosing spondylitis. Arthritis Rheum. 1995;38:499–505.

95. Braun J, Bollow M, Eggens U, Konig H, Distler A, Sieper J. Use of dynamic magnetic resonance imaging with fast imaging in the detection of early and advanced sacroiliitis in spondylarthropathy patients. Arthritis Rheum. 1994;37:1039–1045.

96. Bollow M, Fischer T, Reisshauer H, et al. Quantitative analyses of sacroiliac biopsies in spondyloarthropathies: T cells and macrophages predominate in early and active sacroiliitis—cellularity correlates with the degree of enhancement detected by magnetic resonance imaging. Ann Rheum Dis. 2000;59:135–140.

97. Leirisalo-Repo M, Turunen U, Stenman S, Helenius P, Seppala K. High frequency of silent inflammatory bowel disease in spondylarthropathy. Arthritis Rheum. 1994;37:23–31.

98. Mielants H, Veys EM, Goemaere S, Cuvelier C, De Vos M. A prospective study of patients with spondyloarthropathy with special reference to HLA-B27 and to gut histology. J Rheumatol. 1993;20:1353–1358.

99. Leirisalo-Repo M, Repo H. Gut and spondyloarthropathies. Rheum Dis Clin North Am. 1992;18:23–35.

100. Maki-Ikola O, Leirisalo-Repo M, Turunen U, Granfors K. Association of gut inflammation with increased serum IgA class Klebsiella antibody concentrations in patients with axial ankylosing spondylitis (AS): implication for different aetiopathogenetic mechanisms for axial and peripheral AS? Ann Rheum Dis. 1997;56:180–183.

101. Maki-Ikola O, Nissila M, Lehtinen K, Leirisalo-Repo M, Toivanen P, Granfors K. Antibodies to Klebsiella pneumoniae, Escherichia coli and Proteus mirabilis in the sera of patients with axial and peripheral form of ankylosing spondylitis. Br J Rheumatol. 1995;34:413–417.

102. Purrmann J, Zeidler H, Bertrams J, et al. HLA antigens in ankylosing spondylitis associated with Crohn's disease. Increased frequency of the HLA phenotype B27, B44. J Rheumatol. 1988;15:1658–1661.

103. Lindholm H, Visakorpi R. Late complications after a Yersinia enterocolitica epidemic: a follow up study. Ann Rheum Dis. 1991;50:694–696.

104. Szanto E, Hagenfeldt K. Sacro-iliitis in women—a sequela to acute salpingitis. A follow-up study. Scand J Rheumatol. 1983;12:89–92.

105. Lehtinen K. 76 patients with ankylosing spondylitis seen after 30 years of disease. Scand J Rheumatol. 1983;12:5–11.

106. van der PM, van Denderen JC, van den Brule AJ, et al. Prevalence of Chlamydia trachomatis in urine of male patients with ankylosing spondylitis is not increased. Ann Rheum Dis. 2000;59:300–302.

107. Martínez A, Pacheco-Tena C, Vazquez-Mellado J, Burgos-Vargas R. Relationship between disease activity and infection in patients with spondyloarthropathies. Ann Rheum Dis. 2004; 63: 1338–1340.

108. Lange U, Berliner M, Ludwig M, et al. Ankylosing spondylitis and infections of the female urogenital tract. Rheumatol Int. 1998;17:181–184.

109. Sieper J. Disease mechanisms in reactive arthritis. Curr Rheumatol Rep. 2004;6:110–116.

110. Maksymowych WP. Update in spondylarthropathy. Arthritis Rheum. 2004;51:143–146.

111. Zhang X, Glogauer M, Zhu F, Kim TH, Chiu B, Inman RD. Innate immunity and arthritis: neutrophil Rac and toll-like receptor 4 expression define outcomes in infection-triggered arthritis. Arthritis Rheum. 2005;52:1297–1304.

112. Popov I, Dela Cruz CS, Barber BH, Chiu B, Inman RD. Breakdown of CTL tolerance to self HLA-B*2705 induced by exposure to *Chlamydia trachomatis*. J Immunol. 2002;169:4033–4038.

113. Zhang X, Aubin JE, Kim TH, Payne U, Chiu B, Inman RD. Synovial fibroblasts infected with *Salmonella enterica* serovar Typhimurium mediate osteoclast differentiation and activation. Infect Immun. 2004;72:7183–7189.

114. Olhagen B. Chronic uro-polyarthritis in the male. Acta Med Scand. 1960;168:339–345.

115. Schiefer HG, Weidner W, Krauss H, Gerhardt U, Schmidt KL. Rheumatoid factor-negative arthritis, especially ankylosing spondylitis, and infections of the male urogenital tract. Zentralbl Bakteriol Mikrobiol Hyg [A]. 1983;255:511–517.

116. Claudepierre P, Gueguen A, Ladjouze A, et al. Predictive factors of severity of spondyloarthropathy in North Africa. Br J Rheumatol. 1995;34:1139–1145.

117. Hajjaj-Hassouni N, Maetzel A, Dougados M, Amor B. Comparison of patients evaluated for spondylarthropathy in France and Morocco. Rev Rhum Ed Fr. 1993;60:420–425.

118. Lau CS, Burgos-Vargas R, Louthrenoo W, Mok MY, Wordsworth P, Zeng QY. Features of spondyloarthritis around the world. Rheum Dis Clin North Am. 1998;24:753–770.

119. Huang F, Zhang J, Zhu J, Guo J, Yang C. Juvenile spondyloarthropathies: the Chinese experience. Rheum Dis Clin North Am. 2003;29:531–547.

120. Pacheco-Tena C, Alvarado DLB, Lopez-Vidal Y, et al. Bacterial DNA in synovial fluid cells of patients with juvenile onset spondyloarthropathies. Rheumatology (Oxford). 2001;40:920–927.

121. Lehtinen A, Taavitsainen M, Leirisalo-Repo M. Sonographic analysis of enthesopathy in the lower extremities of patients with spondylarthropathy. Clin Exp Rheumatol. 1994;12:143–148.

122. Balint PV, Kane D, Wilson H, McInnes IB, Sturrock RD. Ultrasonography of entheseal insertions in the lower limb in spondyloarthropathy. Ann Rheum Dis. 2002;61:905–910.

123. Grigoryan M, Roemer FW, Mohr A, Genant HK. Imaging in spondyloarthropathies. Curr Rheumatol Rep. 2004;6:102–109.

124. Hermann KG, Bollow M. Magnetic resonance imaging of the axial skeleton in rheumatoid disease. Best Pract Res Clin Rheumatol. 2004;18:881–907.

6

Inflammatory Bowel Disease Spondyloarthritis: Epidemiology, Clinical Features, and Treatment

Herman Mielants and Filip Van den Bosch

INTRODUCTION

The chronic idiopathic inflammatory bowel diseases (IBDs), ulcerative colitis (UC) and Crohn's disease (CD), are part of the concept of the spondyloarthropathies (SpAs). Other gut diseases that can be associated with joint symptoms, such as Whipple's disease, celiac disease, and arthritis due to intestinal bypass surgery are not considered SpAs any more and will not be reviewed in this chapter.

HISTORICAL ASPECTS

A relationship between the gut and arthritis was postulated by Smith[1] who performed segmental bowel surgery to treat patients with rheumatoid arthritis (RA). Bargen[2] recognized arthritis as a complication of UC. Hench[3] described a peripheral arthritis in patients with IBD and observed the tendency of arthritis to flare with exacerbations of the colitis and to subside with remission of the gut symptoms. Wright and Moll[4] introduced the SpA concept and definitely included IBD in this concept. The group at the University of Ghent[5] demonstrated the strong relationship between gut and joint in different forms of SpA and suggested the presence of subclinical CD in a great number of patients.

EPIDEMIOLOGY AND CLASSIFICATION

The prevalence of UC ranges from 50 to 100 individuals per 100,000 in the general population, and it is more common in whites than in nonwhites and also in a Jewish population. The prevalence of CD has increased during the last few decades to about 75 per 100,000. Ongoing epidemiologic studies suggest that the true prevalence may have been underestimated by 27% to 35%, and these studies suggest the existence of patients with subclinical IBD.[6]

Locomotor involvement in IBD has been divided historically into two patterns: 1) peripheral arthritis and 2) axial involvement, including sacroiliitis with or without spondylitis similar to idiopathic ankylosing spondylitis (AS). Other clinical features mostly typical for the SpAs, such as tendinitis, enthesitis, dactylitis, and clubbing are often present.

The incidence of peripheral arthritis in IBD ranges from 10% to 22% of patients[7,8] with a higher prevalence in patients with CD.[9] The sex ratio is equal, and peak age is between 25 and 44 years. The prevalence of arthritis in IBD increases with the duration of gut disease, going from 12% to 30% in a 20-year follow-up.[10]

The true prevalence of axial involvement is unclear because the onset is often insidious.

Prevalence rates of 10% to 20% for sacroiliitis and 7% to 12% for spondylitis have been reported, although the actual figures are probably higher because of the existence of subclinical axial involvement. With computed tomography (CT) scans, sacroiliitis was detected in 45% of patients with CD with low back pain; most of these instances of sacroiliitis were not recognized on classical radiographs.[11] In a study from an IBD clinic, 30% of patients with IBD had inflammatory low back pain, 33% had unilateral or bilateral sacroiliitis stage II, and in 18% of the patients the sacroiliitis was asymptomatic.[12] Magnetic resonance imaging (MRI) is probably the most sensitive method to detect early or subclinical sacroiliitis or spondylitis,[13] but no systemic MRI studies have yet been performed in IBD. In a series of patients who had CD for at least 5 years, 15 of 42 (36%) had evidence of sacroiliitis on MRI scans and 10 of these patients had frank AS. All the patients with CD who were human leukocyte antigen (HLA)-B27-positive developed AS.[14]

Although it is generally accepted that men are more likely to develop AS (male-to-female ratio is 3:1) in IBD-associated AS, the male-to-female ratio is equal.

Women with IBD and AS have a younger age of onset of AS and more severe disease than male patients. In general, joint disease is more severe, as defined by intake of nonsteroidal inflammatory drugs and a decrease in spinal mobility, in patients with combined IBD and AS than in those with uncomplicated AS.[15]

Using the European Spondylarthropathy Study Group (ESSG) criteria for classification of SpAs[16] and the New York criteria for classification of AS,[17] the diagnosis of SpA was made in 35% of patients and of AS in 10%,[12] whereas in another study these figures were 18% and 3%, respectively.[18]

CLINICAL FEATURES

The clinical features can be subdivided into intestinal symptoms, peripheral arthritis, axial involvement, and extraintestinal and extraarticular features.

Intestinal Symptoms

CD is characterized by the classic triad of abdominal pain, weight loss, and diarrhea. Abdominal pain is common but not severe. Weight loss in the range of 10% to 20% of body weight is common, as are low-grade fever and general debility. At a later stage, fistulae and abscesses may appear. Diarrhea and intestinal blood loss are the most common abdominal manifestations of UC. Diarrhea is almost always present, whereas fever and weight loss are less common. Sometimes it is difficult to distinguish between both diseases, mostly in the presence of isolated colonic involvement.

Peripheral Arthritis

The arthritis is generally pauciarticular and asymmetric and is often transient and migratory. Large and small joints, predominantly of the lower legs, are involved. The arthritis usually is nondestructive and self-limiting, and many attacks subside within 4 to 6 weeks.[19] Recurrences are common. Sausage-like fingers and toes (dactylitis) are common. Enthesopathies, especially inflammation of the Achilles tendon or the insertion of the fascia plantaris, are known manifestations and also may involve the knee or other sites, occurring in about 10% of the patients.[18] Clubbing and, rarely, periostitis may occur in CD. The peripheral arthritis becomes chronic in some patients, and destructive lesions of small joints and hips may occur.

In about 40% of patients with CD and arthritis, during the disease course intestinal symptoms coincide with the joint manifestations and in 40% they antedate them,[18] but the articular symptoms may precede the intestinal symptoms in about 20% of the patients by years.[18,19] In a prospective study of 123 patients with SpAs without clinical signs of gut involvement, 8 (6%) patients developed CD 2 to 9 years after the appearance of the joint symptoms.[20] In UC, there is a more distinct temporal relationship between attacks of arthritis and flares of bowel disease. Surgical removal of diseased colon can induce remission of peripheral arthritis; in CD this treatment has little effect on joint disease.[21]

In an Oxford study,[22] together with the classical pauciarticular group presenting the clinical features mentioned earlier, a second, less common polyarticular subgroup was described. In this subgroup the arthritis persisted for months and years, ran a course independent of IBD, and was not associated with other extraintestinal manifestations. This polyarticular type is rather uncommon,[18] and in a prospective population study of 521 patients with IBD, no patients fulfilled the clinical picture of this type of arthropathy.[19]

Axial Involvement

The clinical picture is mostly indistinguishable from that of uncomplicated AS. The patients complain of inflammatory low back pain, thoracic or cervical pain, buttock pain, and chest pain.

Limitation of lumbar or cervical motion and reduced chest expansion are characteristic clinical signs. Peripheral arthritis can be present, together with the other typical manifestations such as tendinitis or dactylitis. The onset of axial involvement does not parallel that of bowel disease, but frequently precedes it.[7,15] The course also is totally independent of the course of the intestinal disease. Bowel surgery does not alter the course of associated sacroiliitis or spondylitis. Prospectively, all patients with SpAs in whom CD occurred after 2 to 9 years developed axial involvement and fulfilled the criteria for AS.[20]

Extraintestinal and Extraarticular Features

A variety of cutaneous, mucosal, serosal, and ocular manifestations can occur in IBD.

Skin lesions are observed in 10% to 25% of patients. Erythema nodosum parallels the activity of bowel disease, tends to occur in patients with active peripheral arthritis, and is probably a disease-related manifestation.[23] Pyoderma gangrenosum is more severe but a less common manifestation not related to the activity of the bowel and joint disease. Leg ulcers and thrombophlebitis also may occur.

Ocular manifestations, especially anterior uveitis, often occur in IBD (3 to 11%). Uveitis in patients with associated SpAs is often acute in onset, unilateral, and transient, but recurrences are common.[24] In general, the choroid and retina are spared; however, in uncomplicated IBD, lesions are often bilateral, insidious in onset, and chronic in duration.[25] Granulomatous uveitis is rare but may be present in CD. Conjunctivitis and episcleritis also have been observed.

Aphthous ulcerations, mainly affecting the buccal mucosa and tongue, are not uncommon in CD and can parallel disease activity.

Amyloidosis is a well-recognized cause of death in CD,[26] although in clinical series the incidence is only 1%.[26] However, postmortem studies have revealed evidence of amyloid in 25% of patients with CD.

ASSESSMENT OF DISEASE ACTIVITY

Joint disease activity and axial involvement are assessed by the same measurements as those used in different forms of SpAs and AS, such as the Bath Ankylosing Spondylitis Disease Activity Index (BASDAI), the Bath Ankylosing Spondylitis Functional Index (BASFI), the Bath Ankylosing Spondylitis Metrology Index (BASMI), Bath Ankylosing Spondylitis Patient General Score (BAS-G), tender and swollen joint count, enthesitis count, and the different measurements of quality of life presented in other chapters in this textbook. Measurement of disease activity of gut inflammation is performed with the Crohn's Disease Activity Index (CDAI).[27]

IMAGING AND BIOLOGY

There are no diagnostic laboratory tests for the arthritis or spondylitis of IBD. Elevated serum acute-phase reactants (especially C-reactive protein), thrombocytosis (especially in CD), and hypochromic anemia due to chronic blood loss or chronic inflammation are common findings. Rheumatoid factor and antinuclear antibodies are mostly absent.

Anti-*Saccharomyces cerevisiae* antibodies (ASCAs) are considered to be an important marker for CD, although their pathogenic role is not clear.[28] Recently ASCA immunoglobulin A (IgA) levels were found to be significantly higher in SpAs, more specifically in AS than in healthy control subjects and patients with RA,[29] suggesting that this serum marker could identify those patients with SpAs at risk for developing AS.

Results of synovial fluid analysis are consistent with inflammatory arthritis with leucocyte counts ranging from 1,500 to 50,000/mm, predominantly neutrophils. Synovial histologic analysis reveals only nonspecific inflammation, although granulomas have been described. Cultures are negative.

Radiographs of the peripheral joints mostly do not exhibit erosions. Erosive lesions, mainly of the metacarpophalangeal and metatarsal joints, occasionally have been described, differing from those in RA only by their pauciarticular and asymmetric distribution. Adjacent bone proliferation can be present. Destructive lesions of the hip have been reported and related to CD-like lesions on gut biopsy in undifferentiated SpA.[30] The radiographic appearance of the enthesopathies is similar to that found in other SpAs.

The axial involvement of IBD is indistinguishable from that of uncomplicated AS, although the incidence of asymmetric sacroiliitis is higher, and the ankylosis of zygapophyseal joints is more common.[31] As mentioned earlier, asymptomatic sacroiliacal involvement and even spondylitis are common. For further discussion of the use of other techniques such as CT and particularly MRI in the early detection of sacroiliac and axial inflammation, see Chapter 14 on imaging in AS.

Ileocolonoscopy is, of course, the investigation of choice for the diagnosis of IBD as well as for follow-up of the disease. In UC, the mucosa is diffusely involved. The lesions (including superficial ulcerations, edema, friability, and microabscesses) are confined to the colonic mucosa. In CD, the lesions may occur in the entire gastrointestinal (GI) tract, although the terminal ileum and colon are preferentially involved. The lesions are usually ulcerative, but their distribution is patchy. They can occur superficially as in UC, but often are transmural and granulomatous. Aphthoid ulceration, pseudopyloric metaplasia, and sarcoid-like granulomas are virtually pathognomonic findings. Sometimes it is difficult to distinguish between UC and CD especially in patients with isolated colonic involvement.

Numerous ileocolonoscopic studies have demonstrated a high prevalence of gut inflammation in patients with AS and other forms of SpA.[32–36] Other studies have demonstrated gut inflammation in some forms of juvenile chronic arthritis, notably in the pauciarticular late-onset form, which is often associated with HLA-B27 and considered to be a form of SpA.[37] In the follow-up of these children, half of them developed AS (all had gut inflammation at the first examination), and 17% developed CD. In acute anterior uveitis, chronic inflammatory gut lesions were found in 66% of the patients.[38] The histology of the lesions and the patchy distribution resembled those in CD, suggesting that the gut is involved in the pathogenesis of acute anterior uveitis. In psoriatic arthritis (PsA), gut inflammation was demonstrated only in the pauciarticular and axial forms, considered to be part of the SpA concept, and not in the polyarticular form.[39]

The histologic lesions are subdivided into *acute lesions* resembling acute bacterial enteritis and *chronic lesions* resembling the pathologic appearance of chronic idiopathic IBD. The clinical, laboratory, and radiographic disease manifestations in patients with chronic lesions resemble the features of IBD and AS, whereas patients with acute lesions exhibit clinical features of enterogenic reactive arthritis.[40]

GENETICS AND HLA-B27

Substantial evidence favors a genetic cause for IBD. Familial aggregation of CD and UC has been amply documented. Both diseases are believed to be genetically linked, because both occur within the same families, but neither disease has been associated with HLA in family studies. IBD complicated by peripheral arthritis is not associated with HLA-B27. Sacroiliitis and spondylitis in IBD are associated with HLA-B27, but to a lesser degree than in uncomplicated AS (33% versus 85%). Interestingly, patients with AS who lack HLA-B27 have a higher risk of developing IBD than do HLA-B27–positive AS patients.[36,41] On the other hand, more than 50% of the subjects who have HLA-B27 in combination with CD will develop AS.[42]

HLA-BW62 occurs in a high proportion of patients with SpAs who have CD-like lesions on gut biopsy,[43] as well as in patients with proven CD. The B27-B44 phenotype also confers a high risk of development of both CD and AS.[44] In the Oxford study, pauciarticular joint involvement was associated with HLA-B27, B35, and especially DRB1*0103, whereas the polyarticular form was associated only with HLA-B44.[45]

Recently a correlation was reported between mutations in the *NOD2* (*CARD15*) gene, a host defense gene located on chromosome 16, and increased susceptibility for CD.[46,47] The prevalence of this mutation is about 30%.[46–48] The linkage of *CARD15* variants has been related to clinical phenotypes such as younger age at onset, preferential involvement of small bowel,[49,50] or fibrostenosing disease.[51] No association was found with extraintestinal manifestations.

Different investigators have studied the association of *CARD15*/*NOD2* variants in patients with SpAs and found no increased prevalence, concluding that those variants do not affect the risk of development of primary AS.[52–54] By determining *CARD15* variants in patients with CD with or without sacroiliitis, a significant association with these mutations and the presence of sacroiliitis was demonstrated.[55] By studying patients with SpAs who 15 years earlier underwent ileocolonoscopy[36] and comparing the prevalence of *CARD15* mutations of ethnically matched patients with CD and control subjects, these mutations clearly identified a subgroup of patients with SpAs associated with chronic intestinal inflammation prone for evolution to CD.[56]

PATHOLOGY AND THE GUT-JOINT LINK

See Chapter 2 for a discussion on the gut and SpAs.

TREATMENT AND OUTCOME

Nonsteroidal Anti-Inflammatory Drugs

Treatment of peripheral arthritis and spondylitis in patients with IBD is the same as that in AS and SpAs in general. Nonsteroidal anti-inflammatory drugs (NSAIDs) are the first choice, although they may cause an exacerbation of intestinal symptoms in IBD[57] (mainly in UC) or cause ulcerations in the small or large bowel.[58] NSAID-related changes are more common in the proximal parts of the jejunum and ileum than in the terminal ileum and colon.[59]

Virtually all ileocolonoscopic studies in patients with SpAs have demonstrated the absence of any association between the gut lesions and the use of NSAIDs. In the large intestine, NSAIDs, however, may provoke relapse of quiescent IBD, especially in UC,[60] and those prone to relapses have them within a few days after receiving these drugs. The intake of NSAIDs may be associated with an increased risk of emergency admission to the hospital for colitis caused by IBD, particularly among patients with no previous history.[61] Although the new selective cyclooxygenase-2 (COX-2) inhibitors have a proven effect in preventing gastric ulcerations, it is not clear whether these drugs have the same protective effect on the colon, because COX-2 inhibition could have a detrimental role in ulcer healing.[58]

Conventional Disease Modifying Antirheumatic Drugs

Sulfasalazine, which has been successfully used to treat colonic inflammation in UC and CD, has been found to be effective in the treatment of the peripheral arthritis accompanying SpAs,[62] especially if intestinal inflammation is present.[63] It may also have a favorable effect on peripheral arthritis in IBD but will not influence axial symptoms. Although often inducing a clinical remission in SpAs, sulfasalazine does not prevent the development of IBD.[63]

Gold, D-penicillamine, and antimalarial drugs are ineffective. Low-dose methotrexate, successfully used in the treatment of RA and in some cases of refractory IBD,[64] has not yet been proven effective in joint inflammation associated with CD or UC.

Corticosteroids

Intraarticular corticosteroid injections may be beneficial in monoarticular flares. Oral corticosteroids may reduce peripheral synovitis but have no effect on axial symptoms. Their systematic use is justified only if they are required to control the bowel disease. Controlled ileal release budesonide, a corticosteroid that has high affinity for the glucocorticoid receptor but low systemic activity due to extensive first-pass hepatic metabolism may be used as an alternative to prednisone when bowel symptoms are treated; placebo-controlled trials have demonstrated that controlled ileal release budesonide 9 mg/day is effective in patients with mild to moderately active Crohn's ileitis and/or right colon involvement. In an 8-week, placebo-controlled trial, in which patients were randomly assigned to budesonide (3, 9, or 15 mg daily) or placebo, remission occurred in 33, 51, and 43%, respectively, in the budesonide treatment groups compared to 20% in patients receiving placebo.[65] In another study, treatment with budesonide 9 mg once daily for 8 weeks was as effective as treatment with prednisone (40 mg once daily for 2 weeks with gradual tapering) for inducing remission (51% versus 53%) with, however, a safety profile in favor of budesonide.[66] Budesonide was also investigated in RA,[67] in which it was not shown to be superior to conventional prednisone therapy. Thus far, trials in SpAs have not yet been performed, nor has the effect of budesonide on peripheral arthritis or spondylitis been looked at systematically in CD trials.

Conventional Disease Modifying Antirheumatic Drugs Not Yet Evaluated in Spondyloarthropathy

Azathioprine and its principal metabolite 6-mercaptopurine have been used successfully for more than 30 years[68,69] in patients with CD for induction of GI remission in steroid-refractory disease, as a steroid-sparing agent, in fistulizing disease, and for maintenance therapy. A reduction in the dose after 4 years of treatment is often successful for long-term maintenance therapy. However, despite efficacy in RA, the drug has not been studied in relation to the arthritis of CD or UC. Concerning the other SpAs, azathioprine has been used with success in severe Reiter's syndrome,[70] and beneficial effects were reported in a few patients with severe PsA[71] and in one patient with severe and refractory AS (using an intravenous loading dose).[72]

Leflunomide (Arava) is an isoxazole derivative approved for the treatment of RA. It has only been studied in a small, open-label trial of 12 patients with CD who were intolerant of azathioprine[73]: clinical improvement was noted in 8 of 12 patients, suggesting that further study in controlled trials would be warranted. The drug has also been studied in a small, open-label trial of 20 patients with AS: no significant effect was observed for axial disease; a modest improvement was seen in the peripheral arthritis.[74]

Tumor Necrosis Factor-α Blockade in Crohn's Disease and Spondyloarthropathies

It has been demonstrated that treatment with a single infusion of the chimeric monoclonal antibody cA2 (infliximab) directed against tumor necrosis factor-α (TNF-α) was highly effective in the short-term treatment of intestinal involvement in treatment-resistant CD[75,76] (Fig. 6.1), even resulting in the closure of enterocutaneous fistulae.[77] Moreover, the results of the CD clinical trial evaluating infliximab in a new long-term treatment regimen study (ACCENT I) showed that maintenance therapy with infliximab in moderate-to-severe CD prolonged the response and remission of the disease.[78,79]

The first observations that infliximab therapy might be useful for the treatment of resistant peripheral joint and axial manifestations in patients with CD came from an open pilot study[80]: four patients with therapy-resistant or fistulizing CD and concurrent active SpA were treated with 5 mg/kg of infliximab. In addition to remission of gut inflammation, a significant improvement in articular and axial symptoms was observed in all patients. Two patients also had HLA-B27-positive

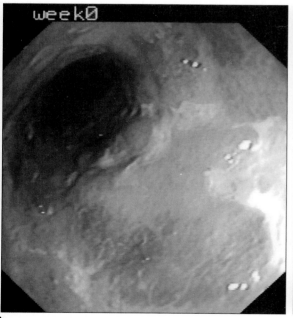
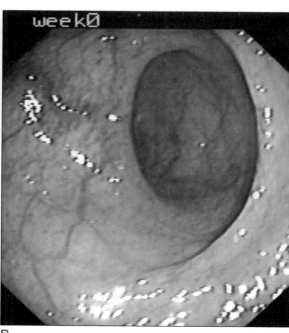

Fig. 6.1 Ileocolonoscopy in Crohn's disease. A: Before treatment with infliximab: presence of important ulcerations. **B:** After treatment with infliximab: disappearance of inflammation and ulcerations.

AS in addition to CD; in one of them and in two other patients the manifestations of SpAs consisted of oligoarticular peripheral arthritis. In all patients, inflammatory variables such as C-reactive protein levels normalized after treatment with infliximab. Axial inflammatory pain disappeared after a single infusion. In two patients peripheral synovitis went into full remission after one infusion, whereas a second treatment was necessary in the third patient. In one patient the disease flared after 3 months, but retreatment with the same dose of infliximab induced a new remission (Fig. 6.2).

As a consequence of these initial findings, TNF-α blockade with infliximab (loading dose regimen 5 mg/kg) was explored in a number of open studies in patients with different forms of active SpAs[81–84]: in total, more than 100 patients with AS have been treated in short-term open studies with infliximab; invariably, a high success rate was reported. A global good response was also observed with a lower dose of 3 mg/kg of infliximab in a small series of patients with AS[85] and in six patients with severe undifferentiated SpA.[86] However, the conventional dose of 5 mg/kg, which is standard in the treatment of CD, appeared to have superior efficacy.

Based on the data of the open studies, two double-blind, placebo-controlled trials were conducted simultaneously in Ghent[87] and Berlin.[88] In these studies the fast and significant improvement of TNF-α blockade was for the first time confirmed in a placebo-controlled way. Although no formal placebo-controlled study has been performed in CD spondyloarthritis, there is little doubt that infliximab is also highly efficacious in this indication. In the previously mentioned ACCENT I trial, which evaluated the efficacy of a retreatment regimen of infliximab in patients with active CD, maintenance therapy turned out to be helpful also for resolving extraintestinal manifestations such as arthritis.[89] Recently, in an Italian open study[90] the efficacy of

a loading dose regimen of 5 mg/kg of infliximab in 24 patients with SpAs associated with active ($n = 16$) or quiescent ($n = 8$) CD was evaluated. Patients were retreated with either 3 mg/kg (for bowel disease remission after the loading dose) or 5 mg/kg when gut symptoms were persisting. The retreatment period varied between 12 and 18 months. Infliximab improved both GI and overall articular symptoms (axial disease, peripheral arthritis, and enthesitis). In patients with inactive CD at baseline, infliximab prevented IBD flares during the follow-up period.

With regard to these findings, a special scientific challenge is the fact that more TNF-α blockers seem to be effective in AS than in IBD. Etanercept is an example of such a drug with discordant efficacy in both diseases. Efficacy measures (both for axial and peripheral disease) in three placebo-controlled trials in which patients with AS were randomly assigned to placebo or subcutaneous etanercept 25 mg twice weekly, improved in the placebo group with the same impressive magnitude as observed with infliximab treatment.[91-93] However, in an 8-week, randomized, double-blind, placebo-controlled trial, etanercept showed no signs of efficacy in patients with active CD.[94] Moreover, Marzo-Ortega et al.[95] treated two patients with CD spondyloarthritis with etanercept and observed complete remission of axial symptoms, whereas their CD either persisted or flared during treatment. The biologic basis of this discrepancy is currently still being researched. Reasons for such a discrepancy may include differences in bioavailability and pharmacodynamics, as well as cell biologic effects (induction of apoptosis) that may differ between different TNF-α blocking agents. For example, there are data suggesting that only infliximab and not etanercept is able to bind to activated peripheral blood and lamina propria lymphocytes derived from the gut of patients with CD.[96] In addition, infliximab but not etanercept induced apoptosis of these lymphocytes, providing a biologic basis, at least in CD, for the difference in the efficacy of infliximab and etanercept.

Other forms of anti-TNF-α therapy are also being evaluated. Preliminary results indicate the efficacy of adalimumab, a fully human monoclonal antibody, in CD,[97] AS,[98] and PsA.[99] CDP571, a humanized, monoclonal chimeric anti-TNF-α antibody, was initially shown to be safe and effective for treatment of patients with CD.[100] However, in a larger, placebo-controlled study,[101] CDP571 turned out to be only modestly effective for short- (week 2) but not long-term (week 28) treatment of unselected patients with moderate-to-severe CD. CDP870, a humanized monoclonal anti-TNF-α antibody attached to polyethylene glycol, showed equivocal results in two recent studies.[102,103] Finally, with onercept, a recombinant form of the natural human soluble p55 TNF receptor, a clinical benefit was suggested in a pilot study involving 12 patients with active CD.[104]

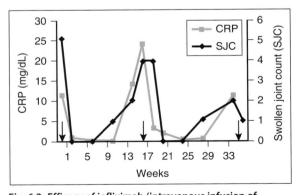

Fig. 6.2 Efficacy of infliximab (intravenous infusion of 5 mg/kg body weight; time point of infusion indicated by *arrows*) in a patient with CD spondyloarthritis. Effect on C-reactive protein (CRP) level and the number of swollen joints (SJC). GI and articular disease flared approximately 3 months after infliximab treatment; retreatment with the same dose induced a new remission.

Thalidomide, a drug with specific immunomodulatory properties, deserves some attention with regard to the discussion on TNF-α blockade. It suppresses the production of TNF-α by monocytes at the transcriptional level, through a reduction of the TNF-α mRNA half-life, and is selective with no significant effects on cytokines such as interleukin (IL)-1, IL-6, and granulocyte-macrophage colony-stimulating factor. It was banned after its use in pregnancy for hyperemesis was found to cause severe birth defects (phocomelia) in children born to mothers exposed to it during their first trimester of pregnancy. Since that time, however, thalidomide has continuously been used under restricted conditions, mainly because of its reported efficacy for rare refractory manifestations, such as erythema nodosum leprosum, chronic cutaneous lupus, Behçet's disease, or chronic graft-versus-host disease.[105] Its safety and efficacy in CD were evaluated in two open-label pilot trials.[106,107] In the first study 12 patients were treated with thalidomide (50 or 100 mg) for 12 weeks; at the end of treatment a clinical response was observed in 70% of patients with clinical remission in 20%. In the second study 14 of 22 patients with refractory CD completed 12 weeks of treatment (200 or 300 mg), all of whom achieved a clinical response; 9 patients were in clinical remission. Side effects included drowsiness, peripheral neuropathy, edema, and dermatitis. As of today, four open-label studies have been performed to test the efficacy of this drug in AS,[108-111] albeit with a limited number of patients: in total 43 patients have been treated with a dose between 100 and 300 mg/day. Duration of treatment was between 6 and 12 months, with the percentage of premature discontinuations ranging between 13% and 42%. Evidence of clinical efficacy was found in 7 of 12 patients in the French studies[108,110] and 21 of 30 in the Chinese study.[111]

Potential New Agents in the Treatment of Crohn's Disease and Spondyloarthropathies

Interleukin-10

IL-10 inhibits effector functions of activated macrophages and monocytes and down-regulates the production of proinflammatory cytokines. The results of clinical studies in CD have so far been inconclusive.[112-115] It is not possible at this time to define exactly the role of IL-10 in the development of SpAs. Key observations on the effect of this cytokine on locomotor manifestations in patients with IBD as well as different types of SpAs are further warranted.

Interleukin-11

The use of recombinant IL-11 (a member of the IL-6 family) has been initiated for severe recurrent thrombocytopenia resulting from chemotherapy. A randomized, controlled trial with IL-11 in patients with active CD not receiving steroids, has demonstrated evidence of benefit and a very good safety profile.[116] The role of IL-11 in SpAs remains to be documented.

Anti-interleukin-12

IL-12 is a key cytokine that drives the inflammatory response mediated by type 1 helper T (Th1) cells. CD is characterized by increased production of IL-12 by antigen-presenting cells in intestinal tissue. In a recent double-blind, placebo-controlled trial the safety and efficacy of a human monoclonal antibody against IL-12 in 79 patients with active CD was evaluated.[117] Uninterrupted treatment for 7 weeks with 3 mg/kg of anti-IL-12 (subcutaneous injection weekly) was found to be safe and resulted in statistically higher response rates compared with placebo. Again, the role of IL-12 in SpAs needs to be further explored.

Intercellular adhesion molecule-1 antisense

The expression of intercellular adhesion molecule-1 (ICAM-1; a member of the immunoglobulin superfamily) can be up-regulated in response to inflammatory mediators. The ligands with which it can interact include the β₂-integrin leucocyte function associated antigen-1 (LFA-1). ICAM-1 and LFA-1 are involved in recruitment and activation of inflammatory cells. In the context of CD, they have been found to be up-regulated on mucosal endothelium and lamina propria mononuclear cells.[118,119]

Initial results in human pilot studies were equivocal.[120,121] A large controlled trial including 299 patients with active, steroid-dependent CD who were randomly assigned to active treatment for 2 or 4 weeks or placebo indicated that at week 14, steroid withdrawal was successful in a significantly higher proportion of patients who received active treatment, suggesting a possible, modest benefit.[122] No data are as yet available about the effect of this compound in SpAs.

Anti-α₄β₇

The α₄β₇ lymphocyte integrin binds to vascular cell adhesion molecule-1 (VCAM-1), fibronectin, and mucosal addressin cell adhesion molecule-1 (MadCAM-1) (expressed selectively on high endothelial venules in mucosal lymphoid tissue and gut lamina propria). α₄-Integrins are involved in leucocyte migration across vascular endothelium. An antibody against α₄ integrin (natalizumab, Antegren) was evaluated in a placebo-controlled trial involving 248 patients with moderate-to-severe CD. Treatment with natalizumab increased the rates of clinical remission, improved the quality of life, increased C-reactive protein levels, and was well tolerated.[123,124] The selective enrichment of α₄β₇ lymphocytes among synovial infiltrates in patients with arthritis and their supposed mucosal origin in SpA arthritis should encourage research on anti-α₄β₇ compounds in SpAs.

GENERAL CONCLUSION

Arthritis and spondylitis are well recognized extraintestinal features of the idiopathic IBDs, and subclinical gut inflammation has been described in the different entities of the SpA concept since the 1980s. Recent immunologic studies (reviewed in Chapter 2) confirm this strong relationship between bowel inflammation in SpAs and CD on the one hand and joint disease (especially peripheral arthropathy) in SpAs on the other hand. In looking at TNF-α blockade with infliximab as a proof of concept, it was found that targeted therapies for CD could also be effective for the treatment of extraintestinal disease manifestations in CD and consequently also for other diseases belonging to the SpA concept. Unraveling the gut-synovium axis could lead to the identification of new therapeutic targets and could contribute to stratification of individual patients in subgroups with an optimal response to a specific therapeutic intervention.

REFERENCES

1. Smith R. Treatment of rheumatoid arthritis by colectomy. Ann Surg. 1922;76:515–578.
2. Bargen JA. Complications and sequelae of chronic ulcerative colitis. Ann Intern Med. 1929;3:335.
3. Hench PS. Acute and chronic arthritis. In: Whipple GH, ed. Nelson's Looseleaf of Surgery. New York, NY: Thomas Nelson Sons; 1935:104.
4. Wright V, Moll JMH. Seronegative polyarthritis. Amsterdam, the Netherlands: North Holland Publishing Company; 1976.
5. Mielants H, Veys EM, Cuvelier C, De Vos M, Botelberghe L. HLA B27 related arthritis and bowel inflammation. Part 2. Ileocolonoscopy and bowel histology in patients with HLA-B27 related arthritis. J Rheumatol. 1985;12:294–298.
6. Mayberry JF, Ballantyne KC, Hardcastle JD, Mangham C, Pye G. Epidemiological study of asymptomatic inflammatory bowel disease: the identification of cases during a screening programme for colorectal cancer. Gut. 1989;30:481–483.
7. Palm O, Moum B, Ongre A, Gran JT. Prevalence of ankylosing spondylitis and other spondylarthropathies among patients with inflammatory bowel disease: a population study (the IBSEN study). J Rheumatol. 2002;29:511–515.
8. Salvarani C, Fornaciari G, Beltrami M, Macchioni PL. Musculoskeletal manifestations in inflammatory bowel disease. Eur J Intern Med. 2000;11:210–214.
9. Gravallese EM, Kantrowitz FG. Arthritic manifestations of inflammatory bowel disease. Am J Gastroenterol. 1988;83:703–709.
10. Veloso FT, Carvalho J, Magro F. Immune-related systemic manifestations of inflammatory bowel disease—a prospective study of 792 patients. J Clin Gastroenterol. 1996;23:29–34.
11. Steer S, Jones H, Hibbert J, et al. Low back pain, sacroiliitis and the relationship with HLA B27 in Crohn's disease. J Rheumatol; 2003 30:518–522.
12. De Vlam K, Mielants H, Cuvelier C, De Keyser F, Veys EM, De Vos M. Spondyloarthropathy is underestimated in inflammatory bowel disease: prevalence and HLA association. J Rheumatol. 2000;27:2860–2865.
13. Braun J, Bollow M, Sieper J. Radiologic diagnosis and pathology of the spondyloarthropathies. Rheum Dis Clin North Am. 1998 24:697–735.
14. Wordworth P. Arthritis and inflammatory bowel disease. Curr Rheumatol Rep. 2000;2:87–88.
15. Brophy S, Pavy S, Lewis P, et al. Inflammatory eye, skin and bowel disease in spondyloarthritis: genetic, phenotypic and environmental factors. J Rheumatol. 2001;28:2667–2673.
16. Dougados M, Van der Linden S, Juhlin R, et al., for the European Spondyloarthropathy Study Group. The European Spondylarthropathy Study Group preliminary criteria for the classification of spondylarthropathy. Arthritis Rheum. 1991;34:1218–1227.
17. Van der Linden S, Valkenburg HA, Cats A. Evaluation of diagnostic criteria for ankylosing spondylitis. A proposal for modification of the New York criteria. Arthritis Rheum. 1984;27:361–368.
18. Salvarani C, Vlachonikolis IG, Van der Heijde DM, et al. Musculoskeletal manifestations in a population based cohort of inflammatory bowel disease patients. Scand J Gastroenterol. 2001;36:1307–1313.
19. Palm O, Moum B, Jahnsen J, Gran JT. The prevalence and incidence of peripheral arthritis in patients with inflammatory bowel disease, a prospective population based study (the IBSEN study). Rheumatology. 2001;40:1256–1261.
20. Mielants H, Veys EM, Cuvelier C, et al. The evolution of spondyloarthropathies in relation to gut histology. III. Relation between gut and joint. J Rheumatol. 1995;22:2279–2284.
21. Isdale A, Wright V. Seronegative arthritis and the bowel. Baillieres Clin Rheumatol. 1989;3:285–301.
22. Orchard TR, Wordsworth BP, Jewell DP. Peripheral arthropathies in inflammatory bowel disease: their articular distribution and natural history. Gut. 1998;42:387–391.
23. Schorr-Lesnick B, Brandt LJ. Selected rheumatologic and dermatologic manifestations of inflammatory bowel disease. Am J Gastroenterol. 1988;83:216–223.
24. Rosenbaum JT. Characterization of uveitis associated with spondyloarthritis. J Rheumatol. 1989;16:792–796.
25. Lyons JL, Rosenbaum JT. Uveitis associated with inflammatory bowel disease compared with uveitis associated with spondyloarthropathy. Arch Ophthalmol. 1997;115:61–64.
26. Greenstein AJ, Janowitz HD, Sachar DB. The extra-intestinal complications of Crohn's disease and ulcerative colitis: a study of 700 patients. Medicine (Baltimore). 1976;55:401–412.
27. Best WR, Becktel JM, Singleton JW, Kern JF Jr. Development of a CD activity index. National Cooperative CD Study. Gastroenterology. 1976;70:439–444.
28. Main J, McKenzie H, Yeaman GR, et al. Antibody to Saccharomyces cerevisiae (Baker's yeast) in Crohn's disease. BMJ 1988;297:1105–1106.
29. Hoffman IE, Demetter P, Peeters M, et al. Anti-Saccharomyces cerevisiae IgA antibodies are raised in ankylosing and undifferentiated spondyloarthropathy. Ann Rheum Dis. 2003;62:455–459.
30. Mielants H, Veys EM, Goethals K, Van der Straeten C, Ackerman C. Destructive hip lesions in seronegative spondyloarthropathies: relation to gut inflammation. J Rheumatol. 1990;17:335–340.
31. Helliwell PS, Hickling P, Wright V. Do the radiological changes of classic ankylosing spondylitis differ from the changes found in spondylitis associated with inflammatory bowel disease, psoriasis and reactive arthritis? Ann Rheum Dis. 1998;57:135–140.
32. Mielants H, Veys EM, Cuvelier C, De Vos M. Course of gut inflammation in spondyloarthropathies and therapeutic consequences. Baillieres Clin Rheumatol. 1996;10;147–164.
33. Grillet B, de Clerck L, Dequeker J, Rutgeerts P, Geboes K. Systematic ileocolonoscopy and bowel biopsy in spondylarthropathy. Br J Rheumatol. 1987;26:338–340.
34. Simenon G, Van Gossum A, Adler M, Rickaert F, Appelboom T. Macroscopic and microscopic gut lesions in seronegative spondyloarthropathies. J Rheumatol. 1990;17:1491–1494.
35. Leirisalo-Repo M, Turunen U, Stenman S, Helenius P, Seppala K. High frequency of silent inflammatory bowel disease in spondylarthropathy. Arthritis Rheum. 1994;37:23–31.
36. Mielants H, Veys EM, Cuvelier C, et al. The evolution of spondyloarthropathies in relation to gut histology. II. Histological aspects. J Rheumatol. 1995;22:2273–2278.
37. Mielants H, Veys EM, Cuvelier C, et al. Gut inflammation in children with late onset pauciarticular juvenile chronic arthritis

and evolution to adult spondyloarthropathy: a prospective study. J Rheumatol. 1993;20:1567–1572.

38. Banares AA, Jover JA, Fernandez-Gutierrez B, et al. Bowel inflammation in anterior uveitis and spondyloarthropathy. J Rheumatol. 1995;22:1112–1117.

39. Schatteman L, Mielants H, Veys EM, et al. Gut inflammation in psoriatic arthritis: a prospective ileocolonoscopic study. J Rheumatol. 1995;22:680–683.

40. Mielants H, Veys EM, Goemaere S, Goethals K, Cuvelier C, De Vos M. Gut inflammation in the spondyloarthropathies: clinical, radiologic, biologic and genetic features in relation to the type of histology: a prospective study. J Rheumatol. 1991;18:1542–1551.

41. Dekker-Saeys AJ, Keat AC. Follow-up study of ankylosing spondylitis over a period of 12 years. Scand J Rheumatol. 1990;87(suppl):120–121.

42. Russell AS, Percy JS, Schlaut J, et al. Transplantation antigens in Crohn's disease: linkage of associated ankylosing spondylitis with HLA-AW27. Am J Dig Dis. 1995;20:359–361.

43. Mielants H, Veys EM, Joos R, Noens L, Cuvekier C, De Vos M. HLA antigens in seronegative spondylarthropathies. Reactive arthritis and arthritis in ankylosing spondylitis: relation to gut inflammation. J Rheumatol. 1987;14:466–471.

44. Purrmann J, Zeidler H, Bertrams J, et al. HLA antigens in ankylosing spondylitis associated with Crohn's disease: increased frequency of the HLA phenotype B27, B44. J Rheumatol. 1988;15:1658–1661.

45. Orchard TR, Thiyagaraja S, Welsh KI, Wordsworth BP, Hill Gston JS, Jewell DP. Clinical phenotype is related to HLA genotype in the peripheral arthropathies of inflammatory bowel disease. Gastroenterology. 2000;118:274–278.

46. Hugot JP, Chamaillard M, Zouali H, et al. Association of NOD2 leucine-rich repeat variants with susceptibility to Crohn's disease. Nature. 2001;411:599–603.

47. Ogura Y, Bonen DK, Inohara N, et al. A frameshift mutation in NOD2 associated with susceptibility to Crohn's disease. Nature. 2001;411:603–606.

48. Hampe J, Cuthbert A, Croucher PJ, et al. Association between insertion mutation in NOD2 gene and Crohn's disease in German and British populations. Lancet. 2001;357:1925–1928.

49. Lesage S, Zouali H, Cezard JP, et al. CARD 15/NOD2 mutational analysis and genotype-phenotype correlation in 612 patients with inflammatory bowel disease. Am J Hum Genet. 2002; 70:845–857.

50. Ahmad T, Armuzzi A, Bunce M, et al. The molecular classification of the clinical manifestations of Crohn's disease. Gastroenterology. 2002;122:854–866.

51. Abreu MT, Taylor KD, Lin YC, et al. Mutations in NOD2 are associated with fibrostenosing disease in patients with Crohn's disease. Gastroenterology. 2002;123:679–688.

52. Miceli-Richard C, Zouali H, Lesage S, et al. CARD 15/NOD2 analyses in spondylarthropathy. Arthritis Rheum. 2002;46:1405–1406.

53. Crane AM, Bradbury L, Van Heel DA, et al. Role of NOD2 variants in spondylarthritis. Arthritis Rheum. 2002;46:1629–1633.

54. Ferreiros-Vidal I, Amarelo J, Barros F, Carracedo A, Gomez-Reino JJ, Gonzalez A. Lack of association of ankylosing spondylitis with the most common NOD2 susceptibility alleles to Crohn's disease. J Rheumatol. 2003;30:102–104.

55. Peeters H, Vander Cruyssen B, Laukens D, et al. Radiologic sacroiliitis, a hallmark of spondylitis is linked with CARD15 gene polymorphisms in patients with Crohn's disease. Ann Rheum Dis. 2004;63:1131–1134.

56. Laukens D, Peeters H, Marichal D, et al. CARD15 gene polymorphisms in patients with spondyloarthropathies identify a specific phenotype previously related to Crohn's disease. Ann Rheum Dis. 2005;64:930–935.

57. Kaufmann HJ, Taubin HL. Nonsteroidal anti-inflammatory drugs activate quiescent inflammatory bowel disease. Ann Intern Med. 1987;107:513–516.

58. Smale S, Natt RS, Orchard TR, Russell AS, Bjarnason I. Inflammatory bowel disease and spondylarthropathy. Arthritis Rheum. 2001;44:2728–2736.

59. Bjarnason I, Hayllar J, MacPherson AJ, Murray FR, McDevitt DG, MacDonald TM. Side effects of nonsteroidal anti-inflammatory drugs on the small and large intestine in humans. Gastroenterology. 1993;104:1832–1847.

60. Rampton DS, McNeil NI, Sarner M. Analgesic ingestion and other factors preceding relapse in ulcerative colitis. Gut. 1983;24:187–189.

61. Evans JM, McMahon AD, Murray FE, McDevitt DG, MacDonald TM. Non-steroidal anti-inflammatory drugs are associated with emergency admission to hospital for colitis due to inflammatory bowel disease. Gut. 1997;40:619–622.

62. Nissila M, Lehtinen K, Leirisalo-Repo M, Luukkainen R, Mutru O, Yli-Kerttula U. Sulfasalazine in the treatment of ankylosing spondylitis. A twenty-six-week, placebo-controlled clinical trial. Arthritis Rheum. 1988;31:1111–1116.

63. Mielants H, Veys EM, Cuvelier C, De Vos M. Course of gut inflammation in spondylarthropathies and therapeutic consequences. Baillieres Clin Rheumatol. 1996;10:147–164.

64. Baron TH, Truss CD, Elson CO. Low-dose oral methotrexate in refractory inflammatory bowel disease. Dig Dis Sci. 1993; 38:1851–1856.

65. Greenberg GR, Feagan BG, Martin F, et al. Oral budesonide for active Crohn's disease. Canadian Inflammatory Bowel Disease Study Group. N Engl J Med. 1994;331:836–841.

66. Bar-Meir S, Chowers Y, Lavy A, et al. Budesonide versus prednisone in the treatment of active Crohn's disease. Gastroenterology. 1998;115:835–840.

67. Kirwan JR, Hällgren R, Mielants H, et al. A randomized placebo controlled 12 week trial of budesonide and prednisolone in rheumatoid arthritis. Ann Rheum Dis. 2004;63:688–695.

68. Willoughby JM, Beckett J, Kumar PJ, Dawson AM. Controlled trial of azathioprine in Crohn's disease. Lancet. 1971;2:944–947.

69. Rhodes J, Bainton D, Beck P, Campbell H. Controlled trial of azathioprine in Crohn's disease. Lancet. 1971;2:1273–1276.

70. Calin A. A placebo controlled cross over study of azathioprine in Reiter's syndrome. Ann Rheum Dis. 1986;45:653–655.

71. Le Quintrec JL, Menkés CJ, Amor B. Severe psoriatic rheumatism. Treatment with azathioprine. Report of 11 cases. Rev Rhum Mal Osteoartic. 1990;57:815–9.

72. Durez P, Horsmans Y. Dramatic response after an intravenous loading dose of azathioprine in one case of severe and refractory ankylosing spondylitis. Rheumatology. 2000;39:182–184.

73. Prajapati DN, Knox JF, Emmons J, Saeian K, Csuka ME, Binion DG. Leflunomide treatment of Crohn's disease patients intolerant to standard immunomodulator therapy. J Clin Gastroenterol. 2003;37:125–128.

74. Haibel H, Rudwaleit M, Braun J, et al. Six months open-label trial of leflunomide in ankylosing spondylitis. Ann Rheum Dis. 2005;64:124–126.

75. van Dullemen HH, van Deventer SJ, Hommes DW, et al. Treatment of Crohn's disease with anti-tumor necrosis factor chimeric monoclonal antibody (cA2). Gastroenterology. 1995; 109:129–135.

76. Targan SR, Hanauer SB, van Deventer SJ, et al. A short-term study of chimeric monoclonal antibody cA2 to tumor necrosis factor alpha for Crohn's disease. Crohn's Disease cA2 Study Group. N Engl J Med. 1997;337:1029–1035.

77. Present DH, Rutgeerts P, Targan S, et al. Infliximab for the treatment of fistulas in patients with Crohn's disease. N Engl J Med. 1999;340:1398–1405.

78. Rutgeerts P, D'Haens G, Targan S, et al. Efficacy and safety of retreatment with anti-tumor necrosis factor antibody (infliximab) to maintain remission in Crohn's disease. Gastroenterology. 1999;117:761–769.

79. Hanauer SB, Feagan BG, Lichtenstein GR, et al. Maintenance infliximab for Crohn's disease: the ACCENT I randomised trial. Lancet. 2002;359:1541–1549.

80. Van Den Bosch F, Kruithof E, De Vos M, De Keyser F, Mielants H. Crohn's disease associated with spondyloarthropathy: effect of TNF-α blockade with infliximab on articular symptoms. Lancet. 2000;356:1821–1822.

81. Van den Bosch F, Kruithof E, Baeten D, De Keyser F, Mielants H, Veys EM. Effects of a loading dose regimen of 3 infusions of chimeric monoclonal antibody to tumour necrosis factor-α (infliximab) in spondyloarthropathy: an open pilot study. Ann Rheum Dis. 2000;59:428–433.

82. Brandt J, Haibel H, Cornely D, et al. Successful treatment of active ankylosing spondylitis with the anti-tumor necrosis

factor—a monoclonal antibody infliximab. Arthritis Rheum. 2000;43:1346–1352.

83. Stone M, Salonen D, Lax M, Payne U, Lapp V, Inman R. Clinical and imaging correlates of response to treatment with infliximab in patients with ankylosing spondylitis. J Rheumatol. 2001; 28:1605–1614.

84. Breban M, Vignon E, Claudepierre P, et al. Efficacy of infliximab in refractory ankylosing spondylitis; results of a six-month open-label study. Rheumatology. 2002;41:1280–1285.

85. Maksymowych W, Jhangri GS, Lambert RG, et al. Infliximab in ankylosing spondylitis: a prospective observational inception cohort analysis of efficacy and safety. J Rheumatol. 2002;29:959–965.

86. Brandt J, Haibel H, Reddig J, Sieper J, Braun J. Successful short term treatment of severe undifferentiated spondyloarthropathy with the anti-tumor necrosis factor—a monoclonal antibody infliximab. J Rheumatol. 2002;29:118–122.

87. Van den Bosch F, Kruithof E, Baeten D, et al. Randomized double-blind comparison of chimeric monoclonal antibody to tumor necrosis factor a (infliximab) versus placebo in active spondylarthropathy. Arthritis Rheum. 2002;46:755–765.

88. Braun J, Brandt J, Listing J, et al. Treatment of active ankylosing spondylitis with infliximab: a randomised controlled multicentre trial. Lancet. 2002;359:1187–1193.

89. Hanauer SB, Lichtenstein GR, Mayer L, et al. Extraintestinal manifestations of Crohn's disease: response to infliximab (Remicade) in the ACCENT I trial through 30 weeks (abstract). Am J Gastroenterol. 2001;96:A26.

90. Generini S, Giacomelli R, Fedi R, et al. Infliximab in spondyloarthropathy associated with Crohn's disease: an open study on the efficacy of inducing and maintaining remission of musculoskeletal and gut manifestations. Ann Rheum Dis. 2004; 63:1664–1669.

91. Gorman JD, Sack KE, Davis JC Jr. Treatment of ankylosing spondylitis by inhibition of tumor necrosis factor α. N Engl J Med. 2002;346:1349–1356.

92. Brandt J, Khariouzov A, Listing J, et al. Six-month results of a double-blind, placebo-controlled trial of etanercept treatment in patients with active ankylosing spondylitis. Arthritis Rheum. 2003;48:1667–1675.

93. Davis JC Jr, Van Der Heijde D, Braun J, et al. Recombinant human tumor necrosis factor receptor (etanercept) for treating ankylosing spondylitis: a randomized, controlled trial. Arthritis Rheum. 2003;48:3230–3236.

94. Sandborn WJ, Hanauer SB, Katz S, et al. Etanercept for active Crohn's disease: a randomised, double-blind placebo-controlled trial. Gastroenterology. 2001;121:1088–1094.

95. Marzo-Ortega H, McGonagle D, O'Connor P, Emery P. Efficacy of etanercept for treatment of Crohn's related spondyloarthritis but not colitis. Ann Rheum Dis. 2003;62:74–76.

96. Van den Brande JM, Braat H, van den Brink GR, et al. Infliximab but not etanercept induces apoptosis in lamina propria lymphocytes from patients with Crohn's disease. Gastroenterology. 2003;124:1774–1785.

97. Sandborn WJ, Hanauer S, Loftus EV Jr, et al. An open-label study of the human anti-TNF monoclonal antibody adalimumab in subjects with prior loss of response or intolerance to infliximab for Crohn's disease. Am J Gastroenterol. 2004;99:1984–1989.

98. Haibel H, Brandt HC, Rudwaleit M, et al. Preliminary results of an open-label, 12-week trial of adalimumab in the treatment of active ankylosing spondylitis (abstract). Ann Rheum Dis. 2004;63(suppl 1):399.

99. Mease P, Gladman D, Ritchlin C, et al. Adalimumab for the treatment of patients with moderately to severely active psoriatic arthritis. Results of a double-blind, randomized, placebo-controlled trial. Arthritis Rheum 2005;52:3279–89.

100. Sandborn WJ, Feagan BG, Hanauer SB, et al. An engineered human antibody to TNF (CDP571) for active Crohn's disease: a randomized double-blind placebo-controlled trial. Gastroenterology. 2001;120:1330–1338.

101. Sandborn WJ, Feagan BG, Radford-Smith G, et al. CDP571, a humanised monoclonal antibody to tumour necrosis factor α, for moderate to severe Crohn's disease: a randomised, double blind, placebo controlled trial. Gut. 2004;53:1485–1493.

102. Schreiber S, Rutgeerts P, Fedorak R, et al. CDP870, a humanized anti-TNF antibody fragment, induces clinical response with remission in patients with active Crohn's disease (abstract). Gastroenterology. 2003;abstract ID 102090.

103. Winter T, Wright J, Ghosh S, et al. Intravenous CDP870, a humanized anti-TNF antibody fragment, in patients with active Crohn's disease-an exploratory study (abstract). Gastroenterology. 2003; Abstract ID 104876.

104. Rutgeerts P, Lemmens L, Van Assche G, et al. Treatment of active Crohn's disease with onercept (recombinant human soluble p55 tumour necrosis factor receptor): results of a randomized, open-label, pilot study. Aliment Pharmacol Ther. 2003;17:185–192.

105. Calabrese L, Fleischer AB. Thalidomide: current and potential clinical applications. Am J Med. 2000;108:487–495.

106. Vasiliauskas EA, Kam LY, Abreu-Martin MT, et al. An open-label pilot study of low-dose thalidomide in chronically active, steroid-dependent Crohn's disease. Gastroenterology. 1999; 117:1278–1287.

107. Ehrenpreis ED, Kane SV, Cohen LB, Cohen RD, Hanauer SB. Thalidomide therapy for patients with refractory Crohn's disease: an open-label trial. Gastroenterology. 1999;117:1271–1277.

108. Breban M, Gombert B, Amor B, Dougados M. Efficacy of thalidomide in the treatment of refractory ankylosing spondylitis. Arthritis Rheum. 1999;42:580–581.

109. Lee L, Lawford R, McNeil HP. The efficacy of thalidomide in severe refractory seronegative spondylarthropathy: comment on the letter by Breban et al. Arthritis Rheum. 2001;44:2456–2457.

110. Breban M, Dougados M. The efficacy of thalidomide in severe refractory seronegative spondylarthropathy: comment on the letter by Breban et al. Reply. Arthritis Rheum. 2001;44:2457–2358.

111. Huang F, Gu J, Zhao W, Zhu J, Zhang J, Yu DT. One-year open-label trial of thalidomide in ankylosing spondylitis. Arthritis Rheum. 2002;47:249–254.

112. Van Deventer SJ, Elson CO, Fedorak RN. Multiple doses of intravenous interleukin 10 in steroid-refractory Crohn's disease. Crohn's Disease Study Group. Gastroenterology. 1997;113:383–389.

113. Schreiber S, Fedorak RN, Nielsen OH, et al. Safety and efficacy of recombinant human interleukin 10 in chronic active Crohn's disease. Crohn's Disease IL-10 Cooperative Study Group. Gastroenterology. 2000;119:1461–1472.

114. Fedorak RN, Gangl A, Elson CO, et al. Recombinant interleukin 10 in the treatment of patients with mild to moderately active Crohn's disease. The Interleukin 10 Inflammatory Bowel Disease Cooperative Study Group. Gastroenterology. 2000;119: 1473–1482.

115. Colombel J, Rutgeerts P, Malchow H, et al. Interleukin 10 (Tenovil) in the prevention of postoperative recurrence of Crohn's disease. Gut. 2001;49:42–46.

116. Sands BE, Winston BD, Salzberg B, et al. Randomized, controlled trial of recombinant human interleukin-11 in patients with active Crohn's disease. Aliment Pharmacol Ther. 2002;16:399–406.

117. Mannon PJ, Fuss IJ, Mayer L, et al. Anti-Interleukin-12 antibody for active Crohn's disease. N Engl J Med. 2004;351:2069–2079.

118. Bernstein CN, Sargent M, Gallatin WM. β2 integrin/ICAM expression in Crohn's disease. Clin Immunol Immunopathol. 1998;86:147–160.

119. Kirman I, Nielsen OH. LFA-1 subunit expression in ulcerative colitis patients. Dig Dis Sci. 1996;41:670–676.

120. Yacyshyn BR, Bowen-Yacyshyn MB, Jewell L, et al. A placebo-controlled trial of ICAM-1 antisense oligonucleotide in the treatment of Crohn's disease. Gastroenterology. 1998;114: 1133–1142.

121. Schreiber S, Nikolaus S, Malchow H, et al. Absence of efficacy of subcutaneous antisense ICAM-1 treatment of chronic active Crohn's disease. Gastroenterology. 2001;120:1339–1346.

122. Yacyshyn BR, Chey WY, Goff J, et al. Double blind, placebo controlled trial of the remission inducing and steroid sparing properties of an ICAM-1 antisense oligodeoxynucleotide, alicaforsen (ISIS 2302), in active steroid dependent Crohn's disease. Gut. 2002;51:30–36.

123. Gordon FH, Lai CW, Hamilton MI, et al. A randomized placebo-controlled trial of a humanized monoclonal antibody to α4 integrin in active Crohn's disease. Gastroenterology. 2001; 121:268–274.

124. Ghosh S, Goldin E, Gordon FH, et al. Natalizumab for active Crohn's disease. N Engl J Med. 2003;348:24–32.

7

Undifferentiated Spondyloarthritis

Henning Zeidler, Jan Brandt, and Sebastian Schnarr

INTRODUCTION

The term *undifferentiated spondyloarthritis* (uSpA) is used to describe manifestations of a spondyloarthritis in patients who do not meet the criteria for any of the well-defined spondyloarthritides. For many reasons uSpA is an essential and very important part of the concept of spondyloarthropathies (SpAs). First of all, a number of epidemiologic, family, and clinical studies described uSpA as the most common or one of the two most common members of the family of SpAs in populations, relatives of patients with ankylosing spondylitis (AS), and the clinical practice of rheumatologists (for review see reference 1). Moreover, the heterogeneity and variability of clinical manifestations and disease course of uSpA raise considerable problems not only for the practitioners of the different medical specialties seen by the patients for their presenting symptoms but also for the rheumatologist because of the difficulties in terminology, classification, and early diagnosis.[2–5] Even if uSpA has been diagnosed, the unpredictable disease course, the disease severity in some patients, and the not uncommon treatment resistance are very challenging for the rheumatologist and other specialists in charge of the management of such conditions. Although an increasing number of original publications deal with uSpA, very few reviews dating back more than a decade and mostly short comments in rheumatologic textbooks are available. The two most extensive chapters devoted entirely to the topic of uSpA date back 15 to 20 years.[6,7] Therefore, in this chapter present knowledge of and future perspectives on uSpA are discussed.

HISTORICAL ASPECTS AND NOMENCLATURE

The existence of patients with signs and symptoms suggestive of AS or SpA, but not fulfilling the classification criteria, was for a long time a common experience in clinical practice but only in the early 1980s was the term *undifferentiated spondyloarthropathy* first used Burns et al. to define the nature and prevalence of manifestations in the first-degree relatives of probands with definite AS and Reiter's syndrome (RS).[8] The original description was published as an abstract and then reported on in more detail in the textbook chapter of Burns and Calin[6] in which they introduced uSpA as a useful addition to the spondylarthropathy nomenclature. The original text is very concise and informative and therefore is cited here:

> Of 599 relatives of 223 consecutively evaluated probands (113 AS and 110 RS) 61 (10 percent) were found to have disease manifestations of a seronegative SpA: 25 AS (41.0 percent), 11 RS (18.0 percent), 5 asymptomatic sacroiliitis (SI) (8.2 percent), and no less than 20 (32.8 percent) with uSpA. The status of the relatives with disease vis-á-vis their diseased probands is outlined in Table 1 [see Table 7.1]. Whereas RS and AS tended to breed true in these family units, relatives with undifferentiated spondyloarthropathy were seen in both groups of probands.
>
> In addition to these 20 first-degree relatives of probands with known AS and RS, an additional 17 patients have been evaluated and diagnosed as uSpA: 14 probands who were initially referred with a working diagnosis of AS, but in whom classic disease by New York criteria was absent, and 3 of their first-degree relatives. These 37 subjects have generally fallen into two categories. The first group are those with symptomatic back pain and a unilateral sacroiliitis on pelvic radiograph. Some of these patients have other enthesopathic features such as asymmetric syndesmophytes, plantar fasciitis, Achilles tendinitis, or heel pain.
>
> The second major group consists of subjects with predominantly peripheral involvement, specifically, (1) dactylitis alone or (2) dactylitis or arthritis in conjunction with one or more of the enthesopathic conditions outlined above.

Historically, the problem of uSpA has well been considered in earlier clinical descriptions and classifications of patients using different terms, such as B27-associated arthritis, HLA-B27–positive oligoarthritis, HLA-B27–related unclassifiable seronegative SpA, persistent yet reversible asymmetric pauciarthritis, seronegative pauciarticular arthritis, syndrome of seronegativity, enthesopathy and arthropathy (SEA syndrome)

TABLE 7.1 DISEASE STATUS OF 61 RELATIVES WITH SPONDYLOARTHRITIS AND THEIR RESPECTIVE PROBANDS

Disease in Relative*	Proband Status	
	AS	RS
AS (25)	18	7 ($P < 0.05$)
RS (11)	0	11 ($P < 0.01$)
AsxSI (5)	1	4 (NS)
uSpA (20)	11	9 (NS)

*Numbers in parentheses indicate the number of relatives with the specific listed. AsxSI, asymptomatic sacroiliitis; uSpA, undifferentiated spondylarthropathy; NS, not significant.
From Burns TM, Calin A. Undifferentiated spondylarthropathy. In: Calin A, ed. Spondylarthropathies. Orlando, FL: Grune & Stratton; 1984:253-264.

in children, late-onset SpA, and finally, the most recent acronym—BASE syndrome (B27, arthritis, sacroiliitis, and extraarticular inflammation).[9–17] The definitions, creation of subgroups, syndromes, and criteria have depended on the particular focus of the investigators' interests, and no consensus definition had emerged before we and others adopted the term *uSpA* and promoted this subset of the wider spectrum of SpAs.[1,17,18–21] Most importantly, the European Spondyloarthropathy Study Group (ESSG) included uSpA in their preliminary criteria for the classification of SpA.[22] From that time on uSpA has been more and more accepted in research and clinical practice as a useful descriptive and working diagnosis in patients with the clinical and radiographic features suggestive of SpA, which do not fulfill the diagnostic criteria for any of the currently established disease categories such as AS, reactive arthritis including RS, psoriatic arthritis (PsA), and the arthritis associated with chronic inflammatory bowel diseases. This definition does not imply a nosologic entity or a uniform syndrome but rather a wide spectrum of disease manifestations, which can be present separately or in various combinations, be intermittent, and have varied expression or severity during a highly variable course of the disease. From a taxonomic point of view uSpA is not a subcategory of the SpA family but is more a provisional diagnosis to differentiate such patients from those with rheumatoid arthritis (RA), connective tissue diseases, and other rheumatic disorders. In this context, *undifferentiated* has several meanings[21]:

1. An early stage of a definite SpA that will later become differentiated into the full clinical picture
2. An abortive form (forme fruste) of a definite SpA not developing into the classical picture of the disease
3. An overlap syndrome that cannot be differentiated into only one definite SpA

4. An unknown, etiologically as-yet-undefined subcategory of SpA that may be differentiated in the future.

Altogether the term *uSpA* refers to the heterogeneity of diseases included and underlines the preliminary state of the classification. Over time the original nomenclature coined by Burns and Calin[6] as *undifferentiated spondyloarthropathy* and referred to by Khan[7] and us[1] with the term *undifferentiated spondyloarthropathies* actually has been modified into *undifferentiated spondyloarthritis* following the European League against Rheumatism (EULAR) proposals for terminology and endorsed by the Assessments in Ankylosing Spondylitis (ASAS) Working Group.[23] Thus, the concept of uSpA now dates back more than 20 years, but the hope of Burns and Calin[6] that these concepts will encourage the following is not outdated:

1. Physicians will feel more comfortable in dealing with patients not characterized by prototypical disease.
2. Patients will not be left in a nondiagnostic limbo and excluded from further study.
3. Investigators can focus on more homogeneous patient populations.
4. Prognosticators will have more complete and relevant subsets on which to base their results.
5. Epidemiologic, etiologic, and therapeutic studies can be directed more precisely to clearly defined entities.

Epidemiology and classification contrast with the high number of epidemiologic studies about AS, only a few studies have been conducted to determine the incidence and prevalence of uSpA. This is because uSpA was not widely recognized as a subset of the SpAs[1] owing to the absence of an internationally accepted definition for uSpA until the 1980s. At that time two sets of criteria were proposed: the Amor criteria based on personal clinical experience[24] and the ESSG criteria based on both clinical and statistical reasoning.[22] Both sets of criteria defined the entire group of patients with SpA with the specific aim of including those with uSpA.

Boyer et al.[25] were some of the first investigators who did a population-based retrospective survey to investigate the prevalence of the whole spectrum of patients with SpAs including uSpA. They used a central database of health records of Alaskan Inupiat Eskimos. Because this Eskimo population has a high prevalence of human leukocyte antigen (HLA)-B27 (25%), a high incidence of SpA was suspected. When the study started, no accepted criteria for uSpA were available, but the criteria used for uSpA were comparable to the Amor and ESSG criteria proposed later. Specifically, Boyer et al. classified patients as having uSpA if they had the presence of objective evidence of inflammation of at least one joint plus at least three of the following features: persistent low back pain and findings consistent with sacroiliitis on examination; asymmetrical joint involvement, predominantly of the lower extremities; sterile knee or ankle effusion characteristic of a nonbacterial inflammation; enthesitis such as plantar fasciitis, Achilles tendinitis, or costochondritis; iritis, conjunctivitis, or uveitis; and a low hemoglobin concentration and an elevated erythrocyte sedimentation rate without evidence of other disease to explain these findings. Among Eskimo men the entire group of SpAs occurred more often than RA and gout. The combined prevalence rate for SpAs in men (1.7%) was more than twice that of RA (0.7%). The prevalence rates of RS (0.6%) and uSpA (0.3%) were high whereas that for AS was surprisingly low (0.1%) (Table 7.2).

In a second study 6 years later the same investigators used the Amor and ESSG criteria for SpAs to define cases.[26] The overall prevalence of SpAs was 2.5%, which was higher than rates observed in the earlier study. One reason might be a more systemic search. Secondly, more women with uSpA or reactive arthritis (ReA) were identified because the subinvestigators had gained acceptance to classify women as having these two diseases. Interestingly, the authors still did not find AS to be a common disorder in this specific population (0.4%).

One of the first studies to determine the overall prevalence of SpA and its subsets among whites was performed in Berlin, Germany[27]; 348 blood donors (50% of whom were HLA-B27 positive) were screened for symptoms of SpA by a mailed questionnaire. A smaller selected group of individuals underwent clinical investigation and had a magnetic resonance imaging (MRI) scan of the sacroiliac joints ($n = 58$). uSpA and AS were classified according to the ESSG and New York criteria. On the basis of a B27 incidence of 9% among the population of Berlin, the estimated prevalence of uSpA was 0.7%, that of AS was 0.9%, and for the whole

group of SpAs was 1.9%.[27] Interestingly, uSpA was the second most common SpA subset.

The higher prevalence of SpAs among Eskimos compared with that in the Berlin population is not surprising, because the B27 molecule is found at a far higher rate in Eskimos than in Western Europeans. However, the reason for the higher percentage of patients with uSpA (and lower percentage of patients with AS) in the Eskimo population compared with that in the Berlin population is not clear. One of the intriguing questions is which and how environmental factors, such as urogenital or enterobacterial infections, influence disease expression,[1] or, from another point of view, which mechanisms protect Eskimos from developing AS. In addition, different methods for ascertaining cases to determine the prevalence of SpAs were used in the Eskimo and Berlin studies. The Eskimo studies were based on the general population that involved unselected individuals, thereby estimating the *true* prevalence, but in a very specific ethnic population with a very high B27 background. The Berlin study used blood donors; thus, it can be argued that participants are not likely to be representative of the general population. They were often selected because of an absence of known disease, and the classic pictures of severe AS might be underrepresented. Thus, estimated prevalence rates might be lower than those being found in the general population. On the other hand, the Berlin study has the advantage of using MRI to potentially detect sacroiliitis earlier then by x-ray films whereby classifying early SpA such as uSpA is more likely.

In another study from Berlin,[28] 170 consecutive patients who presented to the university outpatient clinic with the two leading symptoms of SpAs (inflammatory back pain [IBP] and peripheral asymmetric arthritis of the lower limbs [PALL] were investigated).

TABLE 7.2 INTERNATIONAL COMPARISON OF THE PREVALENCE OF THE WHOLE GROUP OF SPONDYLOARTHRITIDES AND THEIR SUBSETS AS AND uSpA

Race/Country	Method of Ascertaining Patients	Frequency of HLA-B27 in the Population (%)	Prevalence of SpA (%)	Percentage of the Subsets within the SpA Group	
				AS	uSpA
Eskimos[25]	Population survey	25	1.0	10	30
Eskimos[26]	Population survey	25	2.5	15	48
Germany[27]	Blood donor	9	1.9	45	35
Germany[28]	Hospital-based	9	-	30	43
Lebanon[30]	Rheumatological practices	?	8	40	40
Japan[31]	Hospital-based	0.5	0.0095	68	5

Patients underwent clinical examination and pelvic x-ray films if IBP was present. MRI scans of the sacroiliac joints were performed in patients with IBP and indefinite results on sacroiliac x-ray films. Classification was done by using the ESSG criteria for SpAs and the modified New York criteria for AS.

SpA was diagnosed in two-thirds of patients with IBP and PALL. Although one has to recognize that the described cohort presented to a tertiary referral center specializing in inflammatory rather than degenerative rheumatic diseases, this finding supports a high prevalence of SpA found previously on the basis of blood donors as described above. Interestingly, among the SpA subsets, uSpA was classified most often in 43% of the patients followed by AS in 30% (Fig.7.1). Patients with uSpA presented most often with both IBP and PALL (40%), whereas isolated IBP occurred more often in patients with longer disease duration (37%). However, the majority of patients with uSpA and AS in this cohort had a relatively short duration of symptoms with means of 5 and 7 years, respectively. This finding underlines the importance of uSpA because one-third of those may have developed the full picture of AS later in the disease.[29] Moreover MRI scans of the sacroiliac joints were able to detect sacroiliitis in 21 of 32 patients with IBP and unclear x-ray films (66%). Most of them were HLA-B27 positive. That result shows the advantage of MRI technology for detecting sacroiliitis early in B27-positive patients with IBP.

Baddoura et al.[30] performed a study in Lebanon to evaluate the Amor and ESSG criteria. A total of 841 patients presenting to rheumatological practices were classified into the SpA subsets by expert opinion. The ESSG criteria performed somewhat better than the Amor criteria with a sensitivity and a specificity of 91% of 100% versus 77% of 98% in this population that is genetically different from the European population used to develop the criteria. Moreover, the study confirmed the high prevalence of uSpA within the SpA subsets found in the former investigations. AS and uSpA were most common, and both were classified in 40% of the population. Information about the frequency of B27 is not given in this study. Therefore, further explanation for the high prevalence of SpAs in Lebanon is difficult.

One recent study estimated the prevalence of SpA in the Japanese population, known to have a very low frequency of 0.5% for HLA-B27.[31] Surveys were performed in a representative number of rheumatology clinics all over Japan to identify patients with SpA who had presented at a certain time. The prevalence of SpA estimated was rather low (0.0095%); 68.3% of the SpA group were classified as having AS, whereas the frequency of uSpA was 5.4%, much lower than the estimations from the Europe, Lebanon, and Eskimo studies. The investigators postulated that these differences might result from the different genetic and environmental backgrounds and potentially from an insufficient knowledge of SpA classification among the Japanese physicians contributing to the study.

CLINICAL FEATURES

Overall the signs and symptoms of uSpA cover the whole spectrum of the clinical manifestations of sSpAs. Features such as dactylitis, enthesitis, acute anterior uveitis, or mucocutaneous lesions may be the only disease manifestations for an extended period, sometimes in the absence of IBP, sacroiliitis, or peripheral arthritis.

The incidence of different features of uSpA are displayed in Table 7.3. The most important and most common symptom is inflammatory low back pain followed by arthritis and enthesitis. However, the frequencies of these rheumatologic manifestations are highly variable among studies or within cohorts and families. Other features are unilateral or alternating buttock pain, dactylitis, and systemic manifestations such as uveitis, conjunctivitis, mucocutaneous involvement, genitourinary disease, IBD, and cardiac abnormalities.

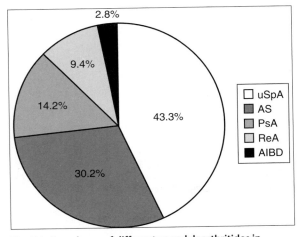

Fig. 7.1 Prevalence of different spondyloarthritides in patients with IBP and peripheral asymmetric arthritis of the lower limbs (*n* =106) presenting to a tertiary referral center classified according to the European Spondyloarthropathy Study Group criteria. AS, ankylosing spondylitis; uSpA, undifferentiated spondyloarthritis; PsA, psoriatic arthritis; ReA, reactive arthritis; AIBD, arthritis associated with inflammatory bowel disease. (From Brandt J, Bollow M, Häberle J, et al. Studying patients with inflammatory back pain and arthritis of the lower limbs clinically and by magnetic resonance imaging: many, but not all patients with sacroiliitis have spondyloarthropathy. Rheumatology (Oxford). 1999;38: 831–836.)

TABLE 7.3 FREQUENCIES OF DIFFERENT SYMPTOMS AND SIGNS IN PATIENTS WITH uSpAS	
Feature	**Percent**
Demographic	
Males	62–88
Mean age at onset (years)	16–23
Clinical	
Low back pain	52–80
Peripheral arthritis	60–100
Polyarthritis	40
Enthesopathy (all)	56
Heel pain	20–28
Mucocutaneous involvement	16
Conjunctivitis/iritis	33
Genitourinary disease	28
Inflammatory bowel disease	4
Cardiac abnormalities	8
Laboratory	
Elevated ESR	19–30
Rheumatoid factor negative	100
HLA-B27 positive	80–84
Radiographic	
Sacroiliitis	16–30
Spinal radiographic changes	20

From Zeidler H, Mau W, Khan MA. Undifferentiated spondyloarthropathies. Rheum Dis Clin North Am. 1992;18:187–202.

Recently, a prospective observational national multi-center study, the German Spondyloarthritis Inception Cohort (GESPIC), was started to better define the frequency of clinical manifestations of SpA in early disease with particular interest for diagnostic purposes.[32] For inclusion in this study patients had to meet either the modified New York or the ESSG classification criteria for AS and for uSpA. Early disease was defined as a maximum duration of symptoms of no longer than 10 years for AS and 5 years for uSpA. Of a total of 311 patients recruited, AS was diagnosed in 190 with a mean duration of 5.8 (+ 2.7) years, and 121 were classified as having uSpA with a mean duration of symptoms of 2.8 (+2.5) years. Most of the patients with uSpA had predominant axial involvement (63%). The frequencies of clinical manifestations at inclusion, at disease onset, and ever for the total population of uSpA and those with predominant axial manifestation (axial uSpA) are given in Figs. 7.2, 7.3, and 7.4, respectively. IBP is by far the most common manifestation at disease onset and during the early disease course, followed by peripheral arthritis and enthesitis equally often in one-third of the patients. Only a small proportion of the patients had dactylitis or uveitis as the initial manifestation or during the disease course. It was concluded from these data that the frequencies of clinical manifestations in early SpA confirm the validity of the estimated frequencies that were used in a recently proposed diagnostic algorithm for preradiographic and early radiographic AS.[33]

Nevertheless, although inflammatory low back pain is the leading clinical feature, the clinician should realize that in early disease, at disease onset, and at inclusion, 31% and 37%, respectively, of the patients had other manifestations associated with SpA. Therefore, in clinical

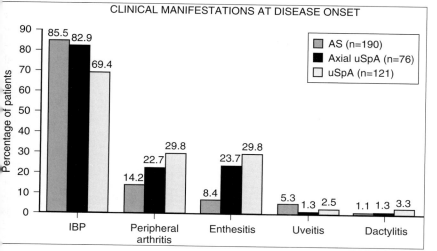

Fig. 7.2 Clinical manifestations at disease onset in AS, uSpA, and uSpA with predominant axial manifestation (axial uSpA). (From Rudwaleit M, Listing J, Märker-Hermann E, et al. Clinical manifestations at disease onset and during the disease course in early spondyloarthritis. Arthritis Rheum. 2004;50(suppl):S617.)

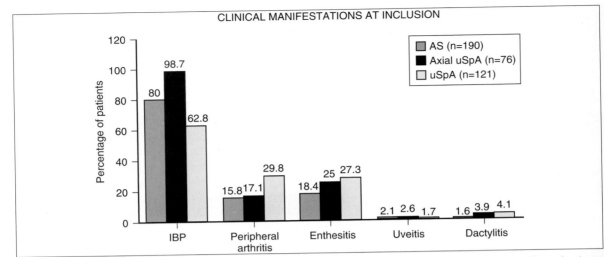

Fig. 7.3 Clinical manifestations at inclusion in the German SpA Cohort Study (GESPIC) in AS, uSpA, and uSpA with predominant axial manifestation (axial uSpA). (From Rudwaleit M, Listing J, Märker-Hermann E, et al. Clinical manifestations at disease onset and during the disease course in early spondyloarthritis. Arthritis Rheum. 2004;50(suppl):S617.)

practice the physician who first sees the patient or the rheumatologist is faced in one-third of the patients with a challenging situation, in that spinal symptoms are not the leading entry criteria for the classification or diagnosis of SpA. To address this issue we review publications in which experiences and data collected from patients with atypical presentations, peripheral arthritis, acute anterior uveitis, lone aortic regurgitation or complete heart block, and juvenile- and late-onset disease and from family studies. Finally, ethnic and geographic differences as well as the relationship

between infections and uSpA will also be reviewed in more detail.

Atypical Clinical Presentation

Sacroiliitis may be asymptomatic, inflammatory low back pain may be absent for a long time, and the disease may evolve over years with atypical, non-inflammatory back pain without significant disability. This finding has been reported in case descriptions,[34,35] but most of the information has been derived from family studies, investigations of patients with anterior

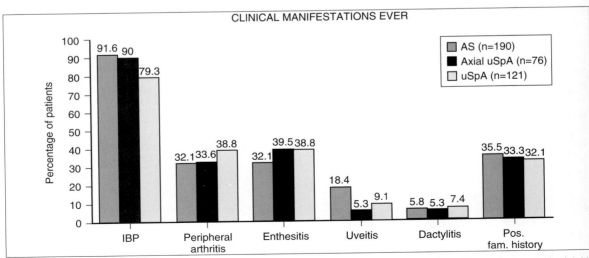

Fig. 7.4 Clinical manifestations ever in AS, uSpA, and uSpA with predominant axial manifestation (axial uSpA). (From Rudwaleit M, Listing J, Märker-Hermann E, et al. Clinical manifestations at disease onset and during the disease course in early spondyloarthritis. Arthritis Rheum. 2004;50(suppl):S617.)

uveitis, and HLA-B27-associated cardiac disease (see later discussion). Three patients reported on by Mader[34] highlight the difficulty in differentiating inflammatory from noninflammatory causes of low back pain in uSpA on clinical grounds alone. One of the patients (a 48-year-old man) denied having significant back pain although he noticed back discomfort and increasing stiffness of the spine and difficulty in performing activities of daily living. The second patient (a 46-year-old man) suffered from occasional back pain of 3 to 4 days' duration over the last few years with exacerbation after physical activity and alleviation by rest. He had no nocturnal pain and morning stiffness of only a few minutes. The third patient (a 46-year-old man) also reported atypical nonirradiating low back pain over many years that was exacerbated by physical activity and alleviated by rest. This pattern of back pain changed into night pain and morning stiffness of 2 hours' duration $1\frac{1}{2}$ years before the diagnosis was made by radiographs of the spine and pelvis showing bilateral sacroiliitis grade 3 to 4 and characteristic syndesmophytes of the lumbar spine.

Peripheral Arthritis

Since recognition of the association between AS and the histocompatibility antigen HLA-B27, numerous investigators have reported that a substantial subgroup of patients formerly classified as having undiagnosed monoarthritis, seronegative peripheral arthritis, or seronegative RA represent the first manifestation of a clinically occult SpA.[9,13,36–47] The peripheral arthritis is mostly monoarticular or oligoarticular, seldom polyarticular, often asymmetric, and mostly affects joints of the lower extremities. Knee, ankle, and wrist are the most frequently involved joints, but any other joint may be affected. When distal arthritis affecting the wrist, ankle, or more distal joints constitutes the main feature, it can be difficult to differentiate uSpA from RA at the beginning of the disease.[44] Moreover, it has been shown that within a group of patients with early seronegative peripheral arthritis of less than 6 months' duration, the clinical manifestations of HLA-B27–associated arthritis are often indistinguishable from those of patients without HLA-B27.[13] A striking prevalence of 83% radiographic sacroiliitis was found in patients who had HLA-B27 compared with 21% in those who did not, despite a paucity of spinal manifestations in both groups.

In one study comparing HLA-B27–positive patients presenting with peripheral arthritis and patients with AS, a significant difference were noted in the distribution of peripheral joint involvement, in the incidence of enthesopathy and uveitis, and in the sex ratio.[41] uSpA was much more commonly seen in women than was AS. The knees, ankles, and small joints were involved more commonly in uSpA, whereas the hip and shoulder joints were involved more commonly in AS. Enthesopathy, predominantly either plantar fasciitis or Achilles tendinitis, was more common in uSpA (54%) than in AS (11%), whereas acute uveitis was much less common in uSpA (2%) than in AS (16%).

Enthesitis

Inflammation at the sites of attachment of a tendon, fascia, ligament, or joint capsule to the bone is a hallmark of SpA.[48] Sometimes peripheral enthesitis may be the main symptom for the patient. Among 150 consecutive patients with SpA, 22% overall and 27% of those with the diagnosis of uSpA had plantar fasciitis and/or Achilles enthesitis.[49] In two series of patients with uSpA, one with juvenile onset and one with late onset, heel enthesitis was the most common peripheral enthesitis followed by enthesitis of the patella, the tibial tubercle, and the base of the fifth metatarsal bone.[50,51] In another series of 476 patients with uSpA followed up for 3 years, peripheral enthesitis was the most common clinical finding in 92%.[52]

Usually enthesitis is seen in conjunction with other clinical features of uSpA, especially peripheral arthritis and dactylitis, but enthesitis may also be the only clinical manifestation for a long time. Long-lasting isolated HLA-B27–associated peripheral enthesitis has been described in adolescents, young and middle-aged adults, and older individuals[51,53,54] at a rate of 9% to 14%. Interestingly, one study from Finland investigating workers in manually strenuous jobs with a history of at least two episodes of humeral epicondylitis showed that 38% of the patients were HLA-B27 positive.[55] Most recently, 33 patients presenting with entheseal pain were studied prospectively, and in 11 of these isolated entheseal SpA was diagnosed with a mean disease duration of 21 months.[56] Among the 11 patients with entheseal SpA, only one was HLA-B27 positive, 8 had more than the 11 tender points needed for a diagnosis of fibromyalgia, 2 experienced inflammatory joint symptoms during the 4 to 6 months of follow-up, and 3 patients had radionuclide scanning and MRI evidence of entheseal inflammation. The feature that best discriminated between entheseal SpA and fibromyalgia was responsiveness to nonsteroidal anti-inflammatory drugs (NSAIDs). How often enthesitis is a single or main manifestation of uSpA has to be investigated further in population-based studies including those using modern imaging techniques such as ultrasonography and MRI.

Uveitis

Uveitis is a prominent feature of different SpAs (see also Chapter 9). Whereas uveitis associated with AS or RS is clinically quite recognizable, uveitis associated with uSpA can be less distinctive in its presentation.[57] In a recent large series of patients with uveitis and HLA-B27–associated uveitis the frequency of uSpA was reported to be 12% to 25% in the whole group of patients in whom SpAs were diagnosed.[57–60] In one study of patients with anterior uveitis referred to an uveitis clinic, undiagnosed uSpA was found in 91% of patients in contrast to other undiagnosed SpAs in 22% to 47% of patients.[57] Acute unilateral anterior uveitis was by far the most common clinical pattern of uveitis. Only one patient with uSpA had bilateral anterior uveitis, and none had panuveitis or chronic anterior uveitis. According to the authors, the patients with uSpA showed a low suspicion of SpA, possibly due to the incomplete clinical spectrum of the disease in these patients; thus, the uveitis episode completed the disease picture and led to the diagnosis of uSpA.[57] Investigators in a recent study who were particularly interested in the prevalence of uSpA in patients with uveitis reported that the rheumatologic manifestations observed in patients with anterior uveitis and uSpA include asymptomatic arthritis and/or IBP, buttock pain, enthesopathy, and a positive family history.[60]

HLA-B27–Associated Cardiac Disease

Some of the SpAs such as AS and RS have long been known to be accompanied by cardiac complications, specifically atrioventricular conduction blocks and lone aortic regurgitation (in contrast with aortic regurgitation combined with a stenotic lesion) (for review see reference 61). During the 1980s, HLA-B27 was found to be an important genetic risk factor for these cardiac conditions, regardless of the presence of the typical extracardiac rheumatic syndromes.[62–68] Subsequently, the concept of *HLA-B27–associated cardiac disease* was developed, supported by immunogenetic, histopathologic, clinical, and electrophysiologic evidence.[61] Both conduction system abnormalities and lone aortic regurgitation have been seen in patients with HLA-B27–related rheumatic and ocular manifestations such as low back pain, peripheral arthralgia/arthritis, conjunctivitis, anterior uveitis, and radiographic sacroiliitis but not fulfilling the criteria for AS or another defined SpAs.[66] Furthermore, an increased frequency of HLA-B27 was found among male, but not female, patients with pacemakers and complete heart block but no evidence of rheumatic disease.[62,69]

Female Sex

Studies performed in Europe, in the United States, and in populations of Alaskan Eskimos demonstrated that uSpA was as common in men as in women or that there was a preponderance of men (male-to-female ratio of 1.8:1) (for review see reference 70), whereas in Northern India females seem to be much less affected by uSpA than males (male-to-female ratio 16:1).[71] The group from India analyzed the profile of uSpA in 25 HLA-B27–positive females compared with that in 38 HLA-B27–positive males with the same disease.[72] Overall the clinical picture in females with uSpA was similar to that in men, albeit with some significant differences. Fewer joints tended to be involved (4.8 versus 7.7), and there was a greater tendency toward asymmetry in females. The mean age at onset was higher at 26 years in females compared with 19 years in males, and the average duration of symptoms before diagnosis was again longer in females (8 years versus 2 years). The authors suggested that the delay in diagnosis in females is due to the presence of a milder form of the disease and/or a low index of suspicion. An alternative explanation is that females may either have less access to or make less use of medical facilities. Genetic and racial differences may also play an important role and should be further investigated in epidemiologic studies comparing the frequency and severity of uSpA in different populations around the world. Interestingly, one report comparing the severity and disease expression of SpA in Alaskan Eskimo men and women showed more women with the diagnosis of uSpA than men.[73] Women with uSpA had evidence suggestive of associated genitourinary or gastrointestinal infection more often than men.

Juvenile- and Late-Onset Disease

Undifferentiated SpA can manifest itself in every age group: infancy, childhood, early adulthood, middle age, and after age 50. In childhood more often than in adults, evidence for well-defined SpAs such as the presence of axial involvement, psoriasis, or other characteristic features, is extremely rare. Most children have a type of uSpA with peripheral arthritis together with enthesitis at onset or the HLA-B27–associated SEA syndrome[15,74] (see also Chapter 8).

Recently, attention has been directed to late-onset uSpA, which is relatively more common than the onset of AS after age 50 (for review see reference 75). In the first study referring to late-onset uSpA, the case histories of 10 HLA-B27–positive men who developed an oligoarthritis together with a large inflammatory pitting edema of the lower extremities after age 50 were reported.[16] They had minimal involvement of the spine, constitutional symptoms, and elevated erythrocyte sedimentation rates (ESRs). Two of the patients presented with bilateral shoulder and hip symptoms mimicking polymyalgia rheumatica. The same pattern of an asymmetrical oligoarthritis of the lower limbs with minimal signs of inflammation at synovial fluid analysis or at synovial biopsy, frequent unilateral edema, marked constitutional signs, and very high ESR was seen in 14 HLA-B27–positive male patients who were hospitalized for seronegative arthritis beginning after age 50.[76]

The largest number of patients with late-onset uSpA was described in a prospective study of consecutive patients collected independently of the modalities of onset and sex.[54] Of 23 patients, only 10 had peripheral arthritis, 3 of whom had ankle or tarsus synovitis together with large inflammatory pitting edema. The spectrum of clinical features is given in Table 7.4, which shows that the clinical spectrum of late-onset uSpA is as broad as it is in other age groups. Inflammatory pitting edema seems to be more common than in younger-onset uSpA but is not always present. In one study the clinical presentation of patients with late-onset SpA (LOSPA) (mean age 65 years) was compared with that of patients with early-onset SpA (EOSPA) (mean age of 27 years).[77] Patients with LOSPA showed a female preponderance and had more cervical and dorsal pain, anterior chest wall involvement, peripheral arthritis, aseptic osteitis, high ESRs, and systemic symptoms such as fever, fatigue, and weight loss. A clear response to NSAID treatment was obtained less often in patients with LOSPA (62%) than in patients with EOSPA (91%).

The diagnosis of late-onset uSpA may be not so difficult in patients who show two or more clinical manifestations of SpA and meet the ESSG or the Amor criteria for SpA. However, one has to consider the possibility that some patients exhibit only one clinical feature for years and that only two-thirds of patients meet the ESSG or Amor criteria for SpA.[54,78] Therefore, sometimes the diagnosis can be difficult and additionally so in elderly patients because they often have several different musculoskeletal problems at the same time. A special aspect of the differential diagnosis is the differentiation from other elderly-onset diseases showing inflammatory swelling with pitting edema of the dorsum of hands or feet, such as the remitting seronegative symmetrical synovitis with pitting edema syndrome, polymyalgia rheumatica, giant cell arteritis, chondrocalcinosis, and others.[75]

Family Studies:

The pivotal study of Burns et al.[8] in first-degree relatives of patients with AS and RS characterized uSpA in families into two groups: 1) predominantly axial involvement with symptomatic back pain and unilateral radiographic sacroiliitis; and 2) predominantly peripheral arthritis, specifically dactylitis alone or dactylitis or arthritis in conjunction with one or more enthesopathic conditions such as asymmetric syndesmophytes, plantar fasciitis, Achilles tendinitis, or heel pain. Additionally, in a report of two independently conducted family studies of HLA-B27–positive probands with AS in the United States and the Netherlands, HLA-B27–positive relatives without radiographic evidence of sacroiliitis who had a history of "chronic inflammatory low back pain" or of "thoracic pain and stiffness" characteristic of SpA were described.[79] From the relative large number of females found with these features of uSpA, it was suggested that women are more likely to manifest this variety of disease.

Other Clinical Features

From systematic investigations using colonoscopy and ileocolonoscopy with biopsies evolved the observation that clinically silent inflammatory gut lesions are present in a large number of patients with uSpA.[80,81] It was concluded that patients with uSpA could be split into three fairly equal subgroups: 1) one subgroup with subclinical inflammatory bowel disease associated with peripheral joint symptoms, 2) one subgroup with a form of enterogenic reactive arthritis, and 3) and one subgroup in which no relationship with the gut could be demonstrated.[80] Two cases of women (one 66 years old and the other 32 years old) with pyoderma gangrenosum and uSpA have been described.[82] Both were HLA-B27 positive and showed the typical clinical features of SpA. One patient developed a self-limiting peripheral arthritis and showed a bilateral grade 2 sacroiliitis. The other woman developed arthritis of the left ankle,

TABLE 7.4 PATTERN OF CLINICAL FEATURES IN LATE-ONSET uSpA	
Age (years)	
At onset	57 (46–72)
At the last examination	62 (48–79)
Sex	11 men; 12 women
HLA-B27	17 positive, 6 negative
Clinical and radiological manifestations	
Only one (n = 4)	2 peripheral arthritis, 2 anterior uveitis
Two (n = 7)	5 enthesitis, 3 peripheral arthritis, 1 dactylitis, 1 inflammatory low back pain, 1 heart involvement, 1 anterior uveitis, 1 osteitis condensans ilii
Three and more (n = 12)	9 inflammatory spinal pain, 9 enthesitis, 7 peripheral arthritis, 6 dactylitis, 3 chest wall pain, 3 pitting edema, 2 buttock pain, 2 anterior uveitis, 9 radiographic sacroiliitis

enthesitis of the heel, the adductor longus, and the levator scapulae muscles, inflammatory low back pain, and a HLA-B27—associated atrioventricular block.

Features of Undifferentiated Spondyloarthropathy Around the World

Reports from patients with SpAs and uSpA in the circumpolar populations, Mexican Mestizos, Asians, and Africans have indicated that ethnic and geographic differences may exist in the prevalence, clinical manifestations, and prognosis of SpAs and uSpA (for review see reference 83). The overall clinical features of uSpA in these populations are similar to those reported in Whites; however, true extraarticular manifestations seem to be less common, e.g., in Thailand extraarticular manifestations have not been observed in uSpA. Interestingly, although many patients with uSpA do not recall any antecedent infection, the increasing number of patients with uSpA recognized in those areas around the world that have a high incidence of bowel infections and infections by arthritogenic bacteria in childhood suggests the possibility that infective agents play a role in initiation and exacerbation of the disease.

Relationship with Infections

Sporadic reports of symptomatic and asymptomatic infections in patients with asymptomatic spondylitis together with data from follow-up studies of patients with ReA and rare coincident cases of AS and ReA suggested a possible relationship between infections and uSpA.[84–91] Therefore, the question was raised whether uSpA may represent a forme fruste of reactive arthritis comparable with undifferentiated oligoarthritis, in which direct or indirect evidence of *Chlamydia, Yersinia,* and *Borrelia* infections were found.[92–96] In a study from India raising this question 64% of the patients with uSpA had elevated immunoglobulin G antibodies to *Salmonella flexneri, Salmonella typhimurium,* or *Chlamydia.*[92] From these data the authors concluded that the patients with uSpA may indeed have ReA in which either the infection was asymptomatic or was too trivial to be remembered by the patient. More recently, the same group of researchers from India reported additional evidence for a potential role of *S. typhimurium* in uSpA by showing positive results for serum antibodies, a peripheral synovial fluid mononuclear cell proliferation assay, and bacterial antigen detection in synovial fluid cells with indirect immunofluorescence.[97] Although all these data are still indirect evidence for a cause-and-effect relationship, future studies searching for bacterial DNA and RNA in the synovial fluid or the synovium may provide the final proof. Interestingly, the most recent investigation from Mexico dealing with this subject reported an association of signs and symptoms of infections with the disease activity of patients with SpAs ($n = 96$) including 32 patients with uSpA.[98] The prevalence of infection, particularly of the gut and upper respiratory tract in AS, was higher in patients with active disease. In uSpA only the prevalence of intestinal infections was higher in those with active disease.

Interestingly, intravesical bacille calmette-guérin, an attenuated live vaccine commonly used as treatment for superficial bladder cancer, also can induce arthritis and in rare HLA-B27–positive individuals may cause clinical findings suggestive of a SpA manifested by dactylitis.[99]

ASSESSMENT OF DISEASE ACTIVITY

Currently no validated instruments exist for the assessment of disease activity in patients with uSpA. In the past such tools were not strongly requested because no studies dealing with uSpA had been performed. In the last several it has become more evident that uSpA is common and is an early form of disease that might develop later into AS.[29] Thus, it becomes obvious that patients with uSpA should be treated, which was done in 270 patients with sulfasalazine (SSZ)[100,101] and in 30 patients with anti-tumor necrosis factor (TNF).[102,106] In these trials the Bath Ankylosing Spondylitis Disease Activity Index (BASDAI), an instrument primarily established for and validated in patients with AS, was used.[107,108] Use of the BASDAI also in patients with uSpA makes sense because the two main and most common symptoms of SpAs, IBP and peripheral arthritis of the lower limbs, are also common in uSpA,[28] and they are a central part of the BASDAI. In the small, open studies that have been performed to investigate the efficacy of the two TNF antagonists, infliximab and etanercept, in patients with uSpA, BASDAI scores showed a reduction of disease activity by more than 50% in most of the patients.[102,106] In the only large, placebo-controlled trial conducted to date, in which 242 patients with uSpA were treated either with SSZ or placebo for 6 months, both groups showed an improvement of disease activity assessed with the BASDAI, but no difference was seen between the groups.[101] Thus, it seems that the BASDAI performed well in patients with uSpA, but further validation is needed.

One disadvantage of the BASDAI is that it is a patient questionnaire and therefore somewhat subjective. Thus more objective measures for the assessment of disease activity such as acute-phase reactants or swollen joint counts and enthesitic regions might be also helpful. For C-reactive protein (CRP) levels and ESRs in uSpA no good data exist to suggest any recommendations.

Swollen joint counts are useful for determining disease activity, but two limitations have to be mentioned: first, the figures for swollen joint counts will be rather small in patients with uSpA because they typically have mono- or oligoarthritis; and second, a relevant proportion might have enthesitis or IBP but no peripheral arthritis.[28] Thus, the swollen joint count indicates only a part of disease activity in some patients.

To assess enthesitis three indices established for AS are available: the Mander Enthesitis Index, the Maastricht Ankylosing Spondylitis Enthesitis Score (MASES), and the Berlin Enthesitis Index.[109–111] The MASES and the index from Berlin are more feasible to use because only 13 and 12 sites, respectively, have to be assessed compared with 30 sites for the Mander Index. It seems to be rational to use one of these indices in uSpA also because the clinical manifestations of enthesitis in uSpA and AS are likely to be similar.

Function is another domain that is influenced by disease activity but also by structural damage. No specific instruments exist to assess function in uSpA. Some investigators have used the Bath Ankylosing Spondylitis Functional Index (BASFI) to measure physical function in uSpA.[112] This index is based on 10 questions about daily functions. Although in patients with AS the restriction in spinal mobility is worse than that in patients with uSpA, the use of the BASFI in the latter might underestimate physical function.

In summary, measures used for AS might be helpful to assess disease activity in patients with uSpA at this time, but as more studies dealing with uSpA are needed in the future, there is also a need for validated instruments for these important group of patients with SpAs.

NATURAL HISTORY

Several years may elapse between the onset of symptoms and the diagnosis of uSpA not only because of the wide range of manifestations, atypical or monosymptomatic presentations, and diversity in severity, but also as a result of the variability of the disease including its self-limited, recurrent, and chronic courses. Moreover, the term *uSpA* is only a working label and provisional diagnosis with the implicit demand for follow-up of each individual patient to establish a final diagnosis or, with a self-limited course, to ascertain remission. Thus, many years may elapse between the classification as uSpA and a definite diagnosis of AS or any other defined SpA. The disease may go into spontaneous remission after a variable time course or evolve over the years with mild clinical manifestations and without significant disability. In contrast, at any point for unknown reasons or sporadically after physical trauma, the clinical manifestations may be aggravated and than evolve

more or less rapidly into the full picture of uSpA.[113,114] A follow-up study of adult patients with unclassified HLA-B27–positive inflammatory diseases first demonstrated that 30% of the patients fulfilled the criteria of AS at reexamination after 28 months[115] (Table 7.5). In further retrospective and prospective studies during the 1980s, the long-term outcome of seronegative oligoarthritis, HLA-B27–associated arthritis, and possible AS was described, and more recently data describing the natural history of patients with the classification of uSpA according to the now widely accepted ESSG criteria became available[29,37,115–122] (Tables 7.5 and 7.6). A significant number of patients with seronegative oligoarthritis, HLA-B27–positive arthritis, and uSpA develop definite AS after variable lengths of follow-up, but the diagnosis may change over time from possible AS into other conditions such as RA, PsA, unclassified arthritis, and degenerative spine disease (Table 7.7).[119] The exact rate of progression into AS is not yet known but could be anywhere between 12% and 68% after 2 years and 11 years, respectively. Alternatively, a proportion of patients have a persistent diagnosis of uSpA over 2 years and even over a decade or longer. Finally, the frequency of natural remissions is also variable, between 10% and 55%, depending on the selection of the patients, different genetic backgrounds, and the time of observation. Although additional follow-up and long-term studies are needed to better establish the natural course of the different patterns of uSpA, most data show a slow progression and relatively benign and indolent character of the disease with mostly good functional status in the long term; e.g., in the report from India 86% of the patients were functionally in class I according to the Steinbrocker classification for RA after a median follow-up of 11 years, and only 14% were in class III.[121] No patient in this study had bamboo spine, but three underwent total hip replacement.

At present, only limited data are available to define the prognosis for and natural history of uSpA in individual patients. Buttock pain and HLA-B27 positivity are weakly associated with progression to a definite SpA.[120] We have shown that one needs an extensive set of criteria (Table 7.8) comprising clinical data (spinal pain, thoracic pain, peripheral arthritis, heel pain, anterior uveitis, and limited motion of cervical or the lumbar spine), elevated ESR, radiologic spinal signs, and HLA-B27 status to predict in patients with possible AS with high discriminatory significance—positive predictive value 76%—the development of AS after 5 and 10 years.[116–119] This set of early diagnostic criteria was more valuable than HLA-B27 determination alone or the criteria without HLA-B27. Furthermore, patients with still-possible AS or uSpA had a higher mean score at the first examination than individuals with other final diagnoses. Nevertheless, more follow-up studies

TABLE 7.5 FOLLOW-UP STUDIES OF HLA-B27–ASSOCIATED ARTHRITIS AND POSSIBLE AS					
Authors	Patients (n)	Follow-up	HLA-B27 Positive	Outcome	Inclusion Criteria
HLA-B27–associated arthritis					
Sany et al., 1980[115]	23	28 months	100%	SpA 30%	Unclassified HLA-B27 inflammatory rheumatic disease
Sambrook et al., 1985[41]	48	5 months–26 years, mean 46 months	100%	SpA 1% Reiter's triad 10% Remission 55%	HLA-B27–positive peripheral arthritis
Blocka and Sibley, 1987[40]	38	25 months	33%	All HLA-B27–positive patients developed SpA or persistent monoarthritis	Chronic monarthritis of undetermined origin
Schattenkirchner and Krüger, 1987[11]	119	2–5 years	100%	SpA 25% Recurrent arthritis 34% Asymptomatic 34%	HLA-B27–positive oligoarthritis
Jänti et al., 2002[122]	47 (from 64)	23 years	37%	63% features of SpA	Seronegative oligoarthritis
Possible AS					
Zeidler et al., 1982[1]	38 (from 86)	4 years	41%	In HLA-B27–positive patients: Radiographic sacroiliitis 62% AS 24% In HLA-B27–negative patients: Radiographic sacroiliitis 28% AS 12%	Possible AS
Zeidler et al., 1985[116]	77 (from 107)	5–6 years	71%	AS 44% Possible AS 38%	Possible AS
Mau et al., 1988[29]	54 (from 88)	10 years	76%	SpA 59% uSpA 19%	Possible AS

TABLE 7.6 FOLLOW-UP STUDIES OF uSpA ACCORDING TO THE ESSG CRITERIA					
Authors	Patients (n)	Follow-up	HLA-B27 Positive	Outcome	Inclusion Criteria
Sampaio-Barros et al., 2001[120]	68	2 years	54%	AS 12% uSpA 75% Remission 13% Psoriatic arthritis 2%	uSpA
Kumar et al., 2001[121]	22 (from 35)	11 years	100%	AS 68% uSpA 18% Remission 10% Psoriatic arthritis 5%	uSpA

TABLE 7.7 DIAGNOSIS OF PATIENTS WITH POSSIBLE AS FOLLOWED OVER 5–6 YEARS AND 10–11 YEARS, RESPECTIVELY

	Phase I (5–6 years)		Phase II (10–11 years)	
	No.	%	No.	%
Definite AS	24	36.5	32	59
Possible AS	28	42.5	10	19
RA	4	6	0	0
Unclassified arthritis	1	1.5	0	0
Psoriatic arthritis	0	0	2	4
Degenerative spine disease	8	12	9	16
Self-limited disease	1	1.5	1	2
Total	66	100	54	100

From Zeidler H, Mau R, Mau W, Freyschmidt J, Majewski A, Deicher H. Evaluation of early diagnostic criteria including HLA-B27 for ankylosing spondylitis in a follow-up study. Z Rheumatol. 1985;44:249–253.

TABLE 7.8 EARLY DIAGNOSTIC CRITERIA FOR AS AND UNDIFFERENTIATED SPONDYLOARTHROPATHIES

	Criteria	Points*
Genetic	HLA-B27 positive	1.5
Clinical	Spinal pain (inflammatory type)	1
	Low back pain, radiating to the buttocks or to the back of the thighs, spontaneously or elicited by stress tests of the sacroiliac joints	1
	Thoracic pain, spontaneous or produced by compression, or limited chest expansion (≥ 2.5 cm)	1
	Peripheral arthritis or heel pain	1
	Anterior uveitis	1
	Limited motion of the cervical or lumbar spine in all planes	1
Laboratory	Elevated ESR: age < 50: male > 15 mm/h, female > 25 mm/h age ≥50: male > 20 mm/h, female > 30 mm/h	1
Radiologic	Spinal signs: syndesmophytes, squaring phenomenon, barrel shaped vertebrae, Romanus or Andersson lesions, involvement of the apophyseal or costotransverse joints	1

Criteria are fulfilled at a total count of ≥3.5 points.
From Zeidler H, Mau R, Mau W, Freyschmidt J, Majewski A, Deicher H. Evaluation of early diagnostic criteria including HLA-B27 for ankylosing spondylitis in a follow-up study. Z Rheumatol. 1985;44:249–253; and Mau W, Zeidler H, Mau R, et al. Evaluation of early diagnostic criteria for ankylosing spondylitis in a 10-year follow-up. Z Rheumatol. 1990;49:82–87.

including new genetic and other markers are needed to elaborate prognostic criteria for remission or chronicity of uSpA.[21,120]

IMAGING

Sacroiliitis is a very common feature of uSpA. Of patients with uSpA, 70% to 80% have IBP, and a high percentage have sacroiliitis.[22,28] However, IBP is not a highly specific indicator of sacroiliitis[27,123]; e.g., in the early and acute stages of sacroiliitis, the diagnosis can be difficult because conventional radiographs may be normal, indicating a need for another valuable imaging technique. The mean time between the first clinical signs of sacroiliitis such as IBP and the development of definite radiologic changes in the sacroiliac joint allowing a diagnosis of AS is between 1 and 9 years.[124] This is one reason that it still takes 7 years before a diagnosis is made in these patients.[125] Rheumatologists should attempt to change this situation because early diagnosis is essential for effective treatment, avoidance of misdiagnosis, and mistreatment.

Magnetic Resonance Imaging

One major item used to differentiate between uSpA and AS beside the clinical picture is a radiograph of the sacroiliac joints. uSpA can only be diagnosed if definite radiologic changes of the sacroiliac joints indicating AS (sacroiliitis equal to or higher than grade 2 bilateral or grade 3 unilateral) by the modified New York criteria[125] have not been established. In patients suspected of having a uSpA, IBP and a radiograph that does not show definite changes of the sacroiliac joint dynamic (gadolinium-enhanced) an MRI scan and the short tau inversion recovery sequence are more sensitive than x-ray films to detect early sacroiliitis.[126,127] Thus, MRI is very helpful for obtaining objective evidence of sacroiliitis in patients without changes on radiographs. An example is shown in Fig. 7.5. Furthermore, the MRI technique, in contrast to radiography, can be used to visualize not only bony changes but also inflammation of the sacroiliac joints or spondylitis and spondylodiscitis.[127] Thus, it is now possible to prove inflammation of the site where IBP is located in patients probably having uSpA who have normal x-ray films. Proven evidence of inflammation by MRI could also be helpful for therapeutic decisions in uSpA. It could be the argument used to recommend infiltration of sacroiliac joints with corticosteroids (which reliably leads to long-term improvement) if sacroiliitis is the major complaint,[128] and a positive MRI result could be an aid in deciding on therapy with the new TNF-blocking agents in selected patients with treatment-refractory uSpA.[103,106,129]

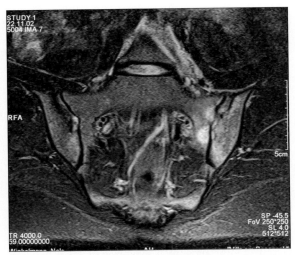

Fig. 7.5 Sacroiliitis detected by MRI in a patient with uSpA without bony changes on the radiograph.

A major general advantage of MRI procedures is the lack of exposure to radiation, which is a recommendation for MRI particularly in young women and children. Disadvantages of MRI are the lack of standardization, the long time necessary to perform the test that not all patients can tolerate, and the high costs.

In summary, MRI is not accepted as a substitute for conventional radiography, but in single patients with mainly early forms of SpAs such as uSpA, it could contribute to the diagnosis.

Scintigraphy

A technique still widely used for imaging of the sacroiliac joints is scintigraphy.[130] Its sensitivity is quite high, but the results are too nonspecific because of the high bone turnover that usually takes place in the region of the sacroiliac joints. An advantage is that inflammation might be detected at different sites of the skeleton. Overall scintigraphy is a useful screening method to detect bony inflammation in uSpA and all other SpAs, but other diagnoses could never be made on the basis of positive scintigram results only.

Ultrasonography

Peripheral enthesitis involvement is a typical manifestation of SpAs, but in some patients it is hard to detect by clinical examination. For the diagnosis of uSpA evidence of enthesitis is one important criterion. In one large study, it was shown that ultrasonography in the B mode combined with power Doppler allowed detection of peripheral enthesitis with abnormal vascularization in all SpA subtypes including uSpA compared with diagnosis in control subjects.[131] However, validation of this technique is necessary to confirm that it might be a potentially useful tool for both the diagnosis and follow-up of SpAs.

TREATMENT AND OUTCOME

Although uSpA is considered to be one of the largest SpA subgroups, there are few data for the treatment of uSpA from clinical trials. Hence, rheumatologists treat patients analogously with patients with AS assuming that uSpA may be a form of early AS. Therefore, the armamentarium of treatments for uSpA is comparable to that for other SpAs and consists of drug therapy, which can be divided into symptomatic pain relief and disease-modifying therapy, physiotherapy, and lifestyle changes.

Spinal Disease

NSAIDs and physiotherapy are the cornerstones of treatment in patients with axial involvement. Intraarticular application of corticosteroids in the sacroiliac joints may be a therapeutic option for patients with NSAID-refractory disease in analogy to treatment for AS.

SSZ is the specific disease-modifying antirheumatic drug (DMARD) that has been evaluated most often for the treatment of SpAs. Recently, the first randomized, controlled study with SSZ in patients with uSpA and early AS (less than 2 years' duration of disease, no syndesmophytes, and no grade 4 sacroiliac changes) was published as an abstract.[101] In this study, 1200 patients received SSZ, and 118 patients received placebo for 6 months. Although the mean BASDAI score dropped significantly until the end of the study, there was no statistical significant difference from the placebo group, except for a subgroup of patients who had only axial involvement without peripheral arthritis. Because the placebo group needed relatively more NSAIDs, the authors concluded that there is a tendency for superior efficacy of SSZ. In summary, the evidence from clinical trials for the treatment of axial inflammation with SSZ in patients with uSpA is weak, and therefore such treatment should be considered only for refractory disease.

The second DMARD occasionally used in SpA is methotrexate (MTX). Until now no results of studies on the treatment of uSpA with MTX have been published, and in AS results from controlled trials with MTX are contradictory.[132–135] Therefore, the use of this drug is still experimental and should be limited to refractory disease. However, a single case report about successful treatment of uSpA coexisting with cutaneous vasculitis showed that MTX therapy might be considered in particular for unusual cases of the disease with organ involvement.[136] With TNF-α being present in sacroiliac joint biopsy specimens from patients with AS who have active sacroiliitis[137] and the dramatic improvement of spinal inflammation in patients with AS with TNF-α-inhibiting therapy,[111,138] this cytokine has been regarded also as a promising target for anti-inflammatory therapy in other spondyloarthritides. Table 7.9 shows an overview of clinical trials with TNF inhibitors in patients with uSpA. So far results for 31 patients with uSpA in six clinical trials have been published. Five of these are open-label trials and the only randomized, placebo-controlled trial deals with a variety of SpA, but includes only 2 patients with uSpA.[102,103,106,139–142]

Infliximab, a chimeric monoclonal antibody, was the first TNF-α inhibitor evaluated in uSpA. Van den Bosch et al.[102,139] treated two patients with uSpA in an open-label trial and another two patients in a randomized, controlled trial together with patients with a variety of other spondyloarthritides. The authors reported that disease activity (according to the BASDAI), patient's and physicians global assessments, pain scores, morning stiffness, and CRP levels significantly improved at week 12. The analysis is not shown for the diagnostic subgroups, but the authors affirm that there were no differences in response among the diagnostic subgroups. At the 1-year follow-up of the open-label trial, 1 patient had to increase the infliximab dosing regimen because of a partial lack of efficacy.[140] Brand et al.[103] were the first to compare a reduced dosage of 3 mg/kg with the standard dose used in AS (5 mg/kg) in 6 patients with uSpA. Although they found a significant treatment response in all patients, the higher dosage was more effective. Recently, Schnarr et al.[141] performed an open label trial with 10 patients with uSpA receiving 5mg/kg of infliximab in weeks 0, 2, and 6. Of the 10 patients,

9 had a history of insufficient treatment with DMARDs. After 12 weeks 8 patients showed reduced pain scores. BASDAI scores for 7 patients improved but only 3 patients achieved an ASAS 20% response rate (ASAS20). Initially elevated ESRs and CRP levels decreased in 5 of 6 and 6 of 7 patients, respectively. Although these data suggest that TNF-α inhibition with infliximab is effective in the treatment of patients with uSpA for 12 weeks, the response rate of uSpA to TNF inhibition in this study is lower than that in other studies. This finding may be due to the mean disease duration of 10 years in which chronic pain disorder might play a significant role in addition to inflammation.

Results from two open-label trials with a total of 11 patients with uSpA in which the TNFp75/Fc-fusion protein etanercept was used are available. Marzo-Ortega et al.[142] published an open study of 10 patients with different SpA subtypes; only 1 of these patients had uSpA. Interestingly, the authors pointed out that the patient with uSpA and a disease duration of 8 months remained in clinical remission more than 9 months after stopping etanercept, which could be an indication for the great potential of TNF-α inhibition, especially in early disease. Brandt et al.[106] treated 10 patients with uSpA with etanercept (25 mg subcutaneously twice weekly) for 3 months followed by a 3-month nontreatment observation period. Of the patients, 60 percent achieved 50 percent improvement in BASDAI scores and the mean BASDAI score at a baseline of 6.1 dropped significantly to 3.5 at week 12. Function, spinal pain, peripheral arthritis, enthesitis, quality of life, and acute-phase reactants improved similarly. After cessation of anti-TNF therapy, 4 of 8 patients had a relapse after

			No. of		
Author	TNF Inhibitor and Dosage	No. of Study Patients	Patients with uSpA	Study Design	Duration
van den Bosch et al., 2000[102]	Infliximab, 5 mg/kg, weeks 0, 2, 6	21	2	Open label	12 weeks*
Brandt et al., 2002[103]	Infliximab, 3 mg/kg vs. 5 mg/kg, weeks 0, 2, 6	6	6	Open label	12 weeks
van den Bosch et al., 2002[139]	Infliximab, 5 mg/kg, weeks 0, 2, 6	40	2	Randomized, controlled trial	12 weeks
Schnarr et al., 2004 (abstract)[141]	Infliximab, 5 mg/kg, weeks 0, 2, 6	10	10	Open label	12 weeks
Marzo-Ortega et al., 2001[142]	Etanercept, 25 mg twice per week	10	1	Open label	6 months
Brandt et al., 2004[106]	Etanercept, 25 mg twice per week	10	10	Open label	12 weeks†

*Kruithof et al., 2002, 1 year follow-up data.
†Followed by a 12-week treatment-free observation period.

TABLE 7.9 CLINICAL TRIALS WITH TNF INHIBITORS IN uSpA

an average of 4.5 weeks. Disease in 2 patients went into long-standing remission.

In summary, the small number of patients with uSpA treated with either infliximab or etanercept provides partial evidence that TNF-α inhibition is effective in controlling spinal inflammation, although no statement about long-term efficacy can be made from these data. Large, placebo-controlled trials with long-term follow up of patients are needed to investigate whether inhibition of proinflammatory cytokines will maintain the structural integrity of joints and spine and prevent progression to AS. Because TNF inhibition is an expensive therapy, it will be a future challenge to identify uSpA subgroups at high risk for functional disability in which early TNF inhibition may be cost-effective.

Anakinra, thalidomide, pamidronate, and radium-224 chloride are other therapeutic options that have been investigated in AS but not in uSpA so use of these drugs should only be considered in patients with refractory disease.

Arthritis and Enthesitis

Enthesitis and asymmetric oligoarthritis are characteristic features of all spondyloarthritides. Standard therapy consists of NSAIDs and physiotherapy. In addition, orthoses are helpful in some patients with enthesitis (e.g., epicondylitis). In refractory disease intraarticular injection and entheseal infiltration with corticosteroids are indicated.[48] As in spinal disease results from clinical trials about the efficacy of SSZ in enthesitis and peripheral arthritis are contradictory.[143-146] The most recent placebo-controlled trial of SSZ in 242 patients with uSpA and early AS did not demonstrate efficacy of SSZ in peripheral arthritis within 6 months.[101] Therefore, the use of SSZ should be reserved for patients with refractory disease that did not adequately respond to NSAIDs and corticosteroid injections.

TNF-α inhibitors are the drugs that unequivocally have the strongest impact on enthesitis and arthritis in patients with SpA.[102,103,106,139-142] All published TNF inhibitor trials ascertain that infliximab and etanercept are equally effective in spinal, entheseal, and peripheral joint inflammation. Because TNF inhibition is an expensive treatment and is accompanied by a higher risk of infection, it should be reserved for patients with severe inflammatory and multilocalized disease that is refractory to standard therapy.

REFERENCES

1. Zeidler H, Mau W, Khan MA. Undifferentiated spondyloarthropathies. Rheum Dis Clin North Am. 1992;18:187–202.
2. Schumacher HR, Bardin T. The spondylarthropathies: classification and diagnosis. Do we need new terminologies? Balliéres Clin Rheumatol. 1998;12:551–565.
3. Berthelot JM, Klarlund M, McGonagle D, et al. Lessons from an international survey of paper cases of 10 real patients from an early arthritis clinic. CRI (Club Rhumatismes et Inflammation) Group. J Rheumatol. 2001;28:975–981.
4. Berthelot JM, Bernelot-Moens HJ, Klarlund M, et al. Differences in understanding and application of 1987 ACR criteria for rheumatoid arthritis and 1991 ESSG criteria for spondylarthropathy. A pilot survey. Clin Exp Rheumatol. 2002;20:145–150.
5. Berthelot JM, Saraux A, Le Henaff C, et al. Confidence in the diagnosis of early spondylarthropathy: a prospective follow-up of 270 early arthritis patients. Clin Exp Rheumatol. 2002;20: 319–326.
6. Burns TM, Calin A. Undifferentiated spondylarthropathy. In: Calin A, ed. Spondylarthropathies. Orlando, FL: Grune & Stratton; 1984:253–264.
7. Khan MA, van der Linden SM. Undifferentiated spondyloarthropathies. In: Khan MA, ed. Ankylosing Spondylitis and Related Spondyloarthropathies. Philadelphia, Pa: Hanley & Belfus; 1990:657–664.
8. Burns T, Marder A, Becks E, et al. Undifferentiated spondylarthritis: a nosological missing link? Arthritis Rheum. 1982; 25 (suppl):142.
9. Nasrallah NS, Masi AT, Chandler RW, Feigenbaum SL, Kaplan SB. HLA-B27 antigen and rheumatoid factor negative (seronegative) peripheral arthritis. Studies in younger patients with early diagnosed arthritis. Am J Med. 1977;63:379–386.
10. Genth E, Peuckert H, Brude E, Hehl M, Hartl W. HLA-B27 positive oligoarthritis. Z Rheumatol. 1978;37:313–328.
11. Schattenkirchner M, Krüger K. Natural course and prognosis of HLA-B27-positive oligoarthritis. Clin Rheumatol 1987;6 (suppl 2): 83–86.
12. Prakash S, Mehra NK, Bhargva S, Malaviya AN. HLA-B27 related 'unclassifiable' seronegative spondyloarthropathies. Ann Rheum Dis. 1983;42:640–643.
13. Bitter T, Jeannet M, de Haller E, Lejeune M. Persistent yet reversible asymmetric pauciarthritis (PRAP): a B27-associated cluster. Ann Rheum Dis. 1979;38(suppl):84–91.
14. Eastmond CJ, Rajah SM, Tovey D, Wright V. Seronegative pauciarticular arthritis and HLA-B27. Ann Rheum Dis. 1980;39:231–234.
15. Rosenberg AM, Petty RE. A syndrome of seronegative enthesopathy and arthropathy in children. Arthritis Rheum. 1982; 25:1041–1047.
16. Dubost JJ, Sauvezie B. Late onset peripheral spondyloarthropathy. J Rheumatol. 1989;16:1214–1217.
17. Thomson GTD, Inman RD. Diagnostic conundra in the spondyloarthropathies: towards a base for revised nosology. J Rheumatol. 1990;17:426–429.
18. Khan MA, van der Linden SM. A wider spectrum of spondyloarthropathies. Semin Arthritis Rheum. 1990;20:107–113.
19. Khan MA, van der Linden SM. Ankylosing spondylitis and other spondyloarthropathies. Rheum Dis Clin North Am. 1990;16: 551–579.
20. Zeidler H. Undifferentiated arthritis and spondylarthropathy as a major problem of diagnosis and classification. Scand J Rheumatol. 1987;65(suppl):54–62.
21. Zeidler H, Werdier D, Klauder A, et al. Undifferentiated arthritis and spondylarthropathy as a challenge for prospective studies. Clin Rheumatol. 1987;6(suppl):112–120.
22. Dougados M, van der Linden S, Juhlin R, et al. The European Spondylarthropathy Study Group preliminary criteria for the classification of spondylarthropathy. Arthritis Rheum. 1991;34:1218–1227.
23. Francois RJ, Eulderink F, Bywaters EG. Commented glossary for rheumatic spinal diseases, based on pathology. Ann Rheum Dis. 1995;54:615–625.
24. Amor B, Dougados M, Mijiyawa M. Criteria of the classification of spondylarthropathies. Rev Rhum Mal Osteoartic. 1990;57:85–89.

25. Boyer GS, Lanier AP, Templin DW. Prevalence rates of spondyloarthropathies, rheumatoid arthritis, and other rheumatic disorders in an Alaskan Inupiat Eskimo population. J Rheumatol. 1988;15:678–683.

26. Boyer GS, Templin DW, Cornoni-Huntley JC, et al. Prevalence of spondyloarthropathies in Alaskan Eskimos. J Rheumatol. 1994; 21:2292–2297.

27. Braun J, Bollow M, Remlinger G, et al. Prevalence of spondylarthropathies in HLA B27-positive and -negative blood donors. Arthritis Rheum. 1998;41:58–67.

28. Brandt J, Bollow M, Häberle J, et al. Studying patients with inflammatory back pain and arthritis of the lower limbs clinically and by magnetic resonance imaging: many, but not all patients with sacroiliitis have spondyloarthropathy. Rheumatology (Oxford). 1999;38:831–836.

29. Mau W, Zeidler H, Mau R, et al. Clinical features and prognosis of patients with possible ankylosing spondylitis. Results of a 10-year followup. J Rheumatol. 1988;15:1109–1114.

30. Baddoura R, Awada H, Okais J, Habis T, Attoui S, Abi Saab M. Validation of the European Spondylarthropathy Study Group and B. Amor criteria for spondyloarthropathies in Lebanon. Rev Rhum Engl Ed. 1997;64:459–464.

31. Hukuda S, Minami M, Saito T, et al. Spondyloarthropathies in Japan: nationwide questionnaire survey performed by the Japan Ankylosing Spondylitis Society. J Rheumatol. 2001; 28:554–559.

32. Rudwaleit M, Listing J, Märker-Hermann E, et al. Clinical manifestations at disease onset and during the disease course in early spondyloarthritis. Arthritis Rheum. 2004;50(suppl):S617.

33. Rudwaleit M, van der Heijde D, Khan MA, Braun J, Sieper J. How to diagnose axial spondyloarthritis early. Ann Rheum Dis. 2004;63:535–543.

34. Mader R. Atypical clinical presentation of ankylosing spondylitis. Semin Arthritis Rheum. 1999;29:191–196.

35. Ferdoutsis M, Bouros D, Meletis G, Patsourakis G, Siafakas NM. Diffuse interstitial lung disease as an early manifestation of ankylosing spondylitis. Respiration. 1995;62:286–289.

36. Arnett FC. Incomplete Reiter's syndrome: clinical comparisons with classical triad. Ann Rheum Dis. 1979;38(suppl 1):73–78.

37. Zeidler H, Wagener P, Eckert G, et al. HLA-B27 in possible ankylosing spondylitis with peripheral arthritis. Rheumatol Int. 1982;2:35–40.

38. Kaarela K, Titinen S, Luukkainen R. Long-term prognosis of monoarthritis, a follow-up study. Scand J Rheumatol. 1983; 12:374–376.

39. Nissilä M, Isomäki H, Kaarela K, Kiviniemi P, Martio J, Sarna S. Prognosis of inflammatory joint disease: a three-year follow-up study. Scand J Rheumatol. 1983;12:33–38.

40. Blocka KLN, Sibley JT. Undiagnosed chronic monoarthritis: clinical and evolutionary profile. Arthritis Rheum. 1987;30:1357–1361.

41. Sambrook P, McGuigan L, Champion D, Edmonds J, Fleming A, Portek I. Clinical features and follow-up study of HLA-B27 positive patients presenting with peripheral arthritis. J Rheumatol. 1985;12:526–528.

42. Hülsemann JL, Zeidler H. Undifferentiated arthritis in an early synovitis out-patient clinic. Clin Exp Rheumatol. 1995;13:37–43.

43. Kvien TK, Glennas A, Melby K. Prediction of diagnosis in acute and subacute oligoarthritis of unknown origin. Br J Rheumatol. 1996;35:359–363.

44. de Saint Pierre V, Saraux A, Lamour A, et al. Spondylarthropathy with distal joint involvement. Scand J Rheumatol. 1996;25: 331–333.

45. Saraux A, Guedes C, Allain J, et al. Valeur diagnostique du phénotype HLA dans les rhumatismes inflammatoires. Press Med. 1997;26:1040–1044.

46. El-Gabalawy HS, Goldbach-Mansky R, Smith D 2nd, et al. Association of HLA alleles and clinical features in patients with synovitis of recent onset. Arthritis Rheum. 1999;42:1696–1705.

47. Inaoui R, Bertin P, Preux PM, Treves R. Outcome of patients with undifferentiated chronic monoarthritis: retrospective study of 46 cases. Joint Bone Spine. 2004;71:209–213.

48. Olivieri I, Barozzi L, Padula A. Enthesiopathy: clinical manifestations, imaging and treatment. BailliÈres Clin Rheumatol. 1998;12:665–681.

49. Gerster JC. Plantar fasciitis and Achilles tendinitis among 150 cases of seronegative spondarthritis. Rheumatol Rehabil. 1980;19:218–222.

50. Olivieri I, Foto M, Ruju GP, Gemignani G, Giustarini S, Pasero G. Low frequency of axial involvement in Caucasian pediatric patients with seronegative enthesopathy and arthropathy syndrome after 5 years of disease. J Rheumatol. 1992;19:469–475.

51. Olivieri I, Padula A, Pierro A, Favaro L, Oranges GS, Ferri S. Late onset undifferentiated seronegative spondyloarthropathy. J Rheumatol. 1995;22:899–903.

52. Rezaian MM, Brent LH. Undifferentiated spondyloarthropathy: three year follow-up study of 476 patients. Arthritis Rheum. 1997;40 (suppl):S227.

53. Olivieri I, Gemignani G, Gherardi S, Grassi L, Ciompi ML. Isolated HLA-B27 Achilles tendinitis. Ann Rheum Dis. 1987;46:626–627.

54. Olivieri I, Pasero G. Longstanding isolated juvenile onset HLA-B27 associated peripheral enthesitis. J Rheumatol. 1987;46: 164–165.

55. Malmivaara A, Viikari-Juntura E, Huuskonen M, et al. Rheumatoid factor and HLA antigens in wrist tenosynovitis and humeral epicondylitis. Scand J Rheumatol. 1995;24:154–156.

56. Godfrin B, Zabraniecki L, Lamboley V, Bertrand-Latour F, Sans N, Fournie B. Spondyloarthropathy with entheseal pain. A prospective study in 33 patients. Joint Bone Spine. 2004;71:557–562.

57. Pato E, Banares A, Jover JA, et al. Undiagnosed spondyloarthropathy in patients presenting with anterior uveitis. J Rheumatol. 2000;27:2198–2202.

58. Tay-Kearney ML, Schwam BL, Lowder C, et al. Clinical features and associated systemic diseases of HLA-B27 uveitis. Am J Ophthalmol. 1996;121:47–56.

59. Monnet D, Breban M, Hudry C, Dougados M, Brezin AP. Ophthalmic findings and frequency of extraocular manifestations in patients with HLA-B27 uveitis. Ophthalmology. 2004;111:802–809.

60. Linder R, Hoffmann A, Brunner R. Prevalence of the spondyloarthritides in patients with uveitis. J Rheumatol. 2004;31: 2226–2229.

61. Bergfeldt L. HLA-B27-associated cardiac disease. Ann Intern Med. 1997;127:621–629.

62. Bergfeldt L. HLA-B27-associated rheumatic diseases with severe cardiac bradyarrhythmias. Clinical features and prevalence in 223 men with permanent pacemakers. Am J Med. 1983;75: 210–215.

63. Bergfeldt L, Möller E. Complete heart block—another HLA-B27 associated disease manifestation. Tissue Antigens. 1983;21:385–390.

64. Bergfeldt L, Edhag O, Rajs J. HLA-B27-associated heart disease. Clinicopathologic study of three cases. Am J Med. 1984;77: 961–967.

65. Qaiyumi S, Hassan ZU, Toone E. Seronegative spondyloarthropathies in lone aortic insufficiency. Arch Intern Med. 1985;145:822–824.

66. Bergfeldt L, Insulander P, Lindblom D, Moller E, Edhag O. HLA-B27: an important genetic risk factor for lone aortic regurgitation and severe conduction system abnormalities. Am J Med. 1988;85:12–18.

67. Sahi SP, Winfield CR. Third-degree heart block developing in an HLA-B27-positive individual with a family history of ankylosing spondylitis. Br J Clin Pract. 1990;44:794–195.

68. Peeters AJ, ten Wolde S, Sedney MI, de Vries RR, Dijkmans BA. Heart conduction disturbance: an HLA-B27 associated disease. Ann Rheum Dis. 1991;50:348–350.

69. Bergfeldt L, Möller E. Pacemaker treated women with heart block have no increase in the frequency of HLA-B27 and associated rheumatic disorders in contrast to men—a sex-linked difference in disease susceptibility. J Rheumatol. 1986:13:941–943.

70. Olivieri I. Undifferentiated seronegative spondyloarthropathy in females. Br J Rheumatol. 1996;35:395–398.

71. Malaviya AN, Mehra NK. Spondyloarthropathies in India. In: Khan MA, ed. Ankylosing Spondylitis and Related Spondyloarthropathies. Spine: State of the Art Reviews. Philadelphia, Pa: Hanley & Belfus, 1990:679–684.

72. Uppal SS, Pande I, Singh G, et al. Profile of HLA-B27 related 'unclassifiable' spondyloarthropathy in females and its comparison with the profile in males. Br J Rheumatol. 1995;34:137–140.

73. Boyer GS, Templin DW, Bowler A, et al. Spondyloarthropathy in the community: differences in severity and disease expression in Alaskan Eskimo men and women. J Rheumatol. 2000;27: 170–176.

74. Prieur A-M. Spondyloarthropathies in childhood. Balliéres Clin Rheumatol. 1998;12:287–307.

75. Olivieri I, Salvarani C, Cantini F, Ciancio G, Padula A. Ankylosing spondylitis and undifferentiated spondyloarthropathies: a clinical review and description of a disease subset with older age at onset. Curr Opin Rheumatol. 2001;13:280–284.

76. Dubost JJ, Ristori JM, Zmantar C, Sauvezie B. Rhumatismes séronégatifs a début tardif: fréquence et atypies des spondylarthropathies. Rev Rhum Mal Osteoartic. 1991;58:577–584.

77. Caplanne D, Tubach F, Le Parc JM. Late onset spondylarthropathy: clinical and biologic comparison with early onset patients. Ann Rheum Dis. 1997;56:176–179.

78. Olivieri I, Oranges GS, Sconosciuto F, Padula A, Ruju GP, Pasero G. Late onset peripheral seronegative spondyloarthropathy: report of two additional cases. J Rheumatol. 1993;20:390–393.

79. Khan MA, van der Linden SM, Kushner I, Valkenburg HA, Cats A. Spondylitic disease without radiologic evidence of sacroiliitis in relatives of HLA-B27 positive ankylosing spondylitis patients. Arthritis Rheum. 1985;28:40–43.

80. Mielants H, Veys EM, Cuvelier C, De Vos M. Subclinical involvement of the gut in undifferentiated spondylarthropathies. Clin Exp Rheumatol. 1989;7:499–504.

81. Altomonte L, Zoli A, Veneziani A, et al. Clinically silent inflammatory gut lesions in undifferentiated spondyloarthropathies. Clin Rheumatol. 1994;13:565–570.

82. Olivieri I, Costa AM, Cantini F, Niccoli L, Marini R, Ferri S. Pyoderma gangrenosum in association with undifferentiated seronegative spondylarthropathy. Arthritis Rheum. 1996;39:1062–1065.

83. Lau CS, Burgos-Vargas R, Louthrenoo W, Mok MY, Wordsworth P, Zeng QY. Features of spondyloarthritis around the world. Rheum Dis Clin North Am. 1998;24:753–770.

84. Rynes RI, Volastro PS, Bartholomew LE. Exacerbation of B27 positive spondyloarthropathy by enteric infections. J Rheumatol. 1984;11:96–97.

85. Golding DN, Robertson MH. Reactive arthritis due to Salmonella schwarzengrund in a patient with asymptomatic spondylitis. Br J Rheumatol. 1985;24:194–196.

86. Paul IR, Mitchell ES, Bell AL. Salmonella reactive arthritis in established ankylosing spondylitis. Ulster Med J 1988;57:215–217.

87. Leirisalo-Repo M, Suoranta H. Ten-year follow-up study of patients with Yersinia arthritis. Arthritis Rheum. 1988;31:533–537.

88. Herrero-Beaumont G, Elswood J, Will R, Armas JB, Calin A. Postsalmonella reactive phenomena in 2 patients with ankylosing spondylitis: no modification of the underlying disease. J Rheumatol. 1990;17:250–251.

89. Gran JT, Paulsen AQ, Gaskjenn H, Schulz T. Reactive arthritis of the cervical spine due to Yersinia enterocolitica in a patient with pre-existing ankylosing spondylitis. Scand J Rheumatol. 1992;21:95–96.

90. Yli-Kerttula T, Tertti R, Toivanen A. Ten-year follow-up study of patients from a Yersinia pseudotuberculosis III outbreak. Clin Exp Rheumatol. 1995;13:333–337.

91. Speed CA, Haslock I. Coincident seronegative spondarthritis: a case report. Clin Rheumatol. 1996;15:301–302.

92. Aggarwal A, Misra R, Chandrasekhar S, Prasad KN, Dayal R, Ayyagari A. Is undifferentiated seronegative spondyloarthropathy a forme fruste of reactive arthritis? Br J Rheumatol. 1997;36:1001–1004.

93. Bas S, Griffais R, Kvien TK, Glennas A, Melby K, Vischer TL. Amplification of plasmid and chromosomal chlamydial DNA on synovial fluid of patients with reactive arthritis and undifferentiated seronegative oligoarthritis. Arthritis Rheum. 1995;38:1005–1013.

94. Erlacher L, Wintersberger W, Menschik M, et al. Reactive arthritis: urogenital swab culture is the only useful method for the detection of the arthritogenic infection in extra-articularly asymptomatic patients with undifferentiated oligoarthritis. Br J Rheumatol. 1995;34:838–842.

95. Sieper J, Braun J, Brandt J, et al. Pathogenetic role of Chlamydia, Yersinia and Borrelia in undifferentiated oligoarthritis. J Rheumatol. 1992;19:1236–1242.

96. Schnarr S, Putschky N, Jendro MC, et al. Chlamydia and Borrelia DNA in synovial fluid of patients with early undifferentiated oligoarthritis: results of a prospective study. Arthritis Rheum. 2001;44:2679–2685.

97. Sinha R, Aggarwal A, Prasad K, Misra R. Sporadic enteric reactive arthritis and undifferentiated spondyloarthropathy: evidence for involvement of Salmonella typhimurium. J Rheumatol. 2003;30:105–113.

98. Martinez A, Pacheco-Tena C, Vazquez-Mellado J, Burgos-Vargas R. Relationship between disease activity and infection in patients with spondyloarthropathies. Ann Rheum Dis. 2004; 63:1338–1340.

99. Schwartzenberg JM, Smith DD, Lindsley HB. Bacillus Calmette-Guérin associated arthropathy mimicking undifferentiated spondyloarthropathy. J Rheumatol. 1999;26:933–935.

100. Brandt J, Buss B, Sieper J, et al. Treatment with sulfasalazine vs azathioprine of ankylosing spondylitis patients with a disease duration <10 years. Arthritis Rheum. 2000;suppl 43:S218.

101. Braun J, Alten R, Burmester G, et al. Efficacy of sulfasalazine in undifferentiated spondyloarthritis and early ankylosing spondylitis: a multicenter randomized controlled trial. Arthritis Rheum. 2004;50:4100 (late-breaking abstract).

102. Van den Bosch F, Kruithof E, Baeten D, De Keyser R, Mielants H, Veys EM. Effects of a loading dose regimen of three infusions of chimeric monoclonal antibody to tumour necrosis factor alpha (infliximab) in spondyloarthropathy: an open pilot study. Ann Rheum Dis. 2000;59:428–433.

103. Brandt J, Haibel H, Sieper J, Braun J. Successful treatment of patients with severe undifferentiated spondyloarthropathy with the anti-TNFα antibody infliximab. J Rheumatol. 2002; 29:118–122.

104. Collantes-Estevez E, Munoz-Villanueva MC, Canete-Crespillo JD, et al. Infliximab in refractory spondyloarthropathies: a multicentre 38 week open study. Ann Rheum Dis. 2003;62:1239–1240.

105. Marzo-Ortega H, McGonagle D, O'Connor P, Emery P. Efficacy of etanercept for treatment of Crohn's related spondyloarthritis but not colitis. Ann Rheum Dis. 2003;62:74–76.

106. Brandt J, Khariouzov A, Listing J, et al. Successful short term treatment of patients with severe undifferentiated spondyloarthritis with the anti-tumor necrosis factor-alpha fusion receptor protein etanercept. J Rheumatol. 2004;31:531–538.

107. Garrett S, Jenkinson TR, Kennedy LG, Whitelock H, Gaisford P, Calin A. A new approach to defining disease status in ankylosing spondylitis. The Bath Ankylosing Spondylitis Disease Activity Index. J Rheumatol. 1994;21:2286–2291.

108. Calin A, Nakache J-P, Gueguen A, Zeidler H, Mielants H, Dougados M. Defining disease activity in ankylosing spondylitis: is a combination of variables (Bath Ankylosing Spondylitis Disease Activity Index) an appropriate instrument? Rheumatology (Oxford). 1999;38:878–882.

109. Mander M, Simpson JM, McLellan A, Walker D, Goodacre JA, Dick WC. Studies with an enthesis index as a method of clinical assessment in ankylosing spondylitis. Ann Rheum Dis. 1987;46:197–202.

110. Heuft-Dorenbosch L, Spoorenberg A, van Tubergen A, et al. Assessment of enthesitis in ankylosing spondylitis. Ann Rheum Dis. 2003;62:127–132.

111. Braun J, Brandt J, Listing J, et al. Treatment of active ankylosing spondylitis with infliximab: a randomised controlled multicentre trial. Lancet. 2002;359:1187–1193.

112. Calin A, Garrett S, Whitelock H, et al. A new approach to defining functional ability in ankylosing spondylitis. The Bath Ankylosing Spondylitis Functional Index. J Rheumatol. 1994;21:2286–2291.

113. Masson G, Thomas P, Bontoux D, Alcalay M. Influence of trauma on initiation of Reiter's syndrome and ankylosing spondylitis. Ann Rheum Dis. 1985;44:860–861.

114. Sandorfi N, Freundlich B. Psoriatic and seronegative inflammatory arthropathy associated with a traumatic onset: 4 cases and a review of the literature. J Rheumatol. 1997;24:187–192.

115. Sany J, Rosenberg F, Panis G, Serre H. Unclassified HLA-B27 inflammatory rheumatic diseases: follow-up of 23 patients. Arthritis Rheum. 1980;23:258–259.

116. Zeidler H, Mau R, Mau W, Freyschmidt J, Majewski A, Deicher H. Evaluation of early diagnostic criteria including HLA-B27 for ankylosing spondylitis in a follow-up study. Z Rheumatol. 1985;44:249–253.

117. Wagener P, Mau W, Zeidler H, Eckert G, Robin-Winn M, Deicher H. HLA-B27 and clinical aspects of ankylosing spondylitis: results of prospective studies. Immunol Rev. 1985;86:93–100.

118. Mau W, Zeidler H, Mau R, Majewski A, Freyschmidt J, Deicher H. Outcome of possible ankylosing spondylitis in a 10 years' follow-up study. Clin Rheumatol. 1987;6(suppl 2):60–66.

119. Mau W, Zeidler H, Mau R, et al. Evaluation of early diagnostic criteria for ankylosing spondylitis in a 10-year follow-up. Z Rheumatol. 1990;49:82–87.

120. Sampaio-Barros PD, Bertolo MB, Kraemer MHS, Marques-Neto JF, Samara AM. Undifferentiated spondyloarthropathies: a 2-year follow-up study. Clin Rheumatol. 2001;20:201–206.

121. Kumar A, Bansal M, Srivastava DN, et al. Long-term outcome of undifferentiated spondylarthropathy. Rheumatol Int. 2001; 20:221–224.

122. Jänti JK, Kaarela K, Lehtinen KES. Seronegative oligoarthritis: a 23-year follow-up study. Clin Rheumatol. 2002;21:353–356.

123. Blackburn WD Jr, Alacrcon GS, Ball GV. Evaluation of patients with back pain of suspected inflammatory nature. Am J Med. 1988;85:766–770.

124. Zink A, Braun J, Listing J, Wollenhaupt J. Disability and handicap in rheumatoid arthritis and ankylosing spondylitis—results from the German rheumatological database. German Collaborative Arthritis Centers. J Rheumatol. 2000;27:613–622.

125. Van der Linden S, Valkenburg HA, Cats A. Evaluation of diagnostic criteria for ankylosing spondylitis: a proposal for modification of the New York criteria. Arthritis Rheum. 1984;27: 361–368.

126. Braun J, Bollow M, Eggens U, Konig H, Distler A, Sieper J. Use of dynamic magnetic resonance imaging with fast imaging in the detection of early and advanced sacroiliitis in spondylarthropathy patients. Arthritis Rheum. 1994;37:1039–1045.

127. Braun J, Bollow M, Sieper J. Radiologic diagnosis and pathology of the spondyloarthropathies. Rheum Dis Clin North Am. 1998;24:697–735.

128. Braun J, Bollow M, Seyrekbasan F, et al. Computed tomography guided corticosteroid injection of the sacroiliac joint in patients with spondyloarthropathy with sacroiliitis: clinical outcome and followup by dynamic magnetic resonance imaging. J Rheumatol. 1996;23:659–664.

129. Braun J, Pham T, Sieper J, Davis J, van der Linden S, Dougados M, et al. International ASAS consensus statement for the use of anti-tumour necrosis factor agents in patients with ankylosing spondylitis. Ann Rheum Dis. 2003;62:817–824.

130. Dequeker J, Goddeeris T, Walravens M, De Roo M. Evaluation of sacro-iliitis: comparison of radiological and radionuclide techniques. Radiology. 1978;128:687–689.

131. D'Agostino M, Said-Nahal R, Hacquard-Bouder C, Brasseur JL, Dougados M, Breban M. Assessment of peripheral enthesitis in the spondylarthropathies by ultrasonography combined with power Doppler. Arthritis Rheum. 2003;48:523–533.

132. Biasi D, Carletto A, Caramaschi P, Pacor ML, Maleknia T, Bambara LM. Efficacy of methotrexate in the treatment of ankylosing spondylitis: a three year open study. Clin Rheumatol. 2000;19:114–117.

133. Roychowdhury B, Bintley-Bagot S, Bulgen DY, Thompson RN, Tunn EJ, Moots RJ. Is methotrexate effective in ankylosing spondylitis? Rheumatology (Oxford). 2002;41:1330–1332.

134. Altan L, Bingol U, Karakoc Y, Aydiner S, Yurkuran M, Yurkuran M. Clinical investigation of methotrexate in the treatment of ankylosing spondylitis. Scand J Rheumatol. 2001;30:255–259.

135. Gonzalez-Lopez L, Garcia-Gonzalez A, Vazquez del Mercado M, Munoz-Valle JF, Gamez-Nava JI. Efficacy of methotrexate in ankylosing spondylitis: a randomized, double blind, placebo controlled trial. J. Rheumatol. 2004;31:1568–1574.

136. Queiro R, De Dios JR. Successful treatment with low-dose weekly methotrexate in a case of undifferentiated spondyloarthropathy coexisting with cutaneous polyarteritis nodosa. Clin Rheumatol. 2002;21:304–305.

137. Braun J, Bollow M, Neure L, et al. Use of immunohistologic and in situ hybridization techniques in the examination of sacroiliac joint biopsy specimens from patients with ankylosing spondylitis. Arthritis Rheum. 1995;38:499–505.

138. Gorman JD, Sack KE, Davis JC Jr. Treatment of ankylosing spondylitis by inhibition of tumor necrosis factor α. N Engl J Med. 2002;346:1349–1356.

139. Van den Bosch F, Kruithof E, Baeten D, et al. Randomized double-blind comparison of chimeric monoclonal antibody to tumor necrosis factor α (infliximab) versus placebo in active spondylarthropathy. Arthritis Rheum. 2002;46:755–765.

140. Kruithof E, Van den Bosch F, Baeten D, et al. Repeated infusions of infliximab, a chimeric anti-TNFα monoclonal antibody, in patients with active spondyloarthropathy: one year follow up. Ann Rheum Dis. 2002, 61:207–212.

141. Schnarr S, Hülsemann JL, Merkesdal S, et al. Anti-tumor necrosis factor-α therapy with the chimeric monoclonal antibody infliximab in severe undifferentiated spondyloarthropathy. Ann Rheum Dis. 2004;63(suppl 1):422.

142. Marzo-Ortega H, McGonagle D, O'Connor P, Emery P. Efficacy of etanercept in the treatment of the entheseal pathology in resistant spondylarthropathy: a clinical and magnetic resonance imaging study. Arthritis Rheum. 2001;44:2112–2117.

143. Burgos-Vargas R, Vazquez-Mellado J, Pacheco-Tena C, Harnandez-Garduno A, Goycochea-Robles MV. A 26 week randomised, double blind, placebo controlled exploratory study of sulfasalazine in juvenile onset spondyloarthropathies. Ann Rheum Dis. 2002;61:941–942.

144. Lehtinen A, Leirisalo-Repo M, Taavitsainen M. Persistence of enthesopathic changes in patients with spondylarthropathy during a 6-month follow-up. Clin Exp Rheumatol. 1995;13: 733–736.

145. Dougados M, van der Linden S, Leirisalo-Repo M, et al. Sulfasalazine in the treatment of spondylarthropathy. A randomized, multicenter, double-blind, placebo-controlled study. Arthritis Rheum. 1995;38:618–627.

146. Clegg DO, Reda DJ, Abdellatif M. Comparison of sulfasalazine and placebo for the treatment of axial and peripheral articular manifestations of the seronegative spondylarthropathies: a Department of Veterans Affairs cooperative study. Arthritis Rheum. 1999;42:2325–2329.

8 The Juvenile-Onset Spondyloarthritides

Rubén Burgos-Vargas

One of the most important groups of rheumatic diseases for specialists in pediatric and adult rheumatology is the juvenile-onset spondyloarthritides. Epidemiologic data in clinical settings and open populations show increased recognition of these disorders. Several follow-up studies have yielded a variety of disease activities and reduced functioning both on a short- and long-term basis. Juvenile-onset spondyloarthritides may have significant effects on the quality of life. The transition from childhood to adulthood can be very painful and the psychologic, social, and economic impacts are very high. There are advances in the understanding of the pathogenesis of these diseases, particularly the involvement of tumor necrosis factor (TNF)-α, and new forms of therapy, mainly TNF-α blockers, make the future for these children very promising.

CONCEPT

The juvenile-onset spondyloarthritides comprise a group of human leukocyte antigen (HLA)-B27–associated disorders that are mainly characterized by enthesitis and arthritis affecting the lower extremities, and, in a variable proportion of patients, the sacroiliac and spinal joints.[1] Additional features include a variety of extraarticular manifestations, and, in some patients, bacterial infections as triggers.

Juvenile-onset spondyloarthritides are closely related to adult-onset diseases. Except for the prevalence of some clinical features at onset and severity throughout the course of the disease, juvenile-onset spondyloarthritides resemble their adult counterparts in most clinical aspects, strength of the HLA-B27 association, and the role of arthritogenic bacteria in their pathogenesis. Not surprisingly, several aspects, from nomenclature to classification and diagnostic criteria reflect to some extent those developed in the adult-onset populations. Today, however, there is some controversy about the concept, definition, and nomenclature that make the issue certainly difficult to understand.

THE JUVENILE-ONSET SPONDYLOARTHRITIDES GROUP

Juvenile-onset spondyloarthritides are characterized by clinical changes that span from childhood to adolescence to adulthood. The course of the disease may evolve from a single episode of monoarthritis to more complex forms of disease, including inflammatory and proliferative phenomena at peripheral and axial entheses and joints accompanied by extraarticular manifestations. During the episodes of disease activity and as result of the long-term structural damage, juvenile onset may lead to diverse degrees of functional and quality-of-life impairment.

The spectrum of the juvenile-onset group is wide and includes undifferentiated conditions and syndromes or diseases that either fulfill specific diagnostic criteria or correspond with the clinical picture of diseases already described in adults.[2] The signs and symptoms that characterize the subgroup of undifferentiated conditions do not allow the diagnosis of specific diseases. The subgroup of undifferentiated spondyloarthritides includes children with isolated arthritis, enthesitis, tendinitis, and dactylitis or combined forms such as the idiopathic form of the seronegative enthesopathy and arthropathy (SEA) syndrome—a term that seems to fit well into enthesitis-related arthritis (ERA).

The subgroup of differentiated disorders includes syndromes and specific diseases that are recognized because of structural changes (e.g., radiographic sacroiliitis, spinal disease, or tarsal ankylosis), extraarticular manifestations (e.g., infectious diarrhea, urethritis, cervicitis, psoriasis, and inflammatory bowel disease [IBD]), or laboratory findings (e.g., bacteriologic or serologic demonstration of infection). This subgroup includes ankylosing spondylitis (AS), reactive arthritis (ReA), and Reiter's syndrome, a subset of psoriatic arthritis (PsA), the arthropathies associated with IBD, specifically Crohn's disease and ulcerative colitis, and rare forms such as ankylosing tarsitis.

In an unknown proportion of patients, symptoms overlap at some time during the course of the disease.

This disease continuum is accompanied by changes in various aspects including the relevance of each manifestation to the clinical picture, the degree of disease activity and damage, and particularly the diagnosis and classification.

EPIDEMIOLOGIC ASPECTS

The prevalence and incidence of juvenile-onset spondyloarthritides, particularly AS in the general population, in multiplex case families, and in groups of children with juvenile arthritis as a whole depend on the prevalence of HLA-B27. Juvenile- or adult-onset spondyloarthritides are seen in approximately 20% of first-degree relatives of patients with juvenile-onset spondyloarthritides.[3,4] The estimated incidence of juvenile-onset spondyloarthritides ranges from 1.44 and 2.10 per 100,000 Canadian and American children,[5-7] but the incidence is higher among Western Canadian Indians,[8,9] particularly the Inuit[10] and is up to 24.0 per 100,000 children in Alaskan Inupiat[11] and Yupik Amerindians.[12] In contrast, their incidence is lower in Costa Rica,[13] Germany[14], Norway,[15,16] and Sweden.[17,18]

The proportion of patients with juvenile-onset spondyloarthritides within the whole group of spondyloarthritides is less than 21% of white people who have AS, but approaches 50% in Mexicans, Indians, North Africans, and Asians.[19-25]

The recognition of juvenile-onset spondyloarthritides in pediatric rheumatology clinics has increased from 0% to 16% in the 1970s to 31% in 1980s.[26] At the end of the 1990s, the juvenile rheumatoid arthritis (JRA)-to-juvenile-onset spondyloarthritides ratio ranged from 1.4:1 to 2.6:1.[5,7,27,28] In long-term follow-up studies of children with HLA-B27 who had juvenile chronic arthritis (JCA) or JRA, 66%[29] and 75%[30] of the children eventually developed AS or undifferentiated spondyloarthritides. However, lower figures (18.5%) have been reported.[31] These variations may result from disease heterogeneity, lack of uniform classification criteria, and methodologic differences.

The prevalence rate of juvenile-onset spondyloarthritides is higher in boys than in girls, particularly in the prepubescent years. The proportion of girls having juvenile-onset spondyloarthritides increases with age and tends to equal that of boys. Although juvenile-onset spondyloarthritides may occur at any age, most cases are found between the ages of 8 and 12 years.

CLASSIFICATION AND DIAGNOSTIC CRITERIA

The term most commonly used to refer to this group of disorders is *juvenile* or *juvenile-onset spondyloarthropathies,* yet the word, *spondyloarthritides,* emphasizes their inflammatory nature. Although not all

children and certainly not all adults develop axial disease, the term seems to be adequate because it maintains consistency with adult-onset nomenclature and classification. Presently, such consistency is a major issue in the transition of these patients from childhood and adolescence to adulthood and the approach taken toward these individuals by society and health policy makers.

The acronym ERA is becoming widely used; however, the concept behind this term does not completely correspond to that of the spondyloarthritides. ERA is one of the seven subgroups of juvenile arthritis defined by the International League of Associations for Rheumatology/World Health Organization group of experts.[32,33] Classification criteria for ERA include the most important features of juvenile-onset spondyloarthritides, but exclusion criteria prevent the classification of a significant proportion of children with spondyloarthritides.[34] Part of the problem is that the criteria for ERA do not include PsA and ReA as part of the spondyloarthritides and limit the use of IBD to being only a descriptor of the disease.

Children with juvenile-onset spondyloarthritides, including those with associated diagnoses as referred to earlier, may be classified according to the criteria of the European Spondyloarthropathy Study Group (ESSG) developed for adult-onset spondyloarthritides.[35] The ESSG criteria have been validated in children[36]; their performance approaches that found in the adult populations, but their sensitivity, positive predictive value, likelihood ratio, and accuracy are lower. Because inflammatory spinal pain is one of two major criteria, the usefulness of the ESSG criteria may be limited.

The distinction between one type of juvenile-onset spondyloarthritis (SA) and another depends on the specificity of clinical, laboratory, and radiographic signs at a given time. The natural course of SA and clinical overlapping may lead to changes in diagnosis and classification from time to time. The recognition, diagnosis, and classification of juvenile-onset spondyloarthritides depend on criteria for adult-onset spondyloarthritides (e.g., AS and ReA), and descriptions of clinical manifestation for adult-onset disease (e.g., ReA, PsA, Reiter's syndrome, Crohn's disease, and ulcerative colitis). Exceptions to this are the recognition of SEA syndrome,[37] which is based on clinical signs, and the development of Vancouver's criteria for PsA in children.[38] Criteria for juvenile AS[39,40] and atypical spondyloarthritides[41] in children have also been developed, but are not in use.

MAJOR CLINICAL FEATURES: ARTHRITIS AND ENTHESITIS

Arthritis and enthesitis occur at peripheral sites in nearly all patients with juvenile-onset spondyloarthritides and at spinal and sacroiliac joint areas in some

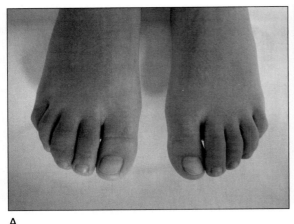 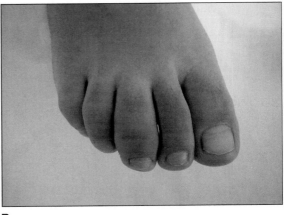

A   B

Fig. 8.1 Asymmetric involvement of the MTP and IP joints of the feet of a 12-year-boy with a very active form of undifferentiated spondyloarthritis. There is dactylitis of the third right toe and metatarsophalangeal swelling of the same foot.

patients.[42–54] The severity, duration, and consequences of arthritis and enthesitis may not parallel each other throughout the clinical course of the disease. Similarly, enthesophyte formation may not be related to the course of synovitis.

Arthritis

Arthritis is the most common sign of juvenile-onset spondyloarthritides. At onset, most patients have unilateral or asymmetric mono- or oligoarthritis involving the knee, midtarsus, and ankle and less commonly the feet metatarsophalangeal (MTP) or interphalangeal (IP) joints, the hips, or any of the upper extremity joints (Fig. 8.1).

The natural course of arthritis is variable. Some patients have a single or very few episodes of mono- or oligoarthritis for 3 to 6 months. Other patients have recurrent episodes of oligo- or polyarthritis for longer periods, followed by partial or complete remission of disease activity, with little or no structural damage at all. Some children have severe and persistent bilateral and symmetric polyarthritis (usually from 5 to 10 joints) and structural damage. The frequency of hip, MTP, and foot IP joint involvement increases along with that of some of the upper extremity joints. The incidence of sacroiliac joint pain, spinal symptoms, and HLA-B27 is higher in these patients. The characteristics of most patients with chronic disease, particularly AS or ankylosing tarsitis, or those with Crohn's disease, ulcerative colitis, and PsA with sacroiliac or spinal involvement correspond to these categories. The highly heterogeneous nature of the natural history of the disease in children, with these variable and sometimes self-limited episodes, has contributed to a lack of a uniform approach to classification.

Enthesitis

Enthesitis, a major component of the juvenile-onset spondyloarthritides, is highly specific for the diagnosis. Like arthritis, peripheral enthesitis occurs predominantly in the lower extremities, particularly in the foot, at single sites at onset, and then at several sites throughout the course of the disease (Fig. 8.2). Foot enthesitis, including tarsal and calcaneal entheses, is one of the most disabling conditions in children with juvenile-onset spondyloarthritides. This can occur at the Achilles tendon and plantar fascia attachments to the posterior and inferior aspect of the calcaneus or along functional entheses such as the longitudinal

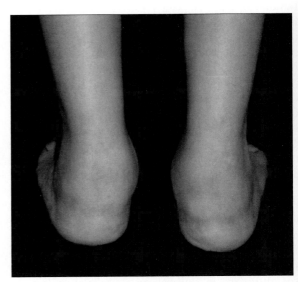

Fig. 8.2 Massive swelling of the ankle and Achilles tendons in a 15-year-old boy with an 8-year history of peripheral arthritis and enthesitis.

apposition of the peroneal and tibialis anterior and posterior, as well as the extensor hallucis longus tendons to the tarsal bones. Soft tissue swelling results from inflammation of tendon sheaths and adjacent bursae. Enthesitis may also occur at the first and fifth metatarsal head entheses, tibial anterior tuberosity, greater trochanter, iliac crest, and ischium. Remarkably, healthy children may complain of pain at entheses sites, particularly around the MTP joints, which make the recognition of enthesitis in such sites quite difficult.[55]

In some patients, the episodes of enthesitis are unique, last longer than those of arthritis (approximately 6–12 months), and involve one or a few entheses. Some children have recurrent episodes of enthesitis followed by partial or complete remission; others develop severe and persistent enthesitis involving many sites, particularly the feet. Persistent enthesitis is associated with bone edema and overgrowth, osteocartilaginous proliferation, enthesophytosis, bone bridging, and ankylosis. Less often, it causes subcortical bone cysts and erosions at tendon attachments.

There seem to be no significant differences in the pattern of arthritis and enthesitis, particularly at peripheral sites, according to diagnosis. Sacroiliac joint and spinal involvement may also be transitory, but in most patients with persistent pain, stiffness, and decreased mobility, structural changes may occur.

Imaging studies of affected sites reveal osteopenia, joint space narrowing, and ankylosis; erosions and destructive changes are rare, but enthesophytosis and bone bridging, particularly in the feet, are commonly seen.[56,57] Marginal or articular surface erosions may be seen in small joints. In contrast to common knowledge, the involvement of the sacroiliac joint may lead to the same changes seen in the adult population, including subchondral sclerosis and irregularities of the articular surface progressing to erosions, joint space narrowing, bone bridging, and complete fusion of the sacroiliac bones. However, syndesmophytosis and ligamentous calcification are nonreversible changes of the spine that become clear many years after onset. Magnetic resonance imaging (MRI) and ultrasound are useful methods for detecting disease activity. The former may show bone edema, which is attributed to inflammation, subtle cartilage and subchondral bone erosions, and enthesophytes.[58,59]

Although there are no specific histologic findings in the synovial membrane of peripheral joints of patients with juvenile-onset spondyloarthritides, there is prominent expression of TNF-α, which correlates with T-cell and macrophages infiltrates.[60] TNF-α expression also correlates with TNF receptor and p55 expression. The synovial membrane may also show high levels of CD8-activated cells, TNF-β, γ-interferon, and interleukins 2, 4, and 6.[60–62] Bacterial DNA from arthritogenic organisms has been identified in the synovial membrane of patients with juvenile-onset AS.[63] Inflammatory infiltrates at the mid-tarsal entheses are not prominent, but bone proliferation predominates.[64]

CONSEQUENCES

Juvenile-onset spondyloarthritides may affect the functional capacity of children, adolescents, and adults. The consequences of disease activity and structural damage and the short- and long-term involvement of the joints and entheses result in diverse degrees of pain, stiffness, loss of movement, functional impairment, and harm to quality of life. Because of the predominant lower limb involvement of juvenile-onset spondyloarthritides, most patients have limitations in walking, standing, climbing stairs, and running. Nearly 60% of children with spondyloarthritides have moderate to severe limitations by 10 years of disease duration.[65–68] Patients with disease activity for 5 years or more have significant functional impairment. The probability of remission reaches only 17% after 5 years of disease duration. In comparison with adults, patients with juvenile-onset AS require more hip replacements and more patients are in functional classes III and IV.[65,69]

CLINICAL PRESENTATIONS

Isolated Forms of Disease

The differentiation of juvenile-onset spondyloarthritides from other forms of arthritis may be quite difficult because of the presentation of isolated signs in many patients.[53,71–75] Peripheral arthritis, specifically monoarthritis or oligoarthritis of the lower extremities, is the most common presentation; rarely does joint disease involve five or more joints at onset. The knees, and less often, the ankles, tarsal joints, and hips are the involved joints in these patients. Most patients seem to have recurrent episodes of pain and swelling sometimes attributed to trauma or extreme exercise.

The long-term follow-up of children with HLA-B27 who have chronic arthritis reveals that between 18.5% and 75% develop spondyloarthritides.[29–31] The demographics, family history, clinical pattern, and HLA type should be considered in the differentiation of spondyloarthritides from other forms of chronic arthritis.[37–41,53] Differential diagnosis from toxic hip synovitis; tuberculosis of the hip and joints and tendons of the fingers; internal derangements of the knee, including meniscus and ligament problems; ankle strain; and bone tumors is also mandatory.

Sacroiliac joint inflammation seen on MRI in children with neither symptoms nor radiographic changes will suggest sacroiliitis,[58,59] but no long-term follow-up of these children has been done. In contrast, children with no bowel symptoms who were followed-up after a subclinical form of nonspecific IBD was diagnosed have an increased incidence of AS throughout follow-up.[76] Enthesitis, tenosynovitis, dactylitis, or hip contractures in children with HLA-B27 have also been found as isolated episodes of disease activity.

Acute uveitis, mucositis, skin disease (excluding psoriasis), or heart disease are likely to occur as unique manifestations of disease in children who later develop spondyloarthritides, but their frequency is unknown. Rarely patients refer to such conditions as the first manifestation of their disease.

Undifferentiated Spondyloarthritides: The Seronegative Enthesopathy Syndrome

Although the term *SEA syndrome* has been replaced by *ERA* and *undifferentiated spondyloarthritides,* it historically represents one of the most important advances in the understanding of juvenile-onset spondyloarthritides.[37] Originally, it referred to the combination of enthesopathy and arthritis or arthralgia as a form of an idiopathic disease or as part of a well-defined SA. The idiopathic form of SEA syndrome is actually an undifferentiated SA. Short- and long-term follow-up of patients with SEA syndrome suggests that most patients with HLA-B27, persistent arthritis, and enthesitis develop AS 5 to 10 years after onset.[48,77–79] The different rates of progression of SEA syndrome to AS depend on case definition and ethnic factors.

Extraarticular manifestations in patients with SEA syndrome or an equivalent disorder include nonspecific IBD, acute uveitis, and systemic symptoms, as well as atlantoaxial subluxation, cardiac conduction disturbances, and pulmonary function test abnormalities.[80–84]

Reactive Arthritis

ReA is a form of arthritis that appears after an infection.[85,86] Although ReA has been described after viral, parasitic, and a number of bacterial infections, use of this term is usually restricted to HLA-B27–associated ReA triggered by arthritogenic bacteria such as *Salmonella, Yersinia, Campylobacter, Shigella,* and *Chlamydia. Reiter's syndrome,* a term not used today (see Chapter 1 of this volume), has been described in children[87,88] and refers to the coincidence of arthritis, conjunctivitis, and urethritis or cervicitis. It is actually a form of ReA with prominent extraarticular manifestations.

The organisms implicated in causing ReA in children are essentially the same as those that trigger ReA in adults, but the relative frequency of each microorganism may differ. For example, the prevalence of ReA triggered by *Salmonella* and *Yersinia* in children is much higher than that triggered by *Chlamydia.* ReA in children rarely develops after epidemics of *Salmonella*

and *Campylobacter,* and their prevalence is lower compared with that found in adults: whereas ReA develops in 5% to 10%[89–91] of children with yersiniosis and 0.5% to 8.0% children after *Salmonella* outbreaks,[92,93] the prevalence in adults with yersiniosis may reach 33%[85] and 3.3% to 13.2% of adults exposed to *Salmonella.*[85] Recently, no single case was found among 286 children with *Salmonella enteritidis* infection.[94]

ReA predominantly involves the joints and entheses of the lower extremities. Some patients with *Salmonella*- and *Yersinia*-induced ReA present with polyarthritis that affects the small joints of the hands. In a number of children, particularly those having HLA-B27, ReA may follow a chronic course and even develop into AS.[86,95–98] The course of ReA, particularly that triggered by *Yersinia* or *Campylobacter* infections, in children without HLA-B27 is rather short and benign.

The infection may be entirely asymptomatic or may produce slight to moderate symptoms up to 4 weeks before onset of arthritis. In some children, infection is only suspected by detecting serum antibodies; in others, the clinical picture may include severe disease.

Children with ReA may have aphthous stomatitis, conjunctivitis, erythema nodosum (particularly in *Yersinia* ReA), circinate balanitis, keratoderma blenor-rhagica (which may clinically and histologically resemble psoriasis) (Fig. 8.3), anterior uveitis, urethritis and cervicitis (particularly in adolescents with sexually acquired ReA), aortic insufficiency, myocarditis, and pericarditis.[86–88,95–99]

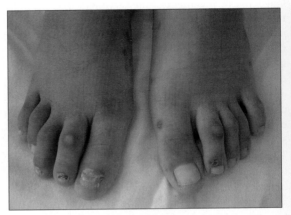

Fig. 8.3 Dorsoplantar aspect of the feet of a 16-year-old patient with chronic reactive arthritis. Although the third digit on the right foot shows some diffuse swelling and hyperpigmentation, the first toe looks atrophic than its counterpart on the left foot. There is nail dystrophy of the first three digits in the right foot (which is more clearly seen on the first toe) and keratoderma blenorrhagic spots over the skin. Interestingly, this patient had recurrent episodes of severe arthritis and enthesitis involving both feet but only recently developed skin lesions.

Juvenile-Onset Ankylosing Spondylitis

The diagnosis of juvenile-onset AS is made according to adult-onset criteria referring to spinal symptoms and radiographic sacroiliitis.[100] Most patients with juvenile-onset AS have isolated conditions, mainly arthritis or SEA syndrome in the initial years and axial disease later on. Few patients present with axial symptoms and radiographic sacroiliitis within 2 to 3 years of disease.[101] Juvenile-onset AS differs from its adult counterpart in clinical features at onset, including a high versus low prevalence of peripheral disease and a low versus high prevalence of axial disease.[19–21,23–25,102] Slight genetic differences have been described,[103–106] but, nevertheless, the prevalence of B27*05 is similar in both groups.[107]

Although the pattern of peripheral enthesopathy and arthropathy is similar to that of other juvenile-onset spondyloarthritides, juvenile-onset AS is characterized by persistent axial involvement (Fig. 8.4).

The prevalence of spinal or sacroiliac joint pain and stiffness, reduced anterior spinal flexion, or chest expansion, increases after 2.5 years of disease and reaches a maximum 5 to 10 years after onset.[53,77] During this period, radiographic sacroiliitis becomes evident in most patients (Fig. 8.5). Less than 15% of patients had axial symptoms in the initial year of disease. Among those who did are a group of children with HLA-B27 who have polyarthritis, enthesitis, axial symptoms, and radiographic sacroiliitis, fulfilling the diagnostic criteria for AS, early in the course of the disease. Axial symptoms first occur in the lumbar and thoracic spine, and less commonly, in the neck and sacroiliac joints.

Of the patients, 5% to 10% have high-grade fever, weight loss, muscle weakness and atrophy, fatigue,

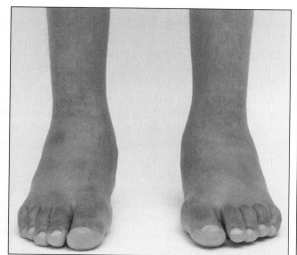

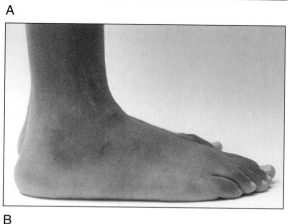

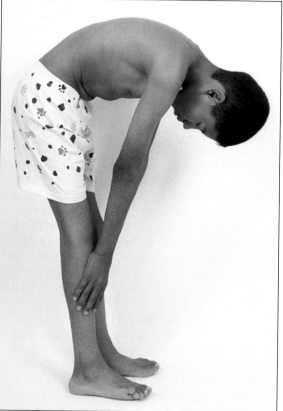

Fig. 8.4 Eleven-year-old boy with juvenile ankylosing spondylitis who, at the age of 7 years, had peripheral arthritis and enthesitis producing diffuse swelling of the tarsal region (**A** and **B**). At the age of 11 years (**C**), he complained of lumbar pain and stiffness, showed reduced anterior spinal flexion, and developed radiographic sacroiliitis.

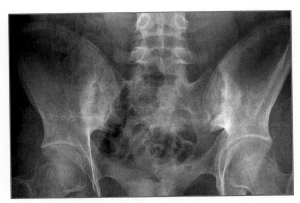

Fig. 8.5 Grade 3 bilateral sacroiliitis in a 14-year-old adolescent with a disease duration of 6 years. There is subchondral sclerosis of the iliac bone, joint surface irregularities, which include some erosions on both sides, and joint space narrowing of the hips.

lymph node enlargement, leukocytosis, and anemia. Up to 27% have one or more attacks of nongranulomatous acute uveitis.[21,39,42,45,46,108] Cardiovascular manifestations are rare but include aortic valve insufficiency, nonspecific conduction disturbances, and fewer miscellaneous findings.[109–111] Amyloidosis may occur in some patients.[42] Atlantoaxial subluxation has been reported.[112,113] Up to 80% of patients with juvenile-onset AS might have nonspecific IBD.[114]

Juvenile-Onset Psoriatic Arthritis

Juvenile-onset PsA is defined as the association, but not necessarily the coincidence, of arthritis and psoriasis in individuals 16 years of age or younger. The majority of patients have oligoarthritis or polyarthritis of the upper and lower extremities resembling neither spondyloarthritides nor JRA.[115–118] Consequently, the concept of juvenile-onset PsA being part of juvenile onset spondyloarthritides or JRA has changed; the disease is now considered to be a special form of arthritis in children.[32,33] According to the Vancouver criteria for diagnosis,[38] the definition might also include patients who have either arthritis or psoriasis and dactylitis, nail pitting, a psoriasis-like rash, or a family history of psoriasis. Nevertheless, a variable proportion of patients with PsA have SA stigmata. As a whole, juvenile-onset PsA is more common in girls than in boys; the age at onset of arthritis is 7 to 11 years and at onset of psoriasis 9 to 13 years, but ranges may be wider. Male gender, age older than 6 years, and spinal disease have been associated with HLA-B27.

Arthritis is the initial manifestation in 50%, psoriasis in 40%, and arthritis and psoriasis in 10% of patients with juvenile-onset PsA. In general, psoriasis appears within 2 years of arthritis, but in some patients the interval is much longer. At onset, 70% of children with juvenile-onset PsA have oligoarthritis.[115–118] The knees, ankles, feet, and proximal IP, distal IP, and proximal and hand IP joints are often affected. Shortly thereafter, most patients develop polyarthritis in the upper and lower extremities. There are several patterns of hand and foot involvement; dactylitis is relatively common. After several years of disease, the frequency of wrist, metacarpophalangeal, MTP, elbow, and less often, hip disease increases.[119,120] The cervical spine is involved more often than other spinal segments. The prevalence of immunogenetic and clinical markers of spondyloarthritides in juvenile-onset PsA is variable. Clinical and radiographic abnormalities of the sacroiliac joints, low back pain, and restricted spinal movements are found in patients with juvenile-onset PsA throughout follow-up. Enthesopathy, HLA-B27, and positive family history are also more common in patients with juvenile-onset PsA.

Systemic manifestations include chronic iridocyclitis in 15% of patients and fever, pericarditis, IBD, or amyloidosis in a few patients.

Arthropathy of Inflammatory Bowel Disease: Crohn's Disease and Ulcerative Colitis

Crohn's disease is a transmural disease that involves the mucosa and regional lymphatics of the colon, distal ileum, and other segments of the digestive tube, with characteristic lesions consisting of noncaseating granulomas. Ulcerative colitis is a diffuse, inflammatory process consisting of neutrophils with crypt abscesses that involves the colonic mucosa. Diagnoses are usually based on clinical, radiographic, endoscopic, and often histopathologic studies. Approximately 18% to 30% of patients with Crohn's disease and 15% of those with ulcerative colitis have onset of disease before age 20.[121,122] The initial symptoms in juvenile-onset Crohn's disease seen most often are abdominal pain, diarrhea, and fever, whereas in juvenile-onset ulcerative colitis these are diarrhea, hematochezia, and abdominal pain. Later, anorexia, abdominal tenderness or a palpable mass, blood in the stools, weight loss, and growth retardation develop in patients with Crohn's disease. Patients with ulcerative colitis often develop abdominal tenderness and leukocytes in the stool. These two types of IBD can be severe and disabling conditions.[123,124]

Children and adolescents with Crohn's disease and ulcerative colitis may have peripheral arthritis and sacroiliac or spinal disease at the time of presentation of gastrointestinal symptoms, or these may develop later.[121,125] The incidence of peripheral arthritis is approximately 9% in patients with Crohn's disease and is approximately 10% to 20% in patients with

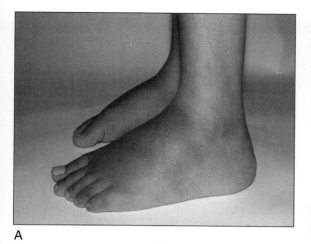

A

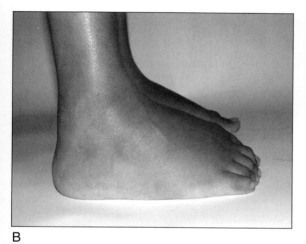

B

Fig. 8.6 Left and right foot of a 10-year-old boy with disease duration of 2 years, which consisted of severe peripheral arthritis and enthesitis. There is impressive tarsal swelling, particularly of the right foot. Radiographically, both feet showed various degrees of ankylosing tarsitis.

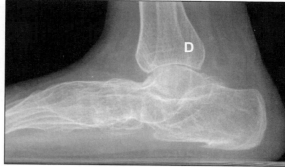

A

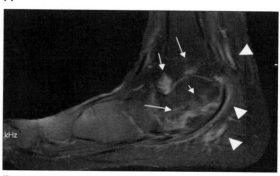

B

Fig. 8.7 Complete fusion of the tarsal bones, generalized osteopenia, and enthesophytosis at the plantar fascia attachment at the calcaneus in a 15-year-old boy with an 8-year history of peripheral arthritis and enthesitis. Magnetic resonance imaging enhanced with gadolineum showing bone edema *(hyperintesive signals, thin arrows)* and soft tissue edema around the *tibialis posterior* tendon and plantar fascia attachment *(short arrow)* indicating the presence of an active inflammatory process despite chronic changes.

ulcerative colitis. Arthritis involves the peripheral joints of the lower extremities and seldom involves those of the upper extremities. Single (about 50% of patients) or recurrent attacks of mono- or oligoarthritis lasting less than 4 weeks occur throughout the course of the disease. Less than 50% of patients with peripheral arthritis have parallel exacerbations of joint disease and gut symptoms. Although some patients have joint erosions and structural changes, this type of arthritis does not typically lead to permanent functional limitation or joint damage.

The peripheral arthritis of these patients does not resemble that of most juvenile-onset spondyloarthritides. Spondylitis and radiographic findings of sacroiliitis are rare, and association with HLA-B27 is found in patients with juvenile-onset Crohn's disease and juvenile-onset ulcerative colitis.

Nonspecific IBD changes occur in up to 80% of patients with juvenile-onset spondyloarthritides and are associated with erosive disease and a high risk of progression to AS.[76,79,114] Although nonspecific IBD rarely causes symptoms, studies of the gut may reveal acute and chronic inflammatory changes in the mucosa and submucosa of the terminal ileum and colon resembling Crohn's disease and ulcerative colitis in more than two thirds of the patients. Conversely, the early stages of Crohn's disease and ulcerative colitis resemble the nonspecific inflammatory changes of the terminal ileum and colon in asymptomatic patients with spondyloarthritides.

Ankylosing Tarsitis

The term *ankylosing tarsitis* refers to a set of clinical and radiographic findings, including some inflammatory (joint synovitis, enthesitis, tenosynovitis, and

TABLE 8.1 PHARMACOLOGIC APPROACH OF JUVENILE-ONSET SPONDYLOARTHRITIDES*		
Drugs[†]	Major Indications	Effect[‡]
Commonly used		
NSAIDs	Pain and swelling Arthritis and enthesitis Peripheral and axial symptoms	Symptomatic relief
Sulfasalazine	Disease activity, peripheral sites	Symptomatic relief, probably, arthritis and enthesitis
	Arthritis and enthesitis Psoriasis Uveitis Intestinal bowel disease	Remission, probably, extraarticular manifestations
Glucocorticoids	Refractory disease activity	Symptomatic relief
Oral prednisone	Arthritis and enthesitis	
Local application (joints, entheses, eyes)	Peripheral and axial symptoms	
	Uveitis	
Intravenous methylprednisolone		
Methotrexate weekly oral or parenteral	Arthritis and enthesitis	No evidence of any efficacy, arthritis and enthesitis
	Psoriasis	Symptomatic relief
	Uveitis	Remission, probably, extraarticular manifestations
Biologics, TNF-α blockers[§]		
Etanercept	Arthritis and enthesitis Extraarticular manifestations	Symptomatic relief Remission, probably
Infliximab	Arthritis and enthesitis Extraarticular manifestations	Symptomatic relief Remission, probably
Occasionally used		
Cyclosporine	Uveitis	Symptomatic relief
	Psoriasis	Remission, probably
Antibiotics	Infection by arthritogenic bacteria	Infection subsides
		No effect on musculoskeletal disease

*The therapeutic approach of this group of diseases has followed the treatment approaches for adult-onset spondyloarthritides and other forms of childhood arthritis and adult-onset spondyloarthritides.
[†]Although most agents are able to reduce disease activity and produce symptomatic relief, nothing is known about long-term effects, particularly any modification of the natural history of the disease.
[‡]Because the natural course of juvenile-onset spondyloarthritides is characterized by recurrent episodes of disease activity and remission, it is still unknown whether any of these drugs do actually induce remission of arthritis, enthesitis, uveitis, psoriasis, or inflammatory bowel disease.
[§]Results of adult-onset spondyloarthritis studies and a few open observations in children indicate a major role of TNF-α blockers in the treatment of these groups of diseases.

bursitis) and proliferative (periostitis, enthesophytosis, and bony ankylosis) manifestations originally described in patients with HLA-B27 who had juvenile-onset spondyloarthritides.[103,126,127] This condition seems equivalent to clinical, radiographic, and perhaps histopathologic features of the spinal and sacroiliac joints in patients with AS. The clinical characteristics of ankylosing tarsitis are midfoot swelling associated with soft tissue swelling around the malleoli, Achilles tendon, and remaining areas of the feet; decreased mobility of tarsal, ankle, and MTP joints; pes planus (and much less often pes cavus); and hyperextension of the MTP joints (Fig. 8.6). Radiographic features include diffuse osteopenia of the tarsal bones, joint space narrowing or ankylosis involving most tarsal joints, bone cysts, erosions, and osseous proliferation at the enthesis (Fig. 8.7). MRI scans show hyperintensive signals in bones, synovial sheaths, bursa, and rarely joint space. Histopathologic findings include slight inflammatory changes, but striking osteocartilaginous proliferation.

Ankylosing tarsitis may occur in patients with undifferentiated juvenile-onset spondyloarthritides or as a stage previous to radiographic sacroiliitis in patients with juvenile-onset AS.

TREATMENT

The therapeutic approach to juvenile-onset spondyloarthritides is based primarily on data derived from other forms of arthritis in children and adult-onset SA studies, as well as personal experiences (Table 8.1). Few studies on the efficacy of certain drugs in the treatment of juvenile-onset spondyloarthritides have been reported. Apart from symptomatic relief, there is no evidence that any treatment, including sulfasalazine, methotrexate, and cyclosporine, may modify disease progression. Reports on the efficacy of etanercept and infliximab in patients with adult-onset spondyloarthritides and in children with juvenile-onset disease show that these are excellent alternatives.

Nonsteroidal anti-inflammatory drugs (NSAIDS), sulfasalazine, and in some patients, glucocorticoids, provide symptomatic relief. Severe disease may not respond to full anti-inflammatory doses of NSAIDS, and, therefore, systemic glucocorticoids may be needed. The effect of intraarticular glucocorticoids in patients with active disease may be limited.

Most patients with juvenile-onset SpA receive sulfasalazine (30–50 mg/kg or less than 2 g/day) as treatment. Although the results reported in open studies are encouraging,[128–132] a 26-week, double-blind comparison with placebo showed favorable results for sulfasalazine for a few parameters.[133] In selected patients, methotrexate may be useful in treating extraarticular manifestations such as IBD, psoriasis, and anterior uveitis. Except for relieving psoriasis and uveitis, there is no clear evidence that methotrexate or cyclosporin has any benefit in the treatment of arthritis and enthesitis in patients with juvenile-onset spondyloarthritides.

In contrast, etanercept and infliximab produce a dramatic improvement in disease activity in patients with undifferentiated spondyloarthritides and juvenile-onset AS.[134–140] Improvement includes a marked reduction in the number of active joints and entheses, pain, and other measures. Despite this response, the TNF-α blockers should be used cautiously because nothing is known about their long-term effects and toxicity and the frequency of infections in children.

Physical and occupational therapy should be mandatory in all patients with juvenile-onset spondyloarthritides.[141] In addition to physical measures to alleviate pain and swelling, it is important to prevent joint contractures and preserve physical functioning. The use of rest, dynamic splints, and exercise programs should be individualized. Special emphasis should be given to exercises that lessen the degree of hip contractures, lower limb muscle weakness, and stiff back.

Surgical treatment is an excellent option for hip disease.[142] Less often, the knees and feet, particularly the MTP joints, are surgically treated. Surgical modalities include soft tissue release, synovectomy, tendon repair, arthroplasty, and joint replacement.

Because juvenile-onset spondyloarthritides may profoundly harm the quality of life of children and adolescents, and, therefore, their transition to adulthood, there are a number of issues to consider.[143] These include the psychologic, educational, and socioeconomic aspects of life. Disease activity and, later, disease damage may affect these individuals' social life, including personal and family activities, education, and employment.

REFERENCES

1. Burgos-Vargas R. The juvenile-onset spondyloarthritides. Rheum Dis Clin North Am. 2002;28:531–560.
2. Burgos-Vargas R, Pacheco TC, Vázquez-Mellado NJ. Juvenile-onset spondyloarthropathies. Rheum Dis Clin North Am. 1997;23:569–598.
3. Ansell BM, Bywaters EG, Lawrence JS. Familial aggregation and twin studies in Still's disease. Juvenile chronic polyarthritis. Rheumatology. 1969;2:37–61.
4. Burgos-Vargas R, Granados J, Castelazo G, et al. The clinical spectrum of ankylosing spondylitis among first degree relatives of patients with juvenile ankylosing spondylitis. Arthritis Rheum. 1990;33(suppl):S158.
5. Malleson PN, Fung MY. Rosenberg AM, for the Canadian Pediatric Rheumatology Association. The incidence of pediatric rheumatic diseases: results from the Canadian Pediatric Rheumatology Association Disease Registry. J Rheumatol. 1996;23:1981–1987.
6. Oen K, Fast M, Post BL. Epidemiology of juvenile rheumatoid arthritis in Manitoba, Canada, 1975–92: cycles in incidence. J Rheumatol. 1995;22:745–750.
7. Denardo BA, Tucker LB, Miller LC, Szer IS, Schaller JG. Demography of a regional pediatric rheumatology patient population. J Rheumatol. 1994;21:1553–1561.
8. Rosenberg AM, Petty R, Oen KG, Schroeder ML. Rheumatic diseases in Western Canadian Indian children. J Rheumatol. 1982;9:589–592.
9. Oen K. Comparative epidemiology of the rheumatic diseases in children. Curr Opin Rheumatol. 2000;12:410–414.
10. Oen K, Postl B, Chalmers IM, et al. Rheumatic diseases in an Inuit population. Arthritis Rheum. 1986;29:65–74.
11. Boyer GS, Lanier AT, Templin DW. Prevalence rates of spondyloarthropathies, rheumatoid arthritis, and other rheumatic disorders in an Alaskan Inupiat Eskimo population. J Rheumatol. 1988;15:678–683.

12. Boyer GS, Lanier AT, Templin DW. Spondyloarthropathy and rheumatoid arthritis in Alaskan Yupik Eskimos. J Rheumatol. 1990;17:489–496.

13. Arguedas O, Fasth A, Andersson-Gare B, Porras O. Juvenile chronic arthritis in urban San José, Costa Rica: a 2 year prospective study. J Rheumatol. 1998;25:1844–1850.

14. Kiessling U, Doring E, Listing J, et al. Incidence and prevalence of juvenile chronic arthritis in East Berlin. 1980–88. J Rheumatol. 1998;25:1837–1843.

15. Kaipainen-Seppanen O, Savvolainen A. Incidence of chronic juvenile rheumatic disease in Finland during 1980–1990. Clin Exp Rheumatol. 1996;14:441–448.

16. Moe N, Rygg M. Epidemiology of juvenile chronic arthritis in northern Norway: a ten-year retrospective study. Clin Exp Rheumatol. 1998;16:99–101.

17. Andersson Gare B, Fasth A, Andersson J, et al. Incidence and prevalence of juvenile chronic arthritis: a population survey. Ann Rheum Dis. 1987;146:277–281.

18. Gäre BA, Fasth A. The natural history of juvenile chronic arthritis: a population based cohort study. I. Onset and disease process. J Rheumatol. 1995;22:295–307.

19. Burgos-Vargas R, Naranjo A, Castillo J, Katona G. Ankylosing spondylitis in the Mexican Mestizo: patterns of disease according to age at onset. J Rheumatol. 1989;16:186–191.

20. Malaviya AN, Mehra NK. Spondyloarthropathies in India. In: Khan MA, ed. Ankylosing Spondylitis and Related Spondyloarthropathies. Spine: State of the Art Reviews. Philadelphia, Pa: Hanley & Belfus; 1990;4:679–684.

21. Claudepierre P, Gueguen A, Ladjouze A, et al. Features associated with juvenile onset spondyloarthropathies in North Africa. Rev Rhum Engl Ed. 1996;63:87–91.

22. Lau CS, Burgos-Vargas R, Louthrenoo W, Mok MY, Wordsworth P, Zheng QY. Features of spondyloarthropathies around the world. Rheum Dis Clin North Am. 1998;24:753–770.

23. Baek HJ, Shin KC, Lee YJ, Kang SW, Lee EB, Yoo CD, Song YW. Juvenile onset ankylosing spondylitis (JAS) has less severe spinal disease course than adult onset ankylosing spondylitis (AAS): clinical comparison between JAS and AAS in Korea. J Rheumatol. 2002;29:1780–1785.

24. Huang F, Zhang J, Zhu J, Guo J, Yang C. Juvenile spondyloarthropathies: the Chinese experience. Rheum Dis Clin North Am. 2003;29:531–547.

25. Aggarwal A, Hissaria P, Misra R. Juvenile ankylosing spondylitis—is it the same disease as adult ankylosing spondylitis? Rheumatol Int. 2005;25:94–96.

26. Rosenberg AM. Analysis of a pediatric rheumatology clinic population. J Rheumatol. 1990;17:827–830.

27. Bowyer S. Roettcher P, members of the Pediatric Rheumatology Database Research Group. Pediatric rheumatology clinic populations in the United States: results of a 3 year survey. J Rheumatol. 1996;23:1968–1974.

28. Symmons DPM, Jones M, Osborne J, Southwood TR, Woo P. Pediatric rheumatology in the United Kingdom: data from the British Pediatric Rheumatology Group National Diagnostic Register. J Rheumatol. 1996;23:1975–1980.

29. Hall MA, Burgos-Vargas R, Ansell BM. Sacroiliitis in juvenile chronic arthritis: a 10-year follow-up. Clin Exp Rheumatol. 1987;5(suppl):65–67.

30. Sheerin KA, Giannini EH, Brewer EJ Jr, Barron KS. HLA-B27-associated arthropathy in childhood: long-term clinical and diagnostic outcome. Arthritis Rheum. 1988;31:1165–1170.

31. Flato B, Smerdel A, Johnston V, et al. The influence of patient characteristics, disease variables, and HLA alleles on the development of radiographically evident sacroiliitis in juvenile idiopathic arthritis. Arthritis Rheum. 2002;46:986–994.

32. Petty RE, Southwood TR, Baum J, et al. Revision of the proposed classification for juvenile idiopathic arthritis: Durban. 1997. J Rheumatol. 1998;25:1991–1994.

33. Petty RE, Southwood TR, Manners P, et al. International League of Associations for Rheumatology classification of juvenile idiopathic arthritis: second revision, Edmonton, 2001. J Rheumatol. 2004;31:390–392.

34. Burgos-Vargas R, Rudwaleit M, Sieper J. The place of juvenile onset spondyloarthropathies in the Durban. 1997 ILAR classification criteria of juvenile idiopathic arthritis. J Rheumatol. 2002;29:869–874.

35. Dougados M, van der Linden S, Juhlin R, et al. The European Spondyloarthropathy Study Group preliminary criteria for the classification of spondyloarthropathy. Arthritis Rheum. 1991;34:1218–1227.

36. Prieur AM, Listrat V, Dougados M, Amor B. Spondyloarthropathies classification criteria in children. Arch Franc Ped. 1993;50:379–385. [in French]

37. Rosenberg AM, Petty RE. A syndrome of seronegative enthesopathy and arthropathy in children. Arthritis Rheum. 1982; 25:1041–1047.

38. Southwood TR, Petty RE, Malleson PN, et al. Psoriatic arthritis in children. Arthritis Rheum. 1989;32:1014–1021.

39. Calabro JJ, Gordon RD, Miller KI. Bechterew's syndrome in children: diagnostic criteria. Scand J Rheumatol. 1980;32(suppl): 45–48.

40. Hafner R. Juvenile spondylo arthritis. Retrospective analysis of 71 patients. Monatsschr Kinderheilkunde. 1987;135:41–49. [in German]

41. Hussein A, Abdul-Khaliqs H, von der Hardt H. Atypical spondyloarthritis in children: proposed diagnostic criteria. Eur J Pediatr. 1989;148:513–517.

42. Ansell BM. Juvenile spondylitis and related disorders. In: Moll JMH, ed. Ankylosing Spondylitis. Edinburgh, Scotland: Churchill Livingstone; 1980.

43. Edstrom G, Thune S, Wittbom-Cigen G. Juvenile ankylosing spondylitis. Acta Rheum Scand. 1960;6:161–173.

44. Jacobs P. Ankylosing spondylitis in children and adolescents. Arch Dis Child. 1963;38:492–499.

45. Schaller JG, Bitnum S, Wedgwood RJ. Ankylosing spondylitis with childhood onset. J Pediatr. 1969;74:505–516.

46. Ladd JR, Cassidy JT, Martel W. Juvenile ankylosing spondylitis. Arthritis Rheum. 1971;14:579–590.

47. Doury P. Infantile and juvenile onset ankylosing spondyloarthritis. Rev Rhum Mal Osteoartic. 1972;39:453–460. [in French]

48. Jacobs JC, Johnston AD, Berdon WE. HLA-B27 associated spondyloarthritis and enthesopathy in childhood: clinical, pathologic and radiographic observations in 58 patients. J Pediatr. 1982;100:5821–5828.

49. Burgos-Vargas R, Madariaga-Ceceňa MA, Katona G. Juvenile ankylosing spondylitis: clinical features in 41 patients. Bol Med Hosp Infant Mex. 1985;42:523–530. [in Spanish]

50. Petty RE, Malleson P. Spondyloarthropathies of childhood. Pediatr Clin North Am. 1986;33:1079–1092.

51. Prieur AM. HLA-B27 associated chronic arthritis in children: review of 65 cases. Scand J Rheumatol. 1987;66(suppl):51–56.

52. Burgos-Vargas R, Petty RE. Juvenile ankylosing spondylitis. Rheum Dis Clin North Am. 1992;18:123–142.

53. Burgos-Vargas R, Vázquez-Mellado J. The early clinical recognition of juvenile-onset ankylosing spondylitis and its differentiation from juvenile rheumatoid arthritis. Arthritis Rheum. 1995;38:835–844.

54. Bywaters EGL. Ankylosing spondylitis in childhood. Clin Rheum Dis. 1976;2:387–396.

55. Sherry DD, Sapp LR. Enthesalgia in childhood: site-specific tenderness in healthy subjects and in patients with seronegative enthesopathic arthropathy. J Rheumatol. 2003;30:1335–1340.

56. Azouz EM, Duffy CM. Juvenile spondyloarthropathies: clinical manifestations and medical imaging. Skeletal Radiol. 1995; 24:399–408.

57. Kleinman P, Rivelis M, Schneider R, Kaye J. Juvenile ankylosing spondylitis. Radiology. 1977;125:775–780.

58. Laxer RM, Babyn P, Liu P, et al. Magnetic resonance studies of the sacroiliac joints in children with HLA-B27 associated seronegative arthropathies. J Rheumatol. 1992;19 (suppl 33):123.

59. Bollow M, Biedermann T, Kannenberg J, et al. Use of dynamic magnetic resonance imaging to detect sacroiliitis in HLA-B27 positive and negative children with juvenile arthritides. J Rheumatol. 1998;25:556–564.

60. Grom AA, Murray KJ, Luyrink L, et al. Patterns of expression of tumor necrosis factor a, tumor necrosis factor β, and their receptors in synovia of patients with juvenile rheumatoid arthritis and juvenile spondylarthropathy. Arthritis Rheum. 1996;39: 1703–1710.

61. Murray KJ, Luyrink L, Grom AA, et al. Immunohistological characteristics of T cell infiltrates in different forms of childhood onset chronic arthritis. J Rheumatol. 1996;23:2116–2124.

62. Murray KJ, Grom AA, Thompson SD, Lieuwen D, Passo MH, Glass DN. Contrasting cytokine profiles in the synovium of different forms of juvenile rheumatoid arthritis and juvenile spondyloarthropathy: prominence of interleukin 4 in restricted disease. J Rheumatol. 1998;25:1388–1398.

63. Pacheco-Tena C, Alvarado de la Barrera C, López-Vidal Y, et al. Bacterial DNA in synovial fluid cells of patients with juvenile onset spondyloarthropathies. Rheumatology. 2001;40:920–927.

64. Jiménez-Balderas FJ, Fernández-Diez J, Fraga A. Tamale foot: deposit of acid mucopolysaccharides in the synovial sheaths of extensor tendons of the foot, resembling tendinitis, in a patient with juvenile ankylosing spondylitis. J Rheumatol. 2000;27: 1788–1791.

65. Calin A, Elswood S. The natural history of juvenile onset ankylosing spondylitis: 24 year retrospective case control study. Br J Rheumatol. 1988;27:91–93.

66. Flato B, Aasland A, Vinje O, Forre O. Outcome and predictive factors in juvenile rheumatoid arthritis and juvenile spondyloarthropathy. J Rheumatol. 1998;25:366–375.

67. Minden K, Kiessling U, Listing J, et al. Prognosis of patients with juvenile chronic arthritis and juvenile spondyloarthropathy. J Rheumatol. 2000;27:2256–2263.

68. Packman JC, Hall MA. Long-term follow-up of 246 adults with juvenile idiopathic arthritis: functional outcome. Rheumatology. 2002;41:1428–1435.

69. García-Morteo O, Maldonado-Cocco JA, Suárez-Almazor ME, Garay E. Ankylosing spondylitis of juvenile onset: comparison with adult onset disease. Scand J Rheumatol. 1983;12:246–248.

70. Ansell BM, Bywaters EGL. Diagnosis of "probable" Still's disease and its outcome. Ann Rheum Dis. 1962;21:253–262.

71. Gerster JC, Piccini P. Enthesopathy of the heels in juvenile onset seronegative B-27 positive spondyloarthropathy. J Rheumatol. 1985;12:310–314.

72. Siegel DM, Baum J. HLA-B27 associated dactylitis in children. J Rheumatol. 1988;15:976–977.

73. Olivieri I, Barbieri P, Gemignani G, Pasero G. Isolated juvenile onset HLA-B27 associated peripheral enthesitis. J Rheumatol. 1990;17:567–568.

74. Olivieri I, Pasero G. Longstanding isolated juvenile onset HLA-B27 associated peripheral enthesitis. J Rheumatol. 1992;19:164–165.

75. Bowyer S. Hip contracture as the presenting sign in children with HLA-B27 arthritis. J Rheumatol. 1995;22:165–167.

76. Mielants H, Veys EM, Cuvelier C, et al. Gut inflammation in children with late onset pauciarticular juvenile chronic arthritis and evolution to adult spondyloarthropathy—a prospective study. J Rheumatol. 1993;20:1567–1572.

77. Burgos-Vargas R, Clark P. Axial involvement in the seronegative enthesopathy and arthropathy syndrome and its progression to ankylosing spondylitis. J Rheumatol. 1989;16:192–197.

78. Olivieri I, Foto M, Ruju GP, Gemignani G, Giustarini S, Pasero G. Low frequency of axial involvement in Caucasian pediatric patients with seronegative enthesopathy and arthropathy syndrome after five years of disease. J Rheumatol. 1992;19:469–475.

79. Cabral DA, Oen KG, Petty RE. SEA syndrome revisited: a longterm followup of children with a syndrome of seronegative enthesopathy and arthropathy. J Rheumatol. 1992;19:1282–1285.

80. Barabino A, Gattorno M, Cabria M, et al. 99mTc-white cell scanning to detect gut inflammation in children with inflammatory bowel diseases or spondyloarthropathies. Clin Exp Rheumatol. 1998;16:327–334.

81. Lionetti P, Pupi A, Veltroni M, et al. Evidence of subclinical intestinal inflammation by 99m technetium leukocyte scintigraphy in patients with HLA-B27 positive juvenile onset active spondyloarthropathy. J Rheumatol. 2000;27:1538–1541.

82. Camiciottoli G, Trapani S, Ermini M, Falcini F, Pistolesi M. Pulmonary function in children affected by juvenile spondyloarthropathy. J Rheumatol. 1999;26:1382–1386.

83. Foster HE, Cairns RA, Burnell RH, et al. Atlantoaxial subluxation in children with seronegative enthesopathy and arthropathy syndrome: two case reports and review of literature. J Rheumatol. 1995;22:548–551.

84. Huppertz H, Voigt I, Muller-Scholden J, Sandhage K. Cardiac manifestations in patients with HLA B27-associated juvenile arthritis. Pediatr Cardiol. 2000;21:141–147.

85. Keat A. Reiter's syndrome and reactive arthritis in perspective. N Engl J Med. 1983;309:1606–1618.

86. Burgos-Vargas R, Vázquez-Mellado J. Reactive arthritides. In: Cassidy JT, Petty RE, eds. Textbook of Pediatric Rheumatology. Philadelphia, Pa: Saunders; 2001:679–689.

87. Singsen BH, Bernstein BH, Koster-King KG, Glovsky MM, Hanson V. Reiter's syndrome in childhood. Arthritis Rheum. 1977; 20(suppl):402–410.

88. Rosenberg AM, Petty RE. Reiter's disease in children. Am J Dis Child. 1979;133:394.

89. Hoogkamp-Korstanje JA, Stolk-Engelaar VM. Yersinia enterocolitica infection in children. Pediatr Infect Dis J. 1995;14:771.

90. Leino R, Mäkela AS, Tiilikainen A, Toivanen A. Yersinia arthritis in children. Scand J Rheumatol. 1980;9:245.

91. Russell AS. Reiter's syndrome in children following infection with Yersinia enterocolitica and Shigella. Arthritis Rheum. 1977;20(suppl):471.

92. Mattila L, Leirisalo-Repo M, Pelkonen P, Koskimies S, Granfors K, Siitonen A. Reactive arthritis following an outbreak of Salmonella bovis morbificans infection. J Infect. 1998;36:289–295.

93. Mattila L, Leirisalo-Repo M, Koskimies S, Gransfors K, Siitonen A. Reactive arthritis following an outbreak of Salmonella infection in Finland. Br J Rheumatol. 1994;33:1136–1141.

94. Rudwaleit M, Richter S, Braun J, Sieper J. Low incidence of reactive arthritis in children following a Salmonella outbreak. Ann Rheum Dis. 2001;60:1055–1057.

95. Hussein A. Spectrum of post-enteric reactive arthritis in childhood. Monatsschr Kinderheilkd. 1987;135:93–98.

96. Cuttica RJ, Scheines EJ, Garay SM, Romanelli MC, Maldonado Cocco JA. Juvenile onset Reiter's syndrome—a retrospective study of 26 patients. Clin Exp Rheumatol. 1992;10(3):285–288.

97. Taccetti G, Trappani S, Ermini M, Falcini F. Reactive arthritis triggered by Yersinia enterocolitica: a review of 18 pediatric cases. Clin Exp Rheumatol. 1994;12:681–685.

98. Kanakoudi-Tsakalidou F, Pardalos G, Prastidou-Gertsi P, Kansouzidou-Kanakoudi A, Tsangaropoulou-Stinga H. Persistent or severe course of reactive arthritis following Salmonella enteritidis infection. Scand J Rheumatol. 1998;27:431–436.

99. Hubscher O, Graci Y, Susini J. Aortic insufficiency in Reiter's syndrome of juvenile onset. J Rheumatol. 1948;11:94–95.

100. Van der Linden S, Valkenburg HA, Cats A. Evaluation of diagnostic criteria for ankylosing spondylitis. A proposal for modification of the New York criteria. Arthritis Rheum. 1984;27: 361–368.

101. Burgos-Vargas R, Vázquez-Mellado J, Cassis N, et al. Genuine ankylosing spondylitis in children: a case control study of patients with definite disease according to current adult-onset criteria shortly after onset. J Rheumatol. 1996;23:2140–2147.

102. Marks S, Bennett M, Calin A. The natural history of juvenile ankylosing spondylitis: a case control study of juvenile and adult onset disease. J Rheumatol. 1982;9:739–741.

103. Burgos-Vargas R, Granados-Arriola J. Ankylosing spondylitis and related diseases in the Mexican Mestizo. In: Khan MA, eds. Ankylosing Spondylitis and Related Spondyloarthropathies. Spine: State of the Art Reviews. Philadelphia, Pa: Hanley & Belfus; 1990;4:665–678.

104. Ploski R, Flato B, Vinje O, Maksymowych W, Forre O, Thorsby E. Association to HLA-DRB1*08, HLA-DPB1*0301 and homozygosity for an HLA-linked proteasome gene in juvenile ankylosing spondylitis. Human Immunol. 1995;44:88–96.

105. Maksymowych P, Luong M, Wong C, et al. The LMP2 polymorphism is associated with susceptibility to acute anterior uveitis in HLA-B27 positive juvenile and adult Mexican individuals with AS. Ann Rheum Dis. 1997;56:807–814.

106. Maksymowych WP, Gorodezky C, Olivo A, et al. HLA-DRB1*09 influences the development of disease in Mexican Mestizo with spondyloarthropathy. J Rheumatol. 1997;24:904–907.

107. López-Larrea C, Gonzalez-Roces S, Peña M, et al. Characterization of B27 haplotypes by oligotyping and genomic sequencing in the Mexican Mestizo population with ankylosing spondylitis: juvenile and adult onset. Human Immunol. 1995;43:174–180.

108. Burgos-Vargas R, Vázquez-Mellado J, Gómez-Gordillo M, Katona G. Uveitis of juvenile ankylosing spondylitis. J Rheumatol. 1988; 15:1039.

109. Gore JE, Vizcarronde FE, Rieffel CN. Juvenile ankylosing spondylitis and aortic regurgitation: a case presentation. Pediatrics. 1982;68:423–425.

110. Stamato T, Laxer RM, de Freitas C, et al. Prevalence of cardiac manifestations of juvenile ankylosing spondylitis. Am J Cardiol. 1995;75:744–746.

111. Jiménez-Balderas FJ, García-Rubi D, Pérez-Hinojosa S, et al. Two-dimensional echo Doppler findings in juvenile and adult onset ankylosing spondylitis with long-term disease. Angiology. 2001;52:543–548.

112. Reid GD, Hill RH. Atlantoaxial subluxation in juvenile ankylosing spondylitis. J Pediatr. 1978;93:531.

113. Thompson CH, Khan MA, Bilenker RM. Spontaneous atlanto-axial subluxation as a presenting manifestation of juvenile ankylosing spondylitis. Spine. 1982;7:78–79.

114. Mielants H, Veys EM, Goemaere S, et al. Gut inflammation in the spondyloarthropathies: clinical, radiologic, biologic, and genetic features in relation to the type of histology: a prospective study. J Rheumatol. 1991;18:1542–1551.

115. Lambert JR, Ansell BM, Stephenson E, et al. Psoriatic arthritis in childhood. Clin Rheum Dis. 1976;2:339–352.

116. Shore A, Ansell BM. Juvenile psoriatic arthritis—an analysis of 60 cases. J Pediatr. 1982;100:529–535.

117. Truckenbrodt H, Häfner R. Psoriatic arthritis in childhood. A comparison with subgroups of chronic juvenile arthritis. Z Rheumatol. 1990;49:88–94.

118. Koo E, Balogh ZS, Gomor B. Juvenile psoriatic arthritis. Clin Rheumatol. 1991;10:245–249.

119. Roberton DM, Cabral DA, Malleson PN, Petty RE. Juvenile psoriatic arthritis: followup and evaluation of diagnostic criteria. J Rheumatol. 1996;23:166–170.

120. Hamilton ML, Gladman DD, Shore A, Laxer RM, Silverman ED. Juvenile psoriatic arthritis and HLA antigens. Ann Rheum Dis. 1990;49:694–697.

121. Burbige EJ, Shi-Shunh H, Bayless TM. Clinical manifestations of Crohn's disease in children and adolescents. Pediatrics. 1975;55:866–871.

122. Hamilton JR, Bruce GA, Abdourhaman M, Gall DG. Inflammatory bowel disease in children and adolescents. Adv Pediatr. 1979;26:311–341.

123. Farmer RG, Michener WM. Prognosis of Crohn's disease with onset in childhood or adolescence. Dig Dis Sci. 1979;24:752–757.

124. Ferguson A, Sedgwick DM. Juvenile-onset inflammatory bowel disease: predictors of morbidity and health status in early adult life. J R Coll Physicians. 1994;28:220–227.

125. Lindsley C, Schaller JG. Arthritis associated with inflammatory bowel disease in children. J Pediatr. 1974;84:16.

126. Burgos-Vargas R. Ankylosing tarsitis: clinical features of a unique form of tarsal disease in the juvenile-onset spondyloarthropathies. Arthritis Rheum. 1991;34(suppl):D196.

127. Pacheco-Tena C, Londoño D, Cazarín-Barrientos J, et al. Development of a radiographic index to assess the tarsal involvement in patients with spondyloarthropathies. Ann Rheum Dis. 2002;61:330–304.

128. Ansell BM, Hall MA, Loftus JK, et al. A multicentre pilot study of sulphasalazine in juvenile chronic arthritis. Clin Exp Rheumatol. 1991;9:201–203.

129. Dulgeroglu M. Sulphasalazine in juvenile rheumatoid arthritis. J Rheumatol. 1988;15:881.

130. Joss R, Veys EM, Myelants H, van Werveke S, Goemaere S. Sulfasalazine treatment in juvenile chronic arthritis: an open study. J Rheumatol. 1991;18:880–884.

131. Suschke HJ. Treatment of juvenile spondyloarthritis and reactive arthritis with sulfasalazine. Monatsschr Kinderheilkd. 1992; 140:658–660.

132. Job-Deslandre C, Menkés CJ. Sulfasalazine treatment for juvenile spondyloarthropathy. Rev Rhum Ed Fr. 1993;60:403–405.

133. Burgos-Vargas R, Vazquez-Mellado J, Pacheco-Tena C, Hernandez-Garduno A, Goycochea-Robles MV. A 26 week randomised, double blind, placebo controlled exploratory study of sulfasalazine in juvenile onset spondyloarthropathies. Ann Rheum Dis. 2002;61:941–942.

134. Tse SML, Babyn P, Boros C, et al. Anti-tumor necrosis factor α therapy leads to improvement of both enthesitis and synovitis in children with juvenile spondyloarthropathy. Arthritis Rheum. 2003;48:S125.

135. Horneff G, Burgos-Vargas R. TNF-α antagonists for the treatment of juvenile-onset spondyloarthritides. Clin Exp Rheumatol. 2002;20(suppl 28):S137–S142.

136. Burgos-Vargas R. Juvenile onset spondyloarthropathies: therapeutic aspects. Ann Rheum Dis. 2002;61(suppl 3):33–39.

137. Schmeling H, Horneff G. Infliximab in two patients with juvenile ankylosing spondylitis. Rheumatol Int. 2004;24:173–176.

138. Henrickson M, Reiff A. Prolonged efficacy of etanercept in refractory enthesitis-related arthritis. J Rheumatol. 2004;31:2055–2061.

139. Horneff G, Schmeling H, Moebius D, et al. Efficacy of etanercept in active refractory juvenile spondylarthropathy. Prospective open study of 40 patients. Presented at the Annual Meeting of the American College of Rheumatology, San Antonio, Tx, October 18, 2004.

140. Tse SML, Burgos-Vargas R, Laxer RM. Anti-tumor necrosis factor α blockade in the treatment of juvenile spondyloarthropathy. Arthritis Rheum. 2005;52:2103–2108.

141. Hebestreit H, Muller-Scholden J, Huppertz HI. Aerobic fitness and physical activity in patients with HLA-B27 positive spondyloarthropathy that is inactive or in remission. J Rheumatol. 1998;25:1626–1633.

142. Sochart DH, Porter ML. Long-term results of total hip replacement in young patients who had ankylosing spondylitis. Eighteen to thirty-year results with survivorship analysis. J Bone Joint Surg Am. 1997;79:1181.

143. Burgos-Vargas R, Pacheco-Tena C, Vázquez-Mellado J. The juvenile onset spondyloarthritides. Rationale for clinical evaluation. Best Pract Res Clin Rheumatol. 2002;16: 551–72.

9 Inflammatory Eye Disease in Spondyloarthritis

Michael S. Wertheim, Tammy M. Martin, and James T. Rosenbaum

REFRESHER IN EYE ANATOMY AND BASIC OPHTHALMOLOGY

The eye has three major anatomical layers: the retina, the uvea, and the corneoscleral shell. The uvea is the middle layer and is richly vascularized. This continuous tract is made up of the iris anteriorly, the ciliary body, and the choroid most posteriorly. Inflammation of the uvea, or uveitis, is defined as inflammation of any or all the parts of this layer. Patients with uveitis may also have inflammation of an adjacent structure such as the retina or vitreous humor.

The nomenclature of uveitis is a contentious issue, with ophthalmologists disagreeing on how the anatomical subsets of uveitis should be classified.[1] Some ophthalmologists use the lens as the defining boundary between anterior and posterior uveitis. In this classification inflammation anterior to the lens is classified as anterior uveitis and any inflammation posterior to the lens is classified as posterior uveitis. Other groups define uveitis slightly differently: anterior uveitis or iritis is defined as inflammation of the iris; inflammation of the ciliary body is known as cyclitis; posterior uveitis or choroiditis is defined as inflammation of the choroid; and if all three uveal components are inflamed, the uveitis is described as a panuveitis.[2] We prefer to define uveitis in the former way using the lens as the boundary for anterior and posterior inflammation, because the differential diagnosis for choroiditis is distinct from the differential diagnosis of a leukocyte infiltrate in the vitreous humor.

The corneoscleral shell is made up of the cornea and sclera anteriorly and only the sclera posteriorly. The sclera functions, in part, as the protective casing of the eye. Inflammation of the sclera is known as scleritis and inflammation of the episclera, the layer above the sclera, is known as episcleritis. Spondyloarthritis (SA) is often associated with anterior uveitis and sometimes associated with scleritis, episcleritis, conjunctivitis, or inflammation in the vitreous humor.

The symptoms of uveitis are different depending on the anatomical site of the inflammation. The sudden onset of anterior uveitis or iritis is associated with a painful, red, watering, photophobic eye and often blurred vision. In contrast, posterior uveitis or choroiditis usually presents with blurred vision and the onset of new floaters in association with minimal or no pain. The floaters indicate inflammatory cells and debris in the vitreous jelly of the eye. On slit-lamp biomicroscopic examination the signs of anterior uveitis include anterior chamber cell, hypopyon (Fig. 9.1), keratic precipitates (Fig. 9.2), and iris to lens adhesions known as posterior synechiae (Fig. 9.3). The signs of posterior uveitis include vitreous cell and debris and retinal or choroidal lesions.

Differentiating scleritis from episcleritis can be difficult on clinical examination alone. The presenting symptoms, however, are quite different. Scleritis usually presents with red, inflamed eyes (Fig. 9.4) associated with deep, boring pain often described as a "bruised" sensation. This pain usually wakes patients

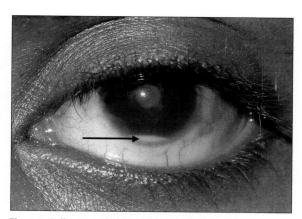

Fig. 9.1 Collection of white cells in the inferior anterior chamber known as a hypopyon (*arrow*) seen in a patient with severe uveitis associated with ReA. (Courtesy of Roger George, MD.)

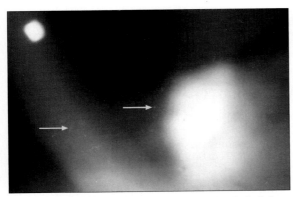

Fig. 9.2 Fine keratic precipitates (KPs) on the endothelial layer of the cornea (*arrows*). These KPs are typical in the uveitides associated with the spondyloarthropathies.

during the night. Episcleritis often presents with sectoral redness. Usually the pain is minimal.

EPIDEMIOLOGY

In the United States uveitis is the cause of 2.8% to 10% of cases of blindness.[3–5] In the largest and most recent study on incidence and prevalence of uveitis, Gritz et al.[6] showed that the incidence of uveitis in a group of patients studied in northern California was 53 per 100,000 person-years and the period prevalence was 115 per 100,000 persons. In the United States approximately 50% of patients with anterior uveitis are HLA-B27 positive.[7] Ninety percent of patients with ankylosing spondylitis (AS) or reactive arthritis (ReA) and anterior uveitis are HLA-B27 positive. Between 20% and 40% of patients who have AS and ReA develop anterior uveitis during the course of their joint disease.[8] Approximately 45% of patients with psoriatic arthropathy (PsA), inflammatory bowel disease (IBD), and anterior uveitis are HLA-B27 positive.[7,9] In a recent study of 175 patients with HLA-B27–associated uveitis it was found that approximately 78% of these patients had extraocular disease that was almost always a SA.[10] The authors of this study recommended that all patients with HLA-B27–associated uveitis be referred for routine rheumatologic examination. Posterior uveitis is rarely associated with HLA-B27 and usually occurs as the residual of a severe episode of anterior and posterior uveitis. Choroiditis is not a feature of the uveitis associated with either AS or ReA.

The incidence of scleritis and episcleritis is far less than that of uveitis. The SAs have each been associated, in varying degrees, with scleritis and episcleritis. The vast majority of occurrences of episcleritis have no systemic association, and the course of the disease is benign and self-limiting. Scleritis has a greater association with systemic disease. Although the most common rheumatologic correlation with scleritis is rheumatoid arthritis, other disease associations include the SAs. In a recent retrospective study, patients with SAs made up 5.8% of all those with scleritis seen at a tertiary referral center.[11] This percentage included IBD (3.3%), AS (1.3%), ReA (0.8%), and PsA (0.4%).[11] It is important to differentiate between scleritis and episcleritis because the treatment, prognosis, and systemic associations differ markedly for these two diseases.

GENETICS

The genetics of uveitis is a subject receiving intense scrutiny. Familial juvenile systemic granulomatosis (also referred to as Blau syndrome or Jabs disease) is a rare, inherited form of uveitis that manifests itself as uveitis, arthritis, and dermatitis.[12–14] The genetic cause of Blau syndrome was discovered in 2001 by Miceli-Richard et al.[15] It was reported that a single amino acid change in a protein known as either nucleotide

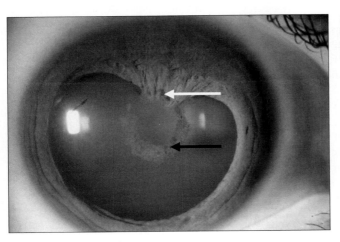

Fig. 9.3 Iris adhesions to the lens. These are known as posterior synechiae (*white arrow*) and pigment deposition on the lens epithelium (*black arrow*) can both be signs of current or previous intraocular inflammation.

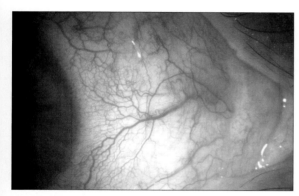

Fig. 9.4 Injection of the scleral vessels in a patient with scleritis.

oligomerization domain 2 (NOD2) or caspase recruitment domain 15 (CARD15) could result in Blau syndrome. Wang et al.[16] further refined this observation in 2002 although in some families with Blau syndrome, a mutation was not detected. Polymorphisms in *CARD15/NOD2* also contribute to susceptibility to Crohn's disease. However, the nucleotide polymorphisms in *CARD15/NOD2* responsible for familial juvenile systemic granulomatosis differ from those associated with Crohn's disease, a granulomatous bowel inflammation.[17,18] *CARD15/NOD2* is located at chromosome 16q12, within a genetic locus that has been implicated in other inflammatory diseases, including psoriasis[19] and systemic lupus erythematosus.[20] More recently, the polymorphisms known to increase the risk of Crohn's disease have not been found to be involved in psoriasis.[21–24] The association of these *CARD15/NOD2* polymorphisms is currently controversial for PsA, with an association found in a Newfoundland cohort but no association in a group of Italian patients.[25,26] It is worth noting that these diseases, including Crohn's disease, have all been associated with uveitis.[27] With this in mind, *CARD15/NOD2* is an excellent candidate gene for scrutiny when one is looking for a genetic predisposition to uveitis. Studies are underway to test the relationship of *CARD15/NOD2* mutations and uveitis. In a small study of 35 patients with Crohn's disease, *CARD15/NOD2* mutations were not detected in the subset of patients with uveitis.[28] This study also indicated that the patients with Crohn's disease and uveitis generally exhibited colonic pathologic changes. The lack of polymorphisms in the patients with uveitis was consistent with published reports that attribute *CARD15/NOD2* polymorphisms to an increased risk of ileal involvement in patients with Crohn's disease.[29,30]

Another approach to studying the genetics of uveitis is to examine the results from studies on patients with spondyloarthropathies (SpAs). These diseases are considered to be multigenic, and it is quite feasible that genetic factors contributing differentially to specific disease manifestations (such as uveitis) will be identified. Genome-wide scans have identified several susceptibility loci for AS[31–33] and for SpAs in general.[34] Recently a genome-wide scan was conducted for acute anterior uveitis (AAU).[35] The most significant linkage was found at the HLA locus, but two other non-HLA regions were demonstrated to have linkage to AAU (chromosomes 1q25-1q31 and 9p21-9p24). These data were directly compared with the AS genome-wide scan conducted by the North American Spondylitis Consortium.[33] The linkage at 1q25-1q31 overlapped with a susceptibility region identified for AS. However, the region on the short arm of chromosome 9 was much stronger for AAU (logarithm of odds [LOD] score 3.72) than that observed for AS (LOD score <1.0).[35] Therefore, this may be the first identification of a uveitis-specific susceptibility locus. A "suggestive" LOD score was obtained for a region overlapping 9p21–9p24 in an Oxford AS cohort.[32]

PATHOGENESIS

As with all inflammatory diseases, pathologic changes are thought to occur in genetically susceptible individuals after exposure to some environmental trigger. The primary feature of uveitis is the infiltration of inflammatory cells into the uveal tissue. The mechanisms involved in uveitis or any other tissue-specific inflammatory manifestation include the activation of monocytes, lymphocytes, granulocytes, antigen-presenting cells, and vascular endothelial cells. These functions are driven in large part by interleukins, chemokines, and adhesion molecules. The environmental trigger may be unknown, a pathogen, or a self-antigen that has become immunogenic (i.e., tolerance has been lost). To make things more complicated (or interesting, depending upon your point of view) a pathogen may express an antigen that mimics a self-antigen. The form of uveitis associated with SA is thought to involve the acquired immune response and be largely T-cell mediated. A role for specific antigens in the initiation of uveitis is generally accepted. The subsequent recruitment of inflammatory cells or recurrent inflammation may not be an antigen-specific response.

To characterize the pathogenesis of uveitis, several avenues of investigation have been explored in humans. These usually involve examination of peripheral blood cells, analysis of proteins in serum, and analysis of cells and proteins in aqueous humor or vitreous from patients with uveitis during active inflammation. A sampling of studies performed on patients with uveitis indicate increased levels of inflammatory cytokines in serum (interleukin [IL]-2, interferon [IFN]-γ, IL-8, and migration inhibitory factor [MIF]), aqueous humor (IL-2, IFN-γ, IL-12, and MIF), and vitreous (IL-12 and MIF).[36–41] In addition to inflammatory cytokines, some chemokines have been implicated in uveitis. For instance, the T-cell–attracting chemokine IFN-γ–inducible protein-10 (IP-10, systematic name CXCL10) is up-regulated in aqueous humor[42] and soluble inter-cellular adhesion molecule-1 (ICAM-1) is increased in serum.[43] Furthermore, the regulatory cytokine, IL-10, is decreased in the aqueous humor[44] of patients with uveitis. The availability of monoclonal antibodies triggered several studies in the 1980s demonstrating that not only were T cells present in aqueous humor but also their numbers t were skewed toward CD4+ T cells (compared with CD8+ T cells); these cells were activated, and the presence of these T cells correlated with disease activity.[45] More refined techniques confirmed these earlier observations and demonstrated that in some studies the majority of T cells in the aqueous humor expressed "memory" markers as well as the Fas antigen, which is involved in apoptosis.[46] In addition, some studies indicated that the infiltrating T cells are characteristic of a predominant Th1 immune response in patients with uveitis.[47]

The investigation of patients with uveitis to determine pathogenic mechanisms is limited because of the risk of collecting biopsy specimens from parts of the eye. Therefore, the analysis of animal models of uveitis has been an important avenue of research. The animal models of uveitis used most commonly are described briefly in the following. However, even though these models have been widely used for uveitis research, none of them is a perfect representation of human disease.

One of the most-studied animal models of uveitis is endotoxin-induced uveitis (EIU), which is typically elicited in either mice or rats but can be induced in several other animal species. In this model, a systemic exposure to bacterial lipopolysaccharide (LPS) activates a leukocytic response that manifests as bilateral uveitis.[48] The inflammation is apparent by 6 hours, generally peaks at 18 to 24 hours, and subsides after 48 hours. The infiltration primarily involves the anterior uveal tract with cells and protein evident in the aqueous humor. The majority of the cellular infiltrates are neutrophils. Our laboratory has demonstrated that uveitis can be induced in rats by infection with *Salmonella* or *Yersinia*.[49] Transgenic rats that express HLA-B27, however, are not more susceptible to this disease.

Another closely related, but less often studied, model is induced by muramyl dipeptide (MDP) in rabbits. MDP is a subunit of peptidoglycan, a component of bacterial cell walls found in both gram-negative and gram-positive organisms. Like LPS, MDP causes a disruption of the blood-aqueous barrier and vascular leakage resulting in increased aqueous humor protein levels.[50] When MDP is administered systemically, the cellular infiltrate is predominantly anterior, is composed of neutrophils, peaks approximately 4 hours after injection, and resolves within 1 to 2 days.[50,51] Uveitis may also occur when MDP is injected directly into the vitreous of rabbits.[52] These two models of acute uveitis (EIU and MDP-induced uveitis) represent activation of the innate immune response and are self-limiting.

A series of animal models involve immunizing animals (usually rats, sometimes mice, and rarely monkeys) against various antigens that result in uveal inflammation. These models involve the acquired immune response, have a time course measured in days to weeks (not hours as in EIU), and are mediated by antigen-specific T cells. As an alternative to immunization, uveitis can be induced with the adoptive transfer of activated, antigen-specific T cells. In all of these models, some species are more susceptible than others, and, within a species, certain inbred strains are more susceptible than others.

Experimental autoimmune uveoretinitis is induced by immunization with different retinal antigens, such as S-antigen, rhodopsin, or interphotoreceptor retinoid-binding protein.[53] Inflammatory cells are typically found in the anterior uveal tract (aqueous humor, iris, and ciliary body), the vitreous, the choroid, and the retina. Because the retinal photoreceptor cells are the major targets of the elicited pathogenic T cells, the retina can be destroyed in animals when inflammation is severe. Because of the posterior involvement, this is not a very representative model of the anterior, recurrent uveitis seen in patients with SA.

Experimental autoimmune anterior uveitis was first described in 1991 and later renamed experimental melanin-induced uveitis when it became apparent that the specific uveitogenic antigens in the heterogenous milieu that was used to immunize animals were melanin-associated compounds.[54,55] The pathogenic T cells target the melanocytes, which reside in uveal tissues. The inflammation is bilateral and anterior, with little retinal involvement. Recently, the antigenic compound responsible for this model has been identified as a particular proteolytic fragment of type I collagen.[56] This fragment of type I collagen is uvea specific presumably because of the unique post-translational glycosylation modifications of the collagen molecule that occur in uveal tissues.

Another model of anterior uveitis occurs in conjunction with experimental autoimmune encephalomyelitis (EAE), a model of multiple sclerosis.[57] EAE is induced by immunization with myelin basic protein, an antigen found on myelinated nerves. In EAE, the central nervous system is targeted with inflammation and damage to the spinal cord. Animals develop a progressive paralysis that is self-limiting and may have a relapsing-remitting course, depending on the experimental conditions. Uveitis may be associated with EAE because myelinated neurons are also found in the uveal tissue, so this becomes a target of the myelin-specific pathogenic T cells. Optic neuritis has also been described in the EAE model.

Uveitis can also be induced by expressing a foreign antigen in the eye, such as hen egg lysozyme, in a mouse whose T cells recognize this antigen.[58]

Multiorgan autoimmunity has been described in mice and humans who fail to express an important thymic transcription factor known as AIRE. Retinitis can be a component of this disease.[59]

CLINICAL FEATURES

Anterior scleritis presents with symptoms of deep, boring ocular pain. The eye is beet red on examination (see Fig. 9.4) and tender to palpation. Scleritis is most commonly anterior but posterior inflammation may also occur. With posterior inflammation the patient may complain of decreased and distorted vision. Posterior scleritis is at times difficult to diagnose, because the eye is often not red in appearance. Diagnosis is usually reached by combining history, ophthalmic examination, and ultrasound imaging of the eye, which shows a thickened posterior sclera (Fig. 9.5). Episcleritis usually presents with minimal or no eye pain and the redness is usually sectoral and confined to the superficial layer (episclera) of the eye.

Conjunctivitis is seen most commonly as part of ReA and rarely as part of the other SAs. ReA involves other mucosal structures as well and may manifest as oral ulcers or penile lesions. The conjunctivitis seen in ReA is classified as a mucopurulent, papillary conjunctivitis and, therefore, can be easily confused with an infectious conjunctivitis or "pink eye."

The clinical courses of uveitis seen in AS and ReA are similar and often differ from the course of eye disease associated with IBD and PsA. We outline these two distinct groups below.

Uveitis Associated with Ankylosing Spondylitis and Reactive Arthritis

The presentation of uveitis associated with AS and ReA is very consistent. Typically the uveitis is anterior and unilateral. The attacks have a sudden onset, are episodic, and have a limited duration, typically less than 2 months.[9] Symptoms include pain, redness, watering, photophobia, and a variable degree of visual loss. Intraocular pressure (IOP) is characteristically lower in the affected eye. This lowering of pressure is in contrast to the typical presentation of another form of anterior uveitis, that due to herpes simplex. The inflammation usually resolves with appropriate therapy within a few months. Recurrent inflammation is common and may affect the contralateral eye. Inflammation in both eyes at the same time is very unusual in AS- and ReA-associated uveitis. Ocular inflammation does not necessarily occur when there is a flare-up of joint disease.

Calin's group[60] studied the relationship between AS and uveitis to try to determine whether uveitis could be used as a prognostic indicator. They compared the relationship between rheumatologic and ophthalmic disease in 1331 patients with AS. A group of patients with AS who had more than five attacks of uveitis was compared to a group of patients with AS and without eye disease. It was found that there is no significant difference between the groups when the severity and duration of rheumatologic disease were compared with the clinical assessment scales available in 1990.[60] However, a subsequent, larger study led by the Calin group demonstrated that AS was significantly more severe as measured by the Bath Ankylosing Spondylitis Radiology Index (BASRI) in patients with AS and uveitis.[61] Therefore, it was concluded that uveitis is a risk factor for a more severe course of AS.

Uveitis Associated with Inflammatory Bowel Disease and Psoriatic Arthritis

Although the SAs have some clinical overlap, the clinical presentation of the uveitis entities are most often distinct when IBD and PsA are compared with AS and ReA. The uveitis in the group with the former can have an insidious onset. Typically it is bilateral and may be anterior or posterior. The duration of the attacks is typically longer and may be more chronic in nature compared with those in the AS and ReA group.[9]

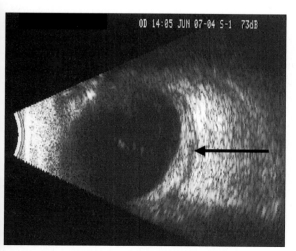

Fig. 9.5 B-scan ultrasound of the right eye showing thickened sclera and fluid behind the sclera (*arrow*) in a patient with posterior scleritis. This is called the T-sign.

Symptoms overlap with those in the AS and ReA group and include pain, redness, watering, photophobia, and decreased vision. Vitreous inflammation will produce floaters or haze. IOP is also characteristically lower in the affected eye. The inflammation is usually chronic and may take many months to resolve. At times the uveitis associated with IBD and PsA may present identically to that associated with AS and ReA.

Bernstein et al.[62] have shown that uveitis was the most common extraintestinal manifestation noted in their cohort of patients with IBD.[62] Crohn's disease is far more likely to present with eye disease than ulcerative colitis.[9] Approximately 5% of patients with IBD develop uveitis during their life, and patients who develop uveitis have an increased risk of developing episcleritis and scleritis.[9]

Queiro et al.[63] showed that the best predictive factors to determine whether patients with psoriasis would develop uveitis are bilateral sacroiliitis, syndesmophyte formation, and a positive HLA-DR13 antigen. This was a small retrospective study of 71 patients with psoriasis. Uveitis is associated with PsA but is not clearly associated with psoriasis itself.[64]

Juvenile Spondyloarthritis and Inflammatory Eye Disease

After juvenile chronic arthritis (JCA), juvenile ankylosing spondylitis (JAS) is the most common juvenile arthritis that presents with uveitis.[65] JAS most typically affects boys in their first decade.[65] As with its adult counterpart approximately 90% of patients are positive for HLA-B27.[65,66] The initial manifestation of ocular disease is a symptomatic, sudden onset, unilateral iritis. Kanski and Shun-Shin[65] suggested that a routine ocular examination in patients with JAS is unnecessary because all attacks of uveitis are symptomatic. Juvenile reactive arthritis is rare and is usually associated with *Salmonella* or *Shigella* infection.

Juvenile psoriatic arthritis tends to affect girls more than boys, and there is no association between any HLA antigen and the eye disease.[65] The course of this uveitis is similar to that of the adult form in that it is more insidious in onset, is bilateral, and has a chronic course. Patients with psoriasis and early-onset arthritis who are antinuclear antigen positive seem to have the same risk of chronic anterior uveitis as those with JCA.[65]

The clinical picture seen in patients with classic uveitis associated with JCA compared with that seen with the other causes of juvenile uveitis is distinct. The uveitis in patients with JCA is usually chronic and anterior. The inflammation is usually bilateral and is characteristically asymptomatic in the early stages of the disease. Therefore, close follow-up of these patients is critical to their long-term care and visual prognosis.

Kanski and Shun-Shin[65] concluded that there is no relationship between the activity of arthritis and iritis. The incidence of cataract, glaucoma, and band keratopathy is much higher in patients with JCA compared with that in children with uveitis associated with another underlying etiology.[65,66]

Ocular Complications Associated with Inflammatory Eye Disease

The potential complications associated with uveitis and scleritis are similar in all forms of SA-associated inflammatory eye disease. Complications can be divided into disease associated and treatment associated. Uveitis can cause cataract formation (Figs. 9.6 and 9.7), decreased IOP (hypotony), iris adhesions to the lens (called posterior synechiae), pigment deposits on the lens (see Fig. 9.3), and macular edema. Cataract formation is common with chronic inflammation but rare with the limited inflammation of HLA-B27–associated uveitis. Band keratopathy (Fig. 9.8) is common in the uveitis associated with JCA but rarely found in association with AS. Glaucoma, i.e., an elevation of IOP that results in damage to the optic nerve, is rare with HLA-B27–associated iritis. Posterior synechiae can form over 360 degrees such that the flow of aqueous humor is impeded. Pressure from the blocked flow of aqueous pushes the iris forward, resulting in a condition called iris bombe. This is a medical emergency that is usually treated by using a laser to create a hole in the iris (an iridotomy) to allow the aqueous humor to flow. The mainstay of treatment of anterior segment inflammation is topical or local corticosteroids (discussed in the next section). The major side effects of topical steroid drops or local steroid injection to the eye are cataract formation, raised IOP, poor wound healing, reduced

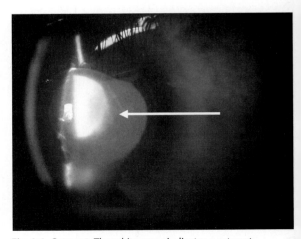

Fig. 9.6 Cataract. The *white arrow* indicates a cataract (opacification of the lens) due to inflammation in a patient with ReA associated uveitis. (Courtesy of Roger George, MD.)

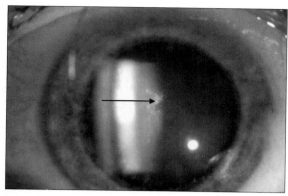

Fig. 9.7 Posterior subcapsular cataract. This is a lens opacity forming on the back surface of the lens, commonly seen in chronic ocular inflammation and with chronic topical steroid application to the eye.

response to an infection, and allergy. Although cataract is correctable by small incision surgery, some of the other potential complications from inflammation and topical or local steroid treatment may be sight threatening.

Treatment

Treatment of inflammatory eye disease can be divided into topical, local, and systemic therapy. Topical therapy for anterior uveitis consists of corticosteroid drops, usually in the form of prednisolone acetate 1% together with a cycloplegic (dilating drop) to prevent the formation of posterior synechiae (see Fig. 9.3) and for pain relief. The anterior uveitis associated with SA typically resolves promptly with the use of steroid drops. Use of the steroid drops is usually tapered over a few weeks to months depending on the individual response.

Local corticosteroid injections around the eye can be an adjunct to therapy. Triamcinolone acetate is the

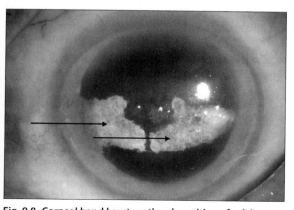

Fig. 9.8 Corneal band keratopathy, deposition of calcium under the corneal epithelium (arrows). This sign is most commonly found in chronic eye inflammation.

steroid most commonly used. The indications for using periocular injections include inflammation that is not responding to topical steroid application, posterior signs of inflammation (macular edema), and previous success using local steroid treatment in specific patients. An intraocular injection involves more risk than a periocular injection. These risks include infections, hemorrhage, retinal detachment, cataract from lens trauma, glaucoma, and sterile inflammation. Accordingly an intraocular triamcinolone injection is almost never indicated for B27-associated iritis.

Oral medication can be used in the treatment of scleritis, episcleritis, and uveitis. Scleritis and episcleritis often respond well to nonsteroidal anti-inflammatory drugs (NSAIDs). Uveitis does not respond to NSAIDs, and the next step in treatment beyond local therapy for this disease and as well as for nonresponsive scleritis is immunosuppressive therapy. This includes the use of oral prednisone, the antimetabolites (methotrexate, azathioprine, or mycophenolate mofetil), T-cell inhibitors (cyclosporine or tacrolimus), and the alkylating agents (chlorambucil and cyclophosphamide). The vast majority of patients with uveitis associated with either AS or ReA have self-limited disease that rarely requires prolonged oral treatment. Oral prednisone is the initial immunosuppressive drug of choice. The recommended initial dose is 1 mg/kg/day with a maximum dose of approximately 60 to 80 mg/day.[67] Therapy is rarely needed for more than 2 weeks. It is rare for the uveitis associated with AS or ReA to enter a chronic phase. The use of oral corticosteroids is unusual, and the use of an additional immunosuppressive drug for this form of uveitis is virtually unheard of in our practice. Occasional patients with uveitis associated with IBD or PsA, however, have a chronic uveitis that requires a steroid-sparing medication. The next immunosuppressive used is usually either an antimetabolite or a T-cell inhibitor. In our practice, methotrexate (oral or subcutaneous) or cyclosporine is the drug of choice. The initial dose of methotrexate is usually about 15 mg/wk with a maximum dose of approximately 25 mg/wk.[67] Patients can take folic acid concurrently with the methotrexate to reduce mucosal toxicity. Cyclosporine is usually started at 2.5 to 5.0 mg/kg/day in a divided dose.[67] These drugs are often combined with a tapering dose of prednisone. If the inflammation is not controlled by this regimen, the use of mycophenolate mofetil (500–1500 mg twice a day) or an alkylating agent (cyclophosphamide [2–3 mg/kg/day] or chlorambucil [0.1–0.2 mg/kg/day]), or a combination of an antimetabolite and a T-cell inhibitor should be considered.[67]

Preventing recurrent attacks is an important, yet difficult, step in the management of inflammatory eye disease. Several studies have been performed to

54. Broekhuyse RM, Kuhlmann ED, Winkens HJ, Van Vugt AH. Experimental autoimmune anterior uveitis (EAAU), a new form of experimental uveitis. I. Induction by a detergent-insoluble, intrinsic protein fraction of the retinal pigment epithelium. Exp Eye Res. 1991;52:465–474.

55. Chan CC, Hikita N, Dastgheib K, Whitcup SM, Gery I, Nussenblatt RB. Experimental melanin-protein-induced uveitis in the Lewis rat. Immunopathologic processes. Ophthalmology. 1994;101:1275–1280.

56. Bora NS, Sohn JH, Kang SG, et al. Type I collagen is the autoantigen in experimental autoimmune anterior uveitis. J Immunol. 2004;17219:7086–7094.

57. Adamus G, Amundson D, Vainiene M, et al. Myelin basic protein specific T-helper cells induce experimental anterior uveitis. J Neurosci Res. 1996;44:513–518.

58. Lai JC, Lobanoff MC, Fukushima A, et al. Uveitis induced by lymphocytes sensitized against a transgenically expressed lens protein. Invest Ophthalmol Vis Sci. 1999;4019:2735–2739.

59. Anderson MS, Venanzi ES, Klein L, et al. Projection of an immunological self shadow within the thymus by the aire protein. Science. 15 2002;298:1395–1401.

60. Edmunds L, Elswood J, Calin A. New light on uveitis in ankylosing spondylitis. J Rheumatol. 1991;18:50–52.

61. Brophy S, Pavy S, Lewis P, et al. Inflammatory eye, skin, and bowel disease in spondyloarthritis: genetic, phenotypic, and environmental factors. J Rheumatol. 2001;2819:2667–2673.

62. Bernstein CN, Blanchard JF, Rawsthorne P, Yu N. The prevalence of extraintestinal diseases in inflammatory bowel disease: a population-based study. Am J Gastroenterol. 2001;96:1116–1122.

63. Queiro R, Torre JC, Belzunegui J, et al. Clinical features and predictive factors in psoriatic arthritis-related uveitis. Semin Arthritis Rheum. 2002;31:264–270.

64. Paiva ES, Macaluso DC, Edwards A, Rosenbaum JT. Characterisation of uveitis in patients with psoriatic arthritis. Ann Rheum Dis. 2000;59:67–70.

65. Kanski JJ, Shun-Shin GA. Systemic uveitis syndromes in childhood: an analysis of 340 cases. Ophthalmology. 1984;9119:1247–1252.

66. Burgos-Vargas R, Petty RE. Juvenile ankylosing spondylitis. Rheum Dis Clin North Am. 1992;18:123–142.

67. Jabs DA, Rosenbaum JT, Foster CS, et al. Guidelines for the use of immunosuppressive drugs in patients with ocular inflammatory disorders: recommendations of an expert panel. Am J Ophthalmol. 2000;130:492–513.

68. Benitez-Del-Castillo JM, Garcia-Sanchez J, Iradier T, Banares A. Sulfasalazine in the prevention of anterior uveitis associated with ankylosing spondylitis. Eye. 2000;14(Pt 3A):340–343.

69. Munoz-Fernandez S, Hidalgo V, Fernandez-Melon J, et al. Sulfasalazine reduces the number of flares of acute anterior uveitis over a one-year period. J Rheumatol. 2003;30:1277–1279.

70. Fries W, Giofre MR, Catanoso M, Lo Gullo R. Treatment of acute uveitis associated with Crohn's disease and sacroiliitis with infliximab. Am J Gastroenterol. 2002;97:499–500.

71. Munoz-Fernandez S, Hidalgo V, Fernandez-Melon J, Schlincker A, Martin-Mola E. Effect of infliximab on threatening panuveitis in Behçet's disease. Lancet. 2001;358:1644.

72. Murphy CC, Ayliffe WH, Booth A, Makanjuola D, Andrews PA, Jayne D. Tumor necrosis factor alpha blockade with infliximab for refractory uveitis and scleritis. Ophthalmology. 2004; 111:352–356.

73. Sfikakis PP, Theodossiadis PG, Katsiari CG, Kaklamanis P, Markomichelakis NN. Effect of infliximab on sight-threatening panuveitis in Behçet's disease. Lancet. Jul 28 2001;358: 295–296.

74. Smith JR, Levinson RD, Holland GN, et al. Differential efficacy of tumor necrosis factor inhibition in the management of inflammatory eye disease and associated rheumatic disease. Arthritis Rheum. 2001;45:252–257.

75. Suhler EB, Smith JR, Lauer AK, et al. A prospective trial of infliximab therapy for patients with refractory uveitis: interim analysis of safety and efficacy outcomes. Invest Ophthalmol Vis Sci. 2004;Session 403 (ARVO E-abstract 3370).

76. El-Shabrawi Y, Hermann J. Anti-tumor necrosis factor-alpha therapy with infliximab as an alternative to corticosteroids in the treatment of human leukocyte antigen B27-associated acute anterior uveitis. Ophthalmology. 2002;10919:2342–2346.

77. Nussenblatt RB, Thompson DJ, Li Z, et al. Humanized anti-interleukin-2 (IL-2) receptor alpha therapy: long-term results in uveitis patients and preliminary safety and activity data for establishing parameters for subcutaneous administration. J Autoimmun. 2003;21:283–293.

78. Jaffe GJ, Ben-Nun J, Guo H, Dunn JP, Ashton P. Fluocinolone acetonide sustained drug delivery device to treat severe uveitis. Ophthalmology. 2000;10719:2024–2033.

79. Jaffe G. Fluocinolone acetonide intravitreal implant for uveitis affecting the posterior segment of the eye. Invest Ophthalmol Vis Sci. 2004;Session 403 (ARVO E-abstract 3369).

10

Epidemiology of Ankylosing Spondylitis and Related Spondyloarthropathies

Nurullah Akkoc and Muhammad Asim Khan

INTRODUCTION

The term *epidemiology* in the traditional sense means the study of the distribution of a disease and the risk factors for its development. In a broader definition, it may also include the scientific methods used to diagnose, analyze, and prevent or control a health problem. The interpretation of any kind of epidemiologic data depends on the nature of the criteria used for case definition, and it is of critical importance when one compares the occurrence rates observed in various studies.

CASE DEFINITION

The diagnosis of ankylosing spondylitis (AS) and related spondyloarthropathies (SpAs) is based on clinical features.[1–6] Although chronic inflammatory back pain and stiffness are usually the first or presenting manifestations of AS, alone they are of limited clinical value in disease diagnosis because a single clinical feature is not sufficient to make the diagnosis. There is no specific diagnostic laboratory test, and a normal erythrocyte sedimentation rate and/or serum C-reactive protein level do not exclude the presence of disease. Radiographic evidence of sacroiliitis is the best nonclinical indicator of the presence of AS and is the most consistent finding. The probability of the disease presence is enhanced when one or more additional features that are typical of AS/SpAs are present. Thus, different sets of classification criteria for AS/SpAs have been established, and they have also been used for diagnostic purposes, although there are as yet no validated *diagnostic* criteria.[7–9]

The first criteria set for the classification of AS was developed at the rheumatic disease conferences in Rome in 1961 (Table 10.1),[7] and it could be considered as epidemiologically useful, because it was possible to make a diagnosis of AS without a radiologic examination of the sacroiliac joints. However, the sensitivity of the clinical components "pain and stiffness in the thoracic region" and "history of evidence of iritis or its sequelae" was found to be quite low when evaluated in a cohort of 27 Pima Indians with definite AS.[10] This led to the development of the New York criteria in 1966, which required the presence of roentgenographic evidence of sacroiliitis (Table 10.2).[8]

In a study including relatives of patients with AS and population control subjects, the New York criterion of "a history of or presence of pain at the dorsolumbar junction or in the lumbar spine" was found to have no discriminating value owing to a lack of specificity.[9] In the same study, the sensitivity of the chest expansion ≤2.5 cm criterion was also found to be very low (15%). Thus, a modification of the New York criteria was proposed with the substitution of the dorsolumbar pain

TABLE 10.1 THE ROME (1961) CLASSIFICATION CRITERIA FOR AS[7]
A. Clinical criteria
Low back pain and stiffness for more than 3 months, not relieved by rest
Pain and stiffness in the thoracic region
Limited motion in the lumbar region
Limited chest expansion
History of evidence of iritis or its sequelae
B. Radiologic criteria
Bilateral sacroiliitis
Definite AS is diagnosed if 4 of 5 clinical criteria are present or bilateral sacroiliitis is associated with any single clinical criterion

TABLE 10.2 THE NEW YORK (1966) CLASSIFICATION CRITERIA FOR AS[8]

A. Clinical criteria

Limitation of motion of the lumbar spine in all three planes (anterior flexion, lateral flexion, and extension)

A history of pain or the presence of pain at the dorsolumbar junction or in the lumbar spine

Limitation of chest expansion to 1 inch (2.5 cm) or less, measured at the level of the 4th intercostal space

B. Radiologic criterion: sacroiliitis (grading on a 0 to 4 scale)

(Normal radiograph of the sacroiliac joints was graded as 0, suspicious changes as grade 1; minimal abnormality as grade 2, small areas showing erosion or sclerosis but no alteration in joint width as grade 3. Unequivocal abnormality, moderate or advanced sacroiliitis with one or more erosions, sclerosis, widening, narrowing or partial or complete ankylosis was considered as grade 4.)

Definite AS if:

a) Bilateral grade 3–4 sacroiliitis in the presence of at least one clinical criterion; or

b) Unilateral grade 3–4 or bilateral grade 2 sacroiliitis with clinical criterion 1 or with both clinical criteria 2 and 3.

Probable ankylosing spondylitis if:

Bilateral grade 3–4 sacroiliitis is present without any clinical criterion

TABLE 10.3 THE MODIFIED NEW YORK (1984) CLASSIFICATION CRITERIA FOR AS[9]

A. Clinical criteria

Low back pain and stiffness for at least 3 months, which improves with exercise, but is not relieved by rest

Limited lumbar spinal motion in sagittal (sideways) and frontal (forward and backward) planes

Chest expansion decreased relative to normal values corrected for age and sex

B. Radiologic criteria

Bilateral sacroiliitis grade 2 to 4

Unilateral sacroiliitis grade 3 or 4

Definite AS, if one radiologic criterion is associated with at least one clinical criterion

Probable AS, if three clinical criteria are present or one radiologic criterion is present without any clinical criterion

TABLE 10.4 AMOR CRITERIA FOR SPONDYLOARTHROPATHY[19]

Parameters*	Scoring
A. Clinical symptoms or past history of	
1. Lumbar or dorsal pain at night or morning stiffness of lumbar or dorsal region	1
2. Asymmetric oligoarthritis	2
3. Buttock pain if alternate buttock pain	1 2
4. Sausage-like toe or digit	2
5. Heel pain or other well-defined enthesitis	2
6. Iritis	2
7. Nongonococcal urethritis or cervicitis within 1 month before the onset of arthritis	1
8. Acute diarrhea within 1 month before the onset of arthritis	1
9. Psoriasis, balanitis, or inflammatory bowel disease (IBD) (ulcerative colitis or Crohn's disease)	2
B. Radiologic findings	
10. Sacroiliitis (bilateral grade 2 or unilateral grade 3)	2
C. Genetic background	
11. Presence of HLA-B27 or family history of ankylosing spondylitis, reactive arthritis, uveitis, psoriasis, or IBD	2
D. Response to treatment	
12. Clear-cut improvement within 48 hours after NSAID intake or rapid relapse of the pain after their discontinuation	2

*A patient is considered to have a spondyloarthropathy if the sum is ≥ 6.

criterion by a slightly modified Rome pain criterion.[9] Moreover, the criterion of ≤2.5 cm chest expansion was changed to limitation of chest expansion compared with age- and sex-adjusted normal values (Table 10.3).[9] The modified New York criteria set has since then been commonly used in clinical practice as well as in several studies.

Sacroiliitis is the hallmark of AS and is a requisite for the diagnosis under the original or the modified New York criteria. However, the assessment of sacroiliac radiographs is not always easy. Radiologic sacroiliitis can easily be missed because of the complex anatomy of the sacroiliac joints; the undulating and oblique articular surfaces make it hard to image these joints on conventional pelvic (anteroposterior) radiographs. Moreover, there is considerable intra- and inter-observer variation in the diagnosis of sacroiliitis on conventional radiographs,[11,12] and formal training in reading plain sacroiliac films does not help in rectifying this problem.[13] This variation may account for some of the disagreement between the various estimates of occurrence of AS.

The radiographic diagnosis is further complicated by the slow evolution of radiologic changes in many patients. Thus, sacroiliac radiographs may be normal in the early phase of the disease[1,3,4,6] and in some patients for many years.[14–18] Therefore, because of the frequent absence of radiographic sacroiliitis in the early stages of the disease and the availability of better methods of imaging, such as magnetic resonance imaging, new, improved criteria are needed, especially for early diagnosis and classification.

Classification criteria that encompass the entire spectrum of SpAs, including the undifferentiated forms, have been developed. These are the Amor criteria (Table 10.4)[19] and the European Spondyloarthropathy Study Group (ESSG) criteria (Table 10.5).[20] In both sets of criteria, the existence of sacroiliitis is included as a component but not as a precondition for diagnosis. These criteria have been validated in various population groups, and their sensitivity and specificity generally exceed 85%.[21–26] However, in a recent study from Spain, only 46.6% of patients who satisfied the ESSG criteria at entry were found by their rheumatologists to have SpA after 5 years of follow-up.[27] The figure for the Amor's criteria was better at 76.5%. Thus, a new approach has been proposed for early diagnosis of axial SpA in patients with inflammatory back pain who lack radiographic sacroiliitis.[28]

DISEASE OCCURRENCE

There are two approaches to define the occurrence of a disease in a defined population: *incidence* and *prevalence*. The incidence of a disease is the number of new cases that occur within a given period of time. Annual incidence of a disease typically refers to incidence per 100,000 people. The concept of prevalence is much simpler, because it is the proportion of diseased individuals in a population.

Occurrences of a disease in the community may be identified through community surveys (community-based studies) or health records (hospital-based studies). Community-based surveys are expensive and very difficult to accomplish for estimating annual incidence rates with any statistical precision, because of the necessity of studying large populations. On the other hand, reliable

TABLE 10.5 THE EUROPEAN SPONDYLOARTHROPATHY STUDY GROUP CRITERIA FOR THE CLASSIFICATION OF SPA[20]	
Criterion	**Definition**
Inflammatory spinal pain	At least four of the following five components: At least 3 months in duration
	Onset before 45 years of age
	Insidious (gradual) onset
	Improved by exercise
	Associated with morning spinal stiffness
OR	
Synovitis	Past or present asymmetric arthritis, or arthritis predominantly in the lower limbs
AND any one (or more) of the following:	
Positive family history	First- or second-degree relatives with AS, psoriasis, acute iritis, ReA, or inflammatory bowel disease
Psoriasis	Past or present, diagnosed by a physician
Inflammatory bowel disease	Past or present ulcerative colitis or Crohn's disease, diagnosed by a physician and confirmed by radiography or endoscopy
Alternate buttock pain	Past or present pain alternating between the two buttocks
Enthesitis	Past or present spontaneous pain or tenderness at examination of the site of the insertion—the Achilles tendon or plantar fascia
Acute diarrhea or urethritis or cervicitis	Episode of diarrhea occurring within 1 month before onset of arthritis
	Nongonococcal urethritis or cervicitis occurring within 1 month before onset of arthritis
Radiographic sacroiliitis	Grades are 0 = normal; 1 = possible; 2 = minimal; 3 = moderate; 4 = completely fused (ankylosed)

estimates of prevalence (the proportion of diseased individuals in a population) can be made with a relatively modest sample size.

There are several problems in performing studies to investigate the occurrence of rheumatic diseases.[29] The community-based prevalence studies are feasible and are more likely to yield all the occurrences in the population compared with the hospital-based studies. However, reliability of community-based studies depends largely on the response rate (response bias). Generally speaking, individuals who are older than age 45 and belong to an upper socioeconomic class and women are more likely to respond if they have the disease under investigation.[30] Young men are less willing to participate in population-based studies[31]; this may be important when one studies the occurrence of AS, which is more prevalent in this group.

Case ascertainment through the review of medical records of the clinical facilities where all the patients in the target population are likely to be seen (hospital-based studies) can be done retrospectively or prospectively.[32] Although it is less costly, the accuracy of this approach is highly dependent on the quality of the records. Moreover, standardization of diagnosis and case verification are difficult to achieve, particularly in retrospective studies, because of the differences in the use of diagnostic tools over time and among physicians. There are several other problems and biases. For example, patients with mild cases may not get referred to the

secondary or tertiary centers (referral bias), or some patients may prefer to seek treatment outside of the recruitment area or from other health care providers and will thus be missed, the so-called "left censorship."

Incidence

There have been only a few reports of the incidence of AS, and these studies are summarized in Table 10.6.[25,33–38] A U.S. study from Rochester, the main city in Olmsted County, Minnesota, was based on medical records and performed in a population that at the time of the study was 99% white and mostly of Scandinavian descent.[33] The case ascertainment was based on the presence of chronic back pain (of at least 3 months' duration), absence of diagnostic criteria for other inflammatory arthropathies or other causes of chronic back pain, and the presence of roentgenographically documented sacroiliitis. The overall annual incidence, adjusted for age and sex, was 6.6 per 100,000 white general population between 1935 and 1973, before human leukocyte antigen (HLA)-B27 typing became available for clinical use.[33] In a subsequent analysis covering the period between 1935 and 1989 an overall annual incidence of 7.3 per 100,000 white population of Rochester was reported, despite the use of different case definition criteria (the modified New York criteria) (Table 10.6). Interestingly, age- and sex-adjusted rates of both studies were remarkably similar and remained quite stable over the period covered by

TABLE 10.6 ANNUAL INCIDENCE RATES OF AS PER 100,000 POPULATION AND MEAN AGES AT ONSET OF DISEASE SYMPTOMS AND AT DIAGNOSIS

Population	Age	Diagnosis	Average Annual Incidence Males	Average Annual Incidence Females	Overall Incidence Adjusted by Age and Sex	Mean Age at Onset of Symptoms	Mean Age at Diagnosis
United States (Rochester, MN)[33]	All ages	Clinical/x-ray	10.7	3.6	6.6	–	–
United States (Rochester, MN)[34]	All ages*	Modified New York	11.7	2.9	7.3	25.1†	30.1†
Finland[35]	≥16	Clinical/x-ray	10.2‡	4.0‡	6.9	28.4§	37.6
Finland[36]	≥16	Clinical/x-ray	8.1‡	4.6‡	6.3	29.6§	39.6
Finland, Kuopio[37]	≥16	Clinical/x-ray	12.3	≤ 8.2	5.8	26.5§	31.5
Greece, Northwest[38]	≥16	Modified New York	2.4	0.5	1.5	30.5	39.8

*Only two of a total of 158 patients with AS, both males, were younger than 15 years of age.[34]
†Median age.
‡Estimated from the data given in the original article according to the composition of the relevant population.
§Estimated from the mean age of diagnosis and mean delay to diagnosis.

both studies, a 55-year period from 1935 through 1989. The age-adjusted incidence of AS is approximately 4 times higher in males than in females.

The city of Rochester and Olmsted County have major advantages for performing population-based studies in that a high proportion of the population seeks health care from a small number of providers joined by a common medical record linkage system.[39] Thus, epidemiologic studies of a wide array of diseases have been possible and have culminated in almost 900 publications since the system was established in 1966.[40]

A study from Finland was performed in a population of about 1 million adults 16 years of age or older, using the records of a nationwide sickness insurance scheme that has provided reimbursement of drugs for patients with certain chronic diseases, including chronic inflammatory rheumatic diseases.[35] The diagnosis of AS was based either on clinical findings and existing documented radiologic examinations or on conclusive clinical findings. The average annual incidence of 6.9 per 100,000 was on the same order of magnitude as the U.S. estimate. The same authors using the same database investigated the incidence of the full spectrum of SpAs as well as that of other chronic inflammatory joint diseases during the year 1995 and compared those with previous data.[36] The annual incidence rates of AS, psoriatic arthritis (PsA), reactive arthritis (ReA), and other forms of SpAs in this study were 6.3, 6.8, 2.2, and 3.3 cases per 100,000 adults, respectively, which make an overall SpA annual incidence rate of 18.8 per 100,000. The incidence remained similar from 1980 through 1995.

A hospital-based study from Kuopio, a city in central Finland, also showed a comparable figure of 5.8 per 100,000 annual incidence rate of AS, which was defined as the presence of back pain for at least 3 months and bilateral sacroiliitis (grade 2 or more) or syndesmophytes or squared vertebrae on radiographs.[37] In this study the incidence of other inflammatory joint diseases was also investigated and the total annual incidence of SpAs was estimated to be 52 per 100,000 in this population (AS, PsA, ReA, and other SpAs).[37] PsA was the subset seen most often with an incidence rate approximately three times higher than that of AS. Although there is a high prevalence of psoriasis (up to 6%) in Finland, the reported incidence of PsA in this study is much higher than that previously reported from Finland and other countries.[36,41,42]

The annual incidence rate of AS is much lower in Greece at 1.5 per 100,000.[38] This rate was determined from a study undertaken in a defined area in the northwestern part of the country, and the patients were collected by review of medical records from two hospitals and eight private practices. Patients were selected on the basis of clinical diagnosis, according to the modified New York criteria for AS. Patients with a history of inflammatory back pain were not further evaluated for AS during the study.

The incidence rate of AS was also reported to be much lower in Japan in two nationwide questionnaire surveys performed in nine districts during a 5-year period (1985 through 1989) for the first survey and a 7-year period (1990 through 1996) for the second survey.[25] Institutions with at least one rheumatologist licensed by the Japanese Orthopedic Association or Japan Rheumatism Association were selected for patient recruitment. Thus, patients with no hospital records were not included. Response rate of the referral institutes was low, with 58% of those selected in the first survey and 74% of those selected in the second survey taking part in the study. The diagnosis of AS was made by the physicians at the institutes according to either the Rome criteria or New York criteria for AS, and the diagnosis of other SpA subsets was based on clinical and radiologic features. No standardization for diagnosis at different institutes was attempted. AS was the predominant SpA subset, consisting of 68.3% of the patients classified as having SpAs. With the assumption that at least one tenth of the patients with real SpAs were identified by the survey, the annual incidence was estimated not to exceed 0.48 per 100,000. The Amor and the ESSG criteria were fulfilled by 84% of the 962 patients of 990 recruited in both surveys and by 84.6% of the 638 patients identified in the second survey, respectively.

These data indicate that the incidence of AS and related SpAs varies across different geographic regions and ethnic groups. However, most studies show three to five times greater incidence among males compared with females. The mean age of onset was in the third decade of life, and the delay in diagnosis ranged from 5 to 10 years (Table 10.6).[25,33–36,38]

Prevalence

There are many more studies on the prevalence rate of AS than on its incidence, for the reasons stated earlier. An important factor that should be considered when one analyzes the prevalence of AS across the world is the distribution of HLA-B27 and its subtypes that may impact the disease prevalence. HLA-B27 is present throughout the world but has a very wide distribution among ethnic groups and geographic regions (Table 10.7),[43] and the disease prevalence seems to roughly correlate directly with that of B27, with some exceptions.[44,45] The highest frequencies of B27 have been reported in the Pawaia tribe in the highlands of Papua New Guinea (53%),[46] the Haida Native Indians on the Queen Charlotte Islands in Western Canada (50%), and among Siberian Eskimos and Chukchis from the Chukotka peninsula in Russia (40%).[47,48] In contrast, B27 is virtually absent among the genetically

TABLE 10.7 HLA-B27 PREVALENCE IN VARIOUS POPULATION GROUPS IN THE WORLD

Population Groups	Prevalence of HLA-B27 (%)*	Population Groups	Prevalence of HLA-B27 (%)*
Caucasoid population groups		**Altaic**	
Ugro-Finnish	12–18	Siberians	6–19
Northern Scandinavians	10–16	Japanese	< 1
Slavic populations	7–14	Ainu (Native Japanese)	4
Western Europeans	6–9	Koreans	3–8
Southern Europeans	2–6	Mongolians	3–9
Sardinians	5	Uygurs, Kazakhs, Turkics, Uzbeks	3–8
Basques	9–14	**Sino-Tibetan**	
Gypsies (Spain)	16–18	Chinese	2–9
Turks	7, 8	Tibetans	12
Arabs,† Jews, Armenians, Iranians	3–5	**Other Asiatic population groups**	
Pakistanis	6–8	Southeast Asians	4–12
Indians (Asian)	2–6	Australian Aborigines	0
Native American populations divided by linguistic groups		Melanesians (Papua New Guinea,[46] Fiji, etc.)	4–53
Eskimo-Aleut	25–40	Polynesians	0–3
Na-Dene (Haida Tlingit Dogrib Navajo)	20–50	Micronesians (Nauru, Guam)	2–5
Amerind		**African population groups**	
North American	7–26	North Africans	1–5
Mexicans Mestizo	3–6	West Africans (Mali, Gambia, Senegal)	2–10
Central American	4–20	Pygmies	7–10
South American	0	Bantu (Nigeria, Southern Africa)	0
North and Central Asiatic linguistic population groups		San (Bushmen)	0
Chukchic	19–40		
Uralic	8–24		

*The numbers are rounded off for simplicity and indicate percentages in healthy control subjects.
†Prevalence of B27 may be much lower (closer to 1%) in the United Arab Emirates and adjacent parts of Saudi Arabia and among Lebanese Maronite Christian Arabs.
Modified from Khan MA. A worldwide overview: the epidemiology of HLA-B27 and associated spondyloarthritides. In: Calin A, Taurog JD, eds. Spondyloarthritides. New York, NY: Oxford University Press; 1998:17–26.

unmixed native populations of Australia, Eastern Polynesia, South America, and the Bantus and Sans (Bushmen) of equatorial and Southern Africa.[49] Approximately 8% of the general population of Western European extraction and 10% to 16% of some of the Scandinavian and Eastern European populations possess HLA-B27 (Table 10.7).[50]

In the previously discussed population-based study from Rochester, Minnesota, a prevalence rate of AS was estimated to be 0.13% (129 cases per 100,000 general population, based on surviving patients).[33] The study covered the period between 1935 through 1973, before the availability in 1974 of HLA-B27 testing to the clinicians, to avoid any diagnostic bias introduced by that test. The authors pointed out that the point prevalence of AS in the 45- to 64-year age group was 0.4%,[33] and this figure is clinically more relevant because 45 years of age is virtually the upper limit of age of onset of AS.[1-6] There was no patient younger than 15 years of age because disease onset at age younger than 15 is very rare, and in a later publication from Rochester only 2 patients with AS, both male, of 158 seen during 55 years (between 1935 and 1989) were younger than 15 years of age.[34]

In the U.S. National Center for Health Statistics survey, Lawrence et al.[51] derived the prevalence of AS from samples from defined populations, such as the previously mentioned data from Rochester,[33] because there was no national data source. However, in the study from Rochester, there were 68 surviving patients with AS, and the total population of Rochester was 52,000 in 1973. So the prevalence rate of 1.29 per 1,000 persons should have been applied to the general population but not for the age group 15 and older as was used by Lawrence et al.[51] They also used population-based data from the Netherlands and the report that only 1.3% of Dutch individuals possessing HLA-B27 develop AS[52]; these are also relatively low figures, as discussed later in this chapter. The diagnosis of AS was based on positive results of a physical examination and radiographic evidence of sacroiliitis, and those with asymptomatic sacroiliitis were excluded. Lawrence et al.[51] applied those results to the 1990 U.S. civilian noninstitutionalized population, based on probability samples of the population. For African-American men, data from medical records of six Veterans Administration Hospitals were relied upon; no data were available for African-American women, for American Indian women, and for the Hispanic and Asian-American populations. Thus, the data used by Lawrence et al.[51] were incomplete and not very robust. They conservatively estimated the prevalence rate for AS to be 0.10% to 0.12% in U.S. population aged 15 years and older.

The overall prevalence rate of SpA (including AS) in the United States was estimated to be 0.21%, but no population-based U.S. study was available for PsA and enteropathic arthritis, and patients with undifferentiated SpAs were not included.[51] Moreover, there were problems with the diagnostic criteria for ReA, and the prevalence estimate was based on data from Navajo Indians (3 cases per 1,000), Alaskan Yupik and Inupiat Eskimos (2 to 10 cases per 1,000), and homosexual men regardless of their human immunodeficiency virus status (3 to 5 cases per 1,000).[51]

The prevalence of AS and related SpAs has been estimated in several European populations using different study designs, such as screening B27-positive individuals, who were most often blood donors or the patients' relatives,[55–59] hospital records,[60] or population surveys in a defined region.[35,52,61–65] This makes it difficult to compare the rates obtained in the various studies, and careful evaluation of the methodologies used is required.

Studies exploring the prevalence of AS using blood donors have shown conflicting results both in B27-positive and -negative subjects. The prevalence ranged from 0% to 20% in B27-positive blood donors and from 0% to 3% in B27-negative donors.[55–57,59,61] Discrepancies among these studies may be due to the small size of the study populations, differences in the selection of patients, and variation in the evaluation of sacroiliac radiographs.[11] Also, one may argue that blood donors are unlikely to be representative of the general population.[60] High prevalence rates have been reported in many blood donor studies,[55,56] including a recent study from Berlin.[62]

In the Berlin study, 348 blood donors, half of them B27-positive, were screened for AS using the modified New York criteria and for SpA using the ESSG criteria. The prevalence rate among the adult Berlin population aged 18 to 65 years was calculated to be 1.9% for SpA and 0.86% for AS on the basis of a B27 frequency of 9.5% in the general population of Berlin.[62] Studies in B27-positive healthy subjects have shown the increased risk of development of AS in the B27-positive relatives of patients compared with other B27-positive persons in the general population.[52,63–65] A Dutch study indicated that about 21% of the B27-positive relatives of B27-positive patients with AS develop the disease.[52]

Several hospital-based studies of populations of European extraction in England, Holland, Norway, Bulgaria, Romania, and the United States have provided prevalence rates that range from 0.1% to 0.8%.[60] However, hospital-based studies may underestimate the true prevalence of AS, because they usually reveal only patients with more severe and typical disease and may not include some patients with mild disease.[16,66] A recent such study showed a very low prevalence rate (0.02%) in northwestern Greece,[38] and the Greeks, like the Italians,[63] also show a weaker association of HLA-B27 (approximately 80%) with AS than Northern Europeans.

Results of population surveys in Europe are shown in Table 10.8; the highest prevalence (1.8%) was observed among Samis (Lapps) living in North Norway.[43,67] There were 11 patients with AS (7 men and 4 women), and only 4 had a prior diagnosis of AS. Moreover, 10 of 11 (91%) were HLA-B27 positive (vs. 24% of the general population), and it was estimated that 6.8% of B27-positive individuals have AS.[43,67]

The prevalence rate was also found to be high among the Scandinavian Caucasian population of northern Norway,[66] where a 16% prevalence of HLA-B27 is seen in the general population.[66,67] In this epidemiologic study, 14,539 of the 21,329 inhabitants of Tromso were surveyed (men aged 20 to 54 years and women aged 20 to 49 years). The complaint of chronic back pain or stiffness was present in 2907 of the 14539 subjects, and 806 of these 2907 subjects were randomly selected for clinical examination. There were 449 individuals who came to be clinically examined for AS, and pelvic radiographs were done in 375 individuals. AS was definitely present in 27 of these 375 subjects with chronic back pain or stiffness. The prevalence of AS was calculated to range between 1.1% and 1.4% (men: 1.9% to 2.2%; women: 0.3% to 0.6%). It was calculated that 6.7% of the B27-positive and 0.2% of B27-negative individuals had AS, and 22.5% of the B27-positive subjects with chronic

TABLE 10.8 POPULATION-BASED SURVEYS OF THE PREVALENCE OF AS IN SOME OF THE EUROPEAN POPULATIONS

Population	Age	Number Studied	Diagnosis	Prevalence (%)			HLA-B27
				AS			
				Males	Females	Total	
Norway, Samis (Lapps)[67]	20–62	836	New York	2.7	1	1.8	24
Norway[66]	20–49 F 20–54 M	14539	New York	1.9–2.2	0.3–0.6	1.1–1.4	16
Finland[35]*	≥30	7217	Clinical/x-ray	0.23[†]	0.08[†]	0.15	12 to 16
Hungary[69]	≥15	6469	New York	0.4	0.08	0.23	13
Greece[72]	≥19	8740	Modified New York	0.4	0.04	0.24	5.4[49]
Turkey[71]	18–40[‡] All males	1436	Clinical/x-ray	0.14	—	—	7 to 8[53,54]

*Men aged 20 to 22 comprised 84% of the sample.
[†]Estimated from the given data in the original article according to the composition of the relevant population.
[‡]See text for data from another study with a prevalence of AS ranging from 0.4% to 1.6%.

back pain or stiffness developed AS. The prevalence of AS in this northern Norwegian population seems to be higher than that of rheumatoid arthritis (RA) because a hospital-based study conducted in Tromso county (with Tromo as the main city) found the prevalence of RA to be between 0.39% and 0.47% among individuals older than 20.[68]

Relatively lower prevalence rates of AS have been reported in the Finnish (0.15%) and Hungarian (0.23%) populations that have 12% to 16% prevalence of HLA-B27[35,69]; the study from Finland was part of the Mini-Finland Health Survey. Higher prevalence rates of 0.4%, 1.6%, and 1% had been reported in an earlier study of three different Finnish population samples consisting of 6,176, 750, and 580 subjects, respectively.[70] However, the diagnosis was based on chest x-ray films in the first two samples and lumbosacral x-ray films were taken only in the third one.

In a Turkish study young men in the army were examined for clinical and radiologic evidence (sacroiliitis) of AS and a 0.14% prevalence was found among very young "healthy" men recruited for army service. Most of them were younger than the peak age of onset of AS, because 84% of them were between 20 and 22 years of age (range 18 to 40).[71] It can also be argued that those with more obvious AS might have been given exemption from military service during the health screening process that is routinely done before recruitment.

The prevalence of SpAs in European populations has been assessed in a few studies[72–76]; results are summarized in Table 10.9. SpA was more common in males in the Greek and Portuguese study, but it was at least as common in females as in males in the French study. Moreover, the French study showed nearly similar rates for SpA and RA.[74] The overall SpA prevalence rates estimated in Greek and French studies were comparable but were markedly less than the prevalence rate of 1.9% found in the aforementioned Berlin study, in which blood donors were screened. The estimated prevalence rate found in the Greek study (0.24%), which used population survey, was markedly greater than the figure reported in another Greek study that was hospital based.

The prevalences of HLA-B27 and AS are high among natives of circumpolar Arctic and Subarctic regions of Eurasia and North America, with the highest prevalence being reported in the Haida Indians living on the Queen Charlotte Islands of British Columbia, Canada. They show a 50% prevalence of HLA-B27, and definite AS has been reported to occur in approximately 10% of the adult Haida male population.[77] Because of the high HLA-B27 frequency, circumpolar populations were studied intensively within the context of a project supported by National Institute of Arthritis and Musculoskeletal and Skin Diseases (NIAMS) from 1989 to 1996, through an interagency agreement with the Indian Health Service (IHS) in Anchorage, Alaska.[78] Over a period of 5 years, cross-sectional data were collected from Inupiat and Yupik Eskimos in four Alaskan regions by U.S. investigators and in four settlements of Siberian Eskimos and Chukchis on Chukotka Peninsula by Russian investigators using the same data collection methods and disease criteria. These collaborative studies have provided most of the data on these populations.

26. Collantes-Estevez E, Cisnal del Mazo A, Munoz-Gomariz E. Assessment of 2 systems of spondyloarthropathy diagnostic and classification criteria (Amor and ESSG) by a Spanish multicenter study. European Spondyloarthropathy Study Group. J Rheumatol. 1995;22:246–251.

27. Collantes E, Veroz R, Escudero A, et al. Can some cases of 'possible' spondyloarthropathy be classified as 'definite' or 'undifferentiated' spondyloarthropathy? Value of criteria for spondyloarthropathies. Spanish Spondyloarthropathy Study Group. Joint Bone Spine. 2000;67:516–520.

28. Rudwaleit M, van der Heijde D, Khan MA, Braun J, Sieper J. How to diagnose axial spondyloarthritis early. Ann Rheum Dis. 2004;63:535–543.

29. Silman A, Hochberg MC. Introduction. In: Silman A, Hochberg MC, eds. Epidemiology of the Rheumatic Diseases. New York, NY: Oxford University Press; 2001:1–3.

30. Criqui MH, Barrett-Connor E, Austin M. Differences between respondents and non-respondents in a population-based cardiovascular disease study. Am J Epidemiol. 1978;108:367–372.

31. Ronmark E, Lundzvist A, Lundback B, Nystrom L. Non-responders to a postal questionnaire on respiratory symptoms and diseases. Eur J Epidemiol. 1999;15:293–299.

32. Symmons DPM. Population studies of musculoskeletal morbidity. In: Silman A, Hochberg MC, eds. Epidemiology of the Rheumatic Diseases. New York, NY: Oxford University Press; 2001:5–28.

33. Carter ET, McKenna CH, Brian DD, Kurland LT. Epidemiology of ankylosing spondylitis in Rochester, Minnesota, 1935–1973. Arthritis Rheum. 1979;22:365–370.

34. Carbone LD, Cooper C, Michet CJ, Atkinson EJ, O'Fallon WM, Melton LJ 3rd. Ankylosing spondylitis in Rochester, Minnesota, 1935–1989. Is the epidemiology changing? Arthritis Rheum. 1992;35:1476–1482.

35. Kaipiainen-Seppanen O, Aho K, Heliovaara M. Incidence and prevalence of ankylosing spondylitis in Finland. J Rheumatol. 1997;24:496–499.

36. Kaipiainen-Seppanen O, Aho K. Incidence of chronic inflammatory joint diseases in Finland in 1995. J Rheumatol. 2000;27:94–100.

37. Savolainen E, Kaipiainen-Seppanen O, Kroger L, Luosujarvi R. Total incidence and distribution of inflammatory joint diseases in a defined population: results from the Kuopio 2000 arthritis survey. J Rheumatol. 2003;30:2460–2468.

38. Alamanos Y, Papadopoulos NG, Voulgari PV, et al. Epidemiology of ankylosing spondylitis in Northwest Greece, 1983–2002. Rheumatology (Oxford). 2004;43:615–618.

39. Kurland LT, Molgaard CA. The patient record in epidemiology. Sci Am. 1981;245:54–63.

40. Melton LJ 3rd. History of the Rochester Epidemiology Project. Mayo Clin Proc. 1996;71:266–274.

41. Soderlin MK, Borjesson O, Kautianen H, Skogh T, Leirisalo-Repo M. Annual incidence of inflammatory joint diseases in a population based study in southern Sweden. Ann Rheum Dis. 2002;61:911–915.

42. Shbeeb M, Uramoto KM, Gibson LE, O'Fallon WM, Gavriel SE. The epidemiology of psoriatic arthritis in Olmsted County, Minnesota USA, 1982–1991. J Rheumatol. 2000;27:1247–1250.

43. Khan MA. A worldwide overview: the epidemiology of HLA-B27 and associated spondyloarthritides. In: Calin A, Taurog JD, eds. Spondyloarthritides. New York, NY: Oxford University Press; 1998:17–26.

44. Nasution AR, Mardjuadi A, Kunmartini S, et al. HLA-B27 subtypes positively and negatively associated with spondyloarthropathy. J Rheumatol. 1997;24:1111–1114.

45. Lopez-Larrea C, Sujirachato K, Mehra NK, et al. HLA-B27 subtypes in Asian patients with ankylosing spondylitis. Evidence for new associations. Tissue Antigens. 1995;45:169–176.

46. Bhatia K, Prasad ML, Barnish G, Koki G. Antigen and haplotype frequencies at three human leucocyte antigen loci (HLA-A, -B, -C) in the Pawaia of Papua New Guinea. Am J Phys Anthropol. 1988;75:329–340.

47. Krylov M, Etdexa S, Alexeeva L, Benevolenskaya L, Arnett FC, Reville JD. HLA class II and HLA-B27 oligotyping in two Siberian native population groups. Tissue Antigens. 1995;46:382–386.

48. Alexeeva L, Krylov M, Vturin V, Mylov N, Erdesz S, Benevolenskaya L. Prevalence of spondyloarthropathies and HLA-B27 in the native population of Chukotka, Russia. J Rheumatol. 1994;21:2298–2300.

49. Khan MA. HLA-B27 and its subtypes in world populations. Curr Opin Rheumatol. 1995;7:263–269.

50. Khan MA, Braun WE, Kushner I, Grecek DE, Muir WA, Steinberg AG. HLA B27 in ankylosing spondylitis: differences in frequency and relative risk in American blacks and Caucasians. J Rheumatol Suppl. 1977;3:39–43.

51. Lawrence RC, Helmick CG, Arnett FC, et al. Estimates of the prevalence of arthritis and selected musculoskeletal disorders in the United States. Arthritis Rheum. 1998;41:778–799.

52. van der Linden SM, Valkenburg HA, de Jongh BM, Cats A. The risk of developing ankylosing spondylitis in HLA-B27 positive individuals. A comparison of relatives of spondylitis patients with the general population. Arthritis Rheum. 1984;27:241–249.

53. Ertem GT, Tanyel E, Tulek N, Ulkar GB, Doganci L. Osteoarticular involvement of brucellosis and HLA-B27 antigen frequency in Turkish patients. Diagn Microbiol Infect Dis. 2004;48:243–245.

54. Gul A, Uyar FA, Inanc M, et al. A weak association of HLA-B*2702 with Behçet's disease. Genes Immun. 2002;3:368–372.

55. Calin A, Fries JF: Striking prevalence of ankylosing spondylitis in "healthy" w27 positive males and females. N Engl J Med. 1975;293:835–839.

56. Cohen LM, Mittal KK, Schmid FR, Rogers LF, Cohen KL. Increased risk for spondylitis stigmata in apparently healthy HL-AW27 men. Ann Intern Med. 1976;84:1–7.

57. Thorel JB, Cavelier B, Bonneau JC, Simmonin JL, Ropartz C, Deshayes P. Study of a population carrying HLA-B27 antigen compared with a population without B27, in the detection of ankylosing spondylitis. Rev Rhum Mal Osteoartic. 1978;45:275–282.

58. Chappel R, Muyelle L, Mortier G, Peetermans M, Brusselaers H. Risk of developing ankylosing spondylitis in "healthy" persons positive for HLA-B27 antigen. Acta Rhumatol. 1979;3:319–328.

59. Christiansen FT, Hawkins BR, Dawkins RL, Owen ET, Potter RM. The prevalence of ankylosing spondylitis among B27 positive normal individuals—a reassessment. J Rheumatol. 1979;6:713–718.

60. Gran JT, Husby G. Ankylosing spondylitis: prevalence and demography. In: Klippel J, Dieppe PA, eds. London, England: Mosby; 1998:6.15:1–6.

61. Alcalay M, Amor B, Haider F, et al. Ankylosing spondylitis and chlamydial infection in apparently healthy HLA-B27 blood donors. J Rheumatol. 1979;6:439–446.

62. Braun J, Bollow M, Remlinger G, et al. Prevalence of spondylarthropathies in HLA-B27 positive and negative blood donors. Arthritis Rheum. 1998;41:58–67.

63. Contu L, Capelli P, Sale S. HLA-B27 and ankylosing spondylitis: a population and family study in Sardinia. J Rheumatol Suppl. 1977;3:18–23.

64. Dawkins RL, et al. Prevalence of ankylosing spondylitis and radiological abnormalities of the sacroiliac joints in HLA-B27 positive individuals. J Rheumatol. 1981;8:1025–1026.

65. LeClercq SA, Russell AS. The risk of sacroiliitis in B27 positive persons: a reappraisal. J Rheumatol. 1984;11:327–329.

66. Gran JT, Husby G, Hordvik M. Prevalence of ankylosing spondylitis in males and females in a young middle-aged population of Tromso, northern Norway. Ann Rheum Dis. 1985;44:359–367.

67. Johnsen K, Gran JT, Dale K, Husby G. The prevalence of ankylosing spondylitis among Norwegian Samis (Lapps). J Rheumatol. 1992;19:1591–1594.

68. Riise T, Jacobsen BK, Gran JT. Incidence and prevalence of rheumatoid arthritis in the county of Tromso, northern Norway. J Rheumatol. 2000;27:1386–1389.

69. Gomor B, Gyodi E, Bakos L. Distribution of HLA-B27 and ankylosing spondylitis in the Hungarian population. J Rheumatol Suppl. 1977;3:33–35.

70. Julkunen H, Korpi J. Ankylosing spondylitis in three Finnish population samples. Prostatovesiculitis and salpingoooophoritis as aetiological factors. Scand J Rheumatol. 1984;52(Suppl):16–18.

71. Yenal O, Usman ON, Yassa K, Uyar A, Agbaba S. Epidemiology of rheumatic syndromes in Turkey. III. Incidence of rheumatic sacroiliitis in men of 20–22 years. Z Rheumatol. 1977;36:294–298.

72. Andrianakos A, Trontzas P, Christoyannis F, et al. Prevalence of rheumatic diseases in Greece: a cross-sectional population based epidemiological study. The ESORDIG Study. J Rheumatol. 2003;30:1589–1601.

73. Bruges-Armas J, Lima C, Peixoto MJ, et al. Prevalence of spondyloarthritis in Terceira, Azores: a population based study. Ann Rheum Dis. 2002;61:551–553.

74. Saraux A, Guedes C, Allain J, et al. Prevalence of rheumatoid arthritis and spondyloarthropathy in Brittany, France. Societe de Rhumatologie de l'Ouest. J Rheumatol. 1999;26:2622–2627.

75. Breban M, Said-Nehal R, Hugot JP, Miceli-Richard C. Familial and genetic aspects of spondyloarthropathy. Rheum Dis Clin North Am. 2003;29:575–594.

76. Saraux A, Guedes C, Allain J, et al. HLA-B27 in French patients with rheumatoid arthritis. Scand J Rheumatol. 1997;26:269–271.

77. Gofton JP, et al. HL-A-27 and ankylosing spondylitis in B.C. Indians. J Rheumatol. 1984;11:572–573.

78. Department of Health and Human Services. National Institute of Arthritis and Musculoskeletal and Skin Diseases. Arctic Research of the United States. 1995;12(Spring/Summer):0.109. Available at: http://www.nsf.gov/pubs/1998/nsf98150/nsf98150.pdf [Last accessed: February 2, 2005].

79. Boyer GS, Templin DW, Cornoni-Huntley JC, et al. Prevalence of spondyloarthropathies in Alaskan Eskimos. J Rheumatol. 1994;21:2292–2297.

80. Boyer GS, Templin DW, Bowler A, et al. Class I HLA antigens in spondyloarthropathy: observations in Alaskan Eskimo patients and controls. J Rheumatol. 1997;24:500–506.

81. Bardin T, Lathrop GM. Postvenereal Reiter's syndrome in Greenland. Rheum Dis Clin North Am. 1992;18:81–93.

82. Khan MA, Epidemiology of HLA-B27 and arthritis. Clin Rheumatol. 1996;15(Suppl 1):10–12.

83. Atkins C, Reuffel L, Roddy J, Platts M, Robinson H, Ward R. Rheumatic disease in the Nuu-Chah-Nulth native Indians of the Pacific Northwest. J Rheumatol. 1988;15:684–690.

84. Benevolenskaia LI, Erdes Sh, Shubin SV, Shokh BN, Mylov NM. The epidemiology of spondylarthropathies among the native inhabitants of Chukotka (Eskimos and Chukchi). 1. The prevalence of spondylarthropathies among the Eskimos and the coast Chukchi. Ter Arkh. 1994;66:12–15.

85. Benevolenskaia LI, Erdes Sh, Krylov MIu, Chekalina NA. The epidemiology of spondyloarthropathies among the native inhabitants of Chukotka. 2. The prevalence of HLA-B27 in the population and among spondyloarthropathy patients. Ter Arkh. 1994;66:41–44.

86. Benevolenskaia LI, Boyer D, Erdes Sh, et al. Comparative study of epidemiology of spondylarthropathies in indigenous population of the Chukot peninsula and Alaska. Ter Arkh. 1998;70:41–46.

87. Silman A. Ankylosing spondylitis and spondyloarthropathies. In: Silman A, Hochberg MC, eds. Epidemiology of the Rheumatic Diseases. New York, NY: Oxford University Press; 2001:100–111.

88. Senna ER, De Barros AL, Silva EO, et al. Prevalence of rheumatic diseases in Brazil: a study using the COPCORD approach. J Rheumatol. 2004;31:594–597.

89. Cardiel MH, Rojas-Serrano J. Community based study to estimate prevalence, burden of illness and help seeking behavior in rheumatic diseases in Mexico City. A COPCORD study. Clin Exp Rheumatol. 2002;20:617–624.

90. Lopez-Larrea C, Gonzalez-Roces S, Pena M, et al. Characterization of B27 haplotypes by oligotyping and genomic sequencing in the Mexican Mestizo population with ankylosing spondylitis: juvenile and adult onset. Hum Immunol. 1995;43:174–180.

91. Gorodezky C. Genetic difference between Europeans and Indians: tissue and blood types. Allergy Proc. 1992;13:243–250.

92. Infante E, Olivo A, Alaez C, et al. Molecular analysis of HLA class I alleles in the Mexican Seri Indians: implications for their origin. Tissue Antigens. 1999;54:35–42.

93. Loeza F, Vargas-Alarcon G, Andrade F, et al. Distribution of class I and class III MHC antigens in the Tarasco Amerindians. Hum Immunol. 2003;63:143–148.

94. Vargas-Alarcon G, Londono JD, Hernandez-Pacheco G, et al. Effect of HLA-B and HLA-DR genes on susceptibility to and severity of spondyloarthropathies in Mexican patients. Ann Rheum Dis. 2002;61:714–717.

95. Arellano J, Vallejo M, Jimenez J, Mintz G, Kretschmer RR. HLA-B27 and ankylosing spondylitis in the Mexican Mestizo population. Tissue Antigens. 1984;23:112–116.

96. Sampaio-Barros PD, Bertolo MB, Kraemer MH, Neto JF, Samara AM. Primary ankylosing spondylitis: patterns of disease in a Brazilian population of 147 patients. J Rheumatol. 2001;28:560–565.

97. Conde RA, Sampaio-Barros PD, Donali EA, et al. Frequency of the HLA-B27 alleles in Brazilian patients with AS. J Rheumatol. 2003;30:2512.

98. Dai SM, Han XH, Zhao DB, Shi YQ, Liu Y, Meng JM. Prevalence of rheumatic symptoms, rheumatoid arthritis, ankylosing spondylitis, and gout in Shanghai, China: a COPCORD study. J Rheumatol. 2003;30:2245–2251.

99. Wigley RD, Zhang NZ, Zeng QY, et al. Rheumatic diseases in China: ILAR-China study comparing the prevalence of rheumatic symptoms in northern and southern rural populations. J Rheumatol. 1994;21:1484–1490.

100. Wu ZB, Zhu P, Wang HK, et al. Prevalence of seronegative spondyloarthritis in the army force of China. Zhonghua Liu Xing Bing Xue Za Zhi. 2004;25:753–755.

101. Chou CT, Pei L, Chang DM, Lee CF, Schumacher HR, Liang MH. Prevalence of rheumatic diseases in Taiwan: a population study of urban, suburban, rural differences. J Rheumatol. 1994; 21:302–306.

102. Chaiamnuay P, Darmawan J, Muirden KD, Assawatanabodee P. Epidemiology of rheumatic disease in rural Thailand: a WHO-ILAR COPCORD study. Community Oriented Programme for the Control of Rheumatic Disease. J Rheumatol. 1998;25:1382–1387.

103. Minh Hoa TT, Darmawan J, Chen SL, Van Hung N, Thi Nhi C, Ngoc An T. Prevalence of the rheumatic diseases in urban Vietnam: A WHO-ILAR COPCORD study. J Rheumatol. 2003; 30:2252–2256.

104. Manahan L, Caragay R, Muirden KD, Allander E, Valkenburg HA, Wigley RD. Rheumatic pain in a Philippine village. A WHO-ILAR COPCORD study. Rheumatol Int. 1985;5:149–153.

105. Yamaguchi A, Tsuchiya N, Mitsui H, et al. Association of HLA-B39 with HLA-B27–negative ankylosing spondylitis and pauci-articular juvenile rheumatoid arthritis in Japanese patients. Evidence for a role of the peptide-anchoring B pocket. Arthritis Rheum. 1995;38:1672–1677.

106. Yamaguchi A, Ogawa A, Tsuchiyz N, et al. HLA-B27 subtypes in Japanese with seronegative spondyloarthropathies and healthy controls. J Rheumatol. 1996;23:1189–1193.

107. Muirden KD. The origins, evolution and future of COPCORD. APLAR J Rheumatol. 1997;1:44–48.

108. Wigley R, Manahan L, Muirden KD, et al. Rheumatic disease in a Philippine village. II: A WHO-ILAR-APLAR COPCORD study, phases II and III. Rheumatol Int. 1991;11:157–161.

109. Feltkamp TE, Mardjuadi A, Huang F, Chou CT. Spondyloarthropathies in eastern Asia. Curr Opin Rheumatol. 2001;13:285–290.

110. Darmawan J, Valkenburg HA, Muirden KD, Wigley RD. Epidemiology of rheumatic diseases in rural and urban populations in Indonesia: a World Health Organization International League Against Rheumatism COPCORD study, stage I, phase 2. Ann Rheum Dis. 1992;51:525–528.

111. Wigley RD. Rheumatic disease in Han Chinese. What have we learned from 19 years of epidemiological study? J Rheumatol. 2003;30:2090–2091.

112. Roberts-Thomson RA, Roberts-Thomson PJ. Rheumatic disease and the Australian aborigine. Ann Rheum Dis. 1999;58:266–270.

113. Minaur N, Sawyers S, Parker J, Darmawan J. Rheumatic disease in an Australian Aboriginal community in North Queensland, Australia. A WHO-ILAR COPCORD survey. J Rheumatol. 2004;31:965–972.

114. Richens J, McGill PE. The spondyloarthropathies. Baillieres Clin Rheumatol. 1995;9:95–109.

115. Al-Rawi ZS, Al-Shakarchi HA, Hasan F, Thewaini AJ. Ankylosing spondylitis and its association with the histocompatibility antigen HLA-B27: an epidemiological and clinical study. Rheumatol Rehabil. 1978;17:72–75.

116. Al-Awadhi AM, Oluis SO, Moussa M, et al. Musculoskeletal pain, disability and health-seeking behavior in adult Kuwaitis using a validated Arabic version of the WHO-ILAR COPCORD Core Questionnaire. Clin Exp Rheumatol. 2004;22:177–183.

117. al Attia HM, Sherif AM, Hossein MM, Ahmed YH. The demographic and clinical spectrum of Arab versus Asian patients with ankylosing spondylitis in the UAE. Rheumatol Int. 1998; 17:193–196.

118. al-Arfaj A. Profile of ankylosing spondylitis in Saudi Arabia. Clin Rheumatol. 1996;15:287–289.

119. Askari A, Al-Bdour MD, Saadeh A, Sawalha AH. Ankylosing spondylitis in north Jordan: descriptive and analytical study. Ann Rheum Dis. 2000;59:571–573.

120. Alharbi SA, Mahmoud FF, Al Awadi A, Al Jumma RA, Khodakhast F, Alsulaiman SM. Association of MHC class I with spondyloarthropathies in Kuwait. Eur J Immunogenet. 1996; 23:67–70.

121. al-Attia HM, al-Amiri N. HLA-B27 in healthy adults in UAE. An extremely low prevalence in Emirian Arabs. Scand J Rheumatol. 1995;24:225–227.

122. Serre JL, Lefranc G, Loiselet J, Jacquard A. HLA markers in six Lebanese religious subpopulations. Tissue Antigens. 1979; 14:251–255.

123. Awadia H, Baddoura R, Naman R, et al. Weak association between HLA-B27 and the spondylarthropathies in Lebanon. Arthritis Rheum. 1997;40:388–389.

124. Davatchi F, Nikbin B, Ala F. Histocompatibility antigens (HLA) in rheumatic diseases in Iran. J Rheumatol Suppl. 1977;3:36–38.

125. Samangooei S, Hakim SM, Khosravi F. Frequency of HLA-alleles B5, B51 and B27 in patients with Behçet's disease from southwest of Iran. Irn J Med Sci 2000;25.

126. Chalmers IM. Ankylosing spondylitis in African Blacks. Arthritis Rheum. 1980;23:1366–1370.

127. Stein M, Davis P, Emmanuel J, West G. The spondyloarthropathies in Zimbabwe: a clinical and immunogenetic profile. J Rheumatol. 1990;17:1337–1339.

128. Mijiyawa M. Ankylosing spondylitis in Togolese patients. Med Trop (Mars). 1993;53:185–189.

129. Lopez-Larrea C, Mijiyawa M, Gonzalez S, et al. Association of ankylosing spondylitis with HLA-B*1403 in a West African population. Arthritis Rheum. 2002;46:2968–2971.

130. Burch VC, Isaacs S, Kalla AA. Ethnicity and patterns of spondyloarthritis in South Africa-analysis of 100 patients. J Rheumatol. 1999;26:2195–2200.

131. Ntsiba H, Bazebissa R. Four first Congolese cases of pelvic ankylosing spondylitis. Bull Soc Pathol Exot. 2003; 96:21–23.

132. Khan MA. Spondyloarthropathies in non-Caucasian populations of the world. Adv Inflamm Res. 1985;9:91–99.

133. Mbayo K, Mbuyi-Muamba JM, Lurhama AZ, Halle L, Kaplan C, Dequeker J. Low frequency of HLA-B27 and scarcity of ankylosing spondylitis in a Zairean Bantu population. Clin Rheumatol. 1998;17:309–310.

134. Okoye RC, Ollier W, Jaraquemada D, et al. HLA-D region heterogeneity in a Nigerian population. Tissue Antigens. 1989;33: 445–456.

135. Brown MA, Jepson A, Young A, Whittle HC, Greenwood BM, Wordsworth BP. Ankylosing spondylitis in West Africans—evidence for a non-HLA-B27 protective effect. Ann Rheum Dis. 1997;56:68–70.

136. Kalidi I, Fofana Y, Rahly AA. Study of HLA antigens in a population of Mali (West Africa). Tissue Antigens. 1988;31:98–102.

137. Hill AV, Allsopp CE, Kwiatkowski D, Anstey NM, Greenwood BM, McMichael AJ. HLA class I typing by PCR: HLA-B27 and an African B27 subtype. Lancet. 1991;337:640–642.

138. Khan MA, Kushner I, Braun WE. Comparison of clinical features in HLA-B27 positive and negative patients with ankylosing spondylitis. Arthritis Rheum. 1977;20:909–912

11 Diagnostic and Classification Criteria

Sandra Guignard, Laure Gossec, and Maxime Dougados

AMOR'S DEVELOPMENT OF SETS OF CRITERIA FOR ANKYLOSING SPONDYLITIS AND SPONDYLOARTHRITIS

Introduction: Ankylosing Spondylitis versus Spondyloarthritides

The concept of spondyloarthritis (SA)[1,2] encompasses several diseases: ankylosing spondylitis (AS), psoriatic arthritis (PsA), reactive arthritis, rheumatic disorders associated with inflammatory bowel disease (IBD), and the undifferentiated forms of the disease. AS is the prototype of this interrelated group of disorders. The subgroups are characterized by axial or peripheral articular involvement, enthesitis, potential extraarticular manifestations, and a high association to a genetic factor of predisposition, the tissue antigen human leukocyte antigen (HLA)-B27. It can be difficult to differentiate these disorders because they may occur simultaneously or sequentially in the same patients and/or their relatives. Moreover, some of the clinical characteristics of these diseases, such as enthesitis and eye involvement, are similar whatever the diagnosis. The monitoring and, to a lesser degree, the treatment of the diseases are related more to their clinical presentation than to a precise diagnosis (e.g., AS or PsA). Classification criteria for SA can also perform well for AS if it is considered as a SA with axial involvement.[3,4]

Thus, there are two different approaches for the development of criteria, one specific for AS and the other more general and related to the concept of spondyloarthritides.

Consequences for the Development of a Set of Criteria: Choice of Patients and Control Subjects

Classification criteria

The main question is whether the objective is to propose a set of criteria for the classification of a patient with SA whatever the clinical presentation or classification of a patient with a disease that is a subgroup of the spondyloarthritides such as AS. It is our opinion that a set of classification criteria for the whole group of spondyloarthritides reflects reality better than different sets of classification criteria for each specific disease.

Indeed, the main requirement for the use of classification criteria is a homogeneous population for clinical and/or biologic research purposes. In particular, a treatment can have different effects based on the clinical presentation (axial symptoms vs. peripheral arthritis vs. enthesopathy). Rather than the use of a set of specific criteria for a disease belonging to the concept of SA, a solution is to specify, for participation in a study, the clinical manifestations allowed or not allowed. For example, for a study of axial manifestations we are more in favor of selecting patients fulfilling Amor's or the European Spondyloarthropathy Study Group (ESSG) criteria *and* having axial symptoms than of including patients only fulfilling the modified New York criteria.[5] In this latter case, the analysis of results is complicated or even impossible because a patient can fulfill the modified New York criteria (which rely heavily on radiographic evidence of spinal involvement) but complain only of peripheral arthritis at the time of the study if no further definition of active axial involvement were allowed.

Diagnostic criteria

Here, the main question is whether a set of criteria has a specific symptom as an entry parameter (e.g., back pain, peripheral arthritis, or heel pain) or if the set of criteria is valid for any inaugural symptom. The issue of diagnostic criteria involves separating the patient from the background population, not distinguishing one disease from another.

It is the opinion of the authors that for diagnostic purposes a specific set of criteria for each of the main rheumatologic manifestations will be more relevant with a detailed (weighted) description of the entry parameter.

List of Parameters: Clinical Features and Radiologic Aspects Potentially of Interest for Integration in a Set of Criteria

We will enumerate here some characteristic features of spondyloarthropathies that can potentially be entered into sets of criteria. Our objective is not to detail the different features of SA but to try to extract from epidemiologic studies the features that are either both sensitive and specific or at the least very specific and therefore of interest for integration in a set of criteria.

For this purpose, the main clinical and radiologic manifestations will be evaluated. We will also present the potential role for new imaging techniques.

Axial involvement
Inflammatory spinal pain
Inflammatory back pain in AS has an insidious onset, starts in the lumbar region, is associated with morning stiffness, improves with exercise, and generally occurs before the age of 40. This symptom is considered relevant if it is present for at least 3 months.[6] It is the hallmark of AS and is used in all sets of criteria.

Ankylosis
Ankylosis is the consequence of the ossification of ligaments and vertebrocostal and sternocostal joints. Spinal mobility is impaired, associated with abnormal posture and an increased risk of fracture. Ankylosis is characteristic of advanced disease,[7] and it is thus not useful in diagnostic criteria. However, some elements related to ankylosis such as limited spinal mobility are used in classification criteria.

Sacroiliitis
Inflammatory sacroiliac pain is typical of AS and is always considered for diagnostic criteria. Radiologic sacroiliitis is one of the most important elements of the classification criteria for AS because of its particularly high specificity.[8] However, radiologic evidence of sacroiliitis appears after 2 to 5 years of evolution and is characteristic of more advanced disease. Pelvic radiographs are usually normal when early SA is suspected.[7–9] Thus, findings in patients with an undifferentiated SA or at onset of their disease may not fulfill radiographic criteria. Furthermore, because of the major interobserver variability in interpreting and grading radiographic sacroiliac joints and the difficulty in identifying abnormalities in younger (teen-aged) subjects, sacroiliitis is sometimes difficult to assess. For this reason, some criteria have been based on bilateral or high-grade sacroiliitis.

Perspectives
Magnetic resonance imaging (MRI) is helpful in detecting early changes that cannot be identified by radiography, particularly bone edema,[10,11] but its role in diagnosis is still under investigation. Tomodensitometry and MRI perform equally well in staging of erosions and osteosclerosis.[12]

Anterior chest wall and root joints
Anterior chest wall pain is the result of manubriosternal, sternoclavicular, and costosternal arthritis and may lead to reduced chest expansion in advanced forms of AS. It is used in most criteria for AS.

Peripheral articular involvement
Peripheral arthritis is less common than axial involvement in AS. A typical feature is dactylitis (sausage-like digit). Asymmetrical, mono- or oligoarthritis of the lower limbs may also be seen. Although these forms of arthritis are not very specific for AS, they may be associated with axial ankylosis and can be useful in classification criteria for AS.

Perspectives
In the future, the use of ultrasonography to explore inflammatory joints might be of interest to differentiate primary synovial (rheumatoid-like) arthritis from entheseal (SA-like) arthritis.[13]

Enthesitis
Enthesitis is the painful inflammation of the entheses and affects the heel, iliac crest, anterior tibial tuberosity, or anterior chest wall. Entheses are a target area of SA and enthesitis seems interesting for use in criteria. However, entheseal abnormalities in SA are not detected by clinical examination. Compared with ultrasonography, clinical examination has a low sensitivity (22.6%) and a moderate specificity (79.7%) for the detection of enthesitis at the lower limbs.[14]

Perspectives
1. An ultrasonographic quantitative score of lower limb enthesitis has been proposed, but further studies are required to validate it in SA.[14] A systematic ultrasonographic evaluation of the heel area in patients complaining of back pain might be of interest to differentiate patients with AS from patients with mechanical back pain.[15]
2. The role of MRI is currently under evaluation. MRI can detect entheseal abnormalities consisting of perientheseal bone marrow edema, which is maximal at the entheseal insertion.[16] Nevertheless, compared with ultrasonography, MRI is not sensitive in detecting early changes of enthesitis. Fatty degeneration appears late in MRI, whereas it is detected earlier using ultrasonography. Ultrasonography also performs better than MRI in detecting early calcification processes at the insertion site.[16] It is possible that ultrasonography will appear in future sets of criteria, if further studies confirm its properties.

Family history and genetic background
HLA-B27
This genetic susceptibility factor is common to all spondyloarthritides and was observed in 88% to 95% of patients with AS.[17,18] This antigen in found in 6% to 8% of the white population, and therefore approximately 6% to 8% of the population with mechanical back

pain will be HLA-B27 positive. In different studies, HLA-B27 sensitivity varies from 83% to 96%,[19,20] and its specificity ranges from 91% to 96%.[20,21] Therefore, it is clearly an interesting and important feature for sets of criteria.

Perspectives

In recent immunologic studies different HLA-B27 subtypes have been found. Some of these subtypes may have a protective effect against SA (HLA-B*2709, for instance).[22] Further investigations are required to determine whether these subtypes could be of interest in diagnosing or classifying AS.

Family studies

Multiple occurrences of AS in the same family were first reported by Bremner et al.[23] The risk of development of AS in these families was 20 to 40 times higher than that in the general population. Interrogating the patient about his/her family history is part of some sets of criteria in AS.

Extraarticular features

Extraarticular features of spondyloarthritides include IBD, psoriasis, urethritis, and acute anterior uveitis. Uveitis is the most common extraarticular feature in patients with AS (prevalence of 40% in patients with AS).[24] The definition of acute anterior uveitis consists of a painful red eye of at least 2 days' duration and/or necessitating local treatment with corticosteroids. The most specific eye involvement in SA is an acute, recurrent, and alternate anterior uveitis.[25]

AVAILABLE SETS OF CRITERIA: DESCRIPTION AND EVALUATION

Introduction

To understand the current problem of defining the diagnosis of AS, it is interesting to review the successive stages in rheumatologic concepts over the last 40 years. In the 1950s, the problem involved the identification of AS from among the whole group of rheumatic diseases and in particular rheumatoid arthritis. At that time, an inflammatory rheumatologic disorder different from rheumatoid arthritis and involving axial manifestations was individually identified as "seronegative" arthritis. In the 1960s, axial involvement was the main clinical manifestation emphasized. Classification criteria for AS were first specified at the Rome conference in 1963[17] and were later evaluated in Blackfoot and Pima Indians.[26] This led to modifications, resulting in the New York criteria formulated in 1966.[27] In 1977, a definition of inflammatory back pain useful for screening patients with AS was proposed.[6] In 1984,

modified New York criteria were published[5] with the objective of better sensitivity.

While these criteria were being developed, the concept of SA was emerging.[1,2] This concept considers the spectrum of these diseases rather than each individual diagnosis and classification (Table 11.1) and led to the development of classification criteria for the entire group of patients with SA, among whom are patients with AS. The specific aim of the Amor[28] and ESSG[29] classification criteria was to include individuals with undifferentiated SA. Amor's classification criteria were formulated based on personal clinical experience.[28] The ESSG classification criteria were based on both clinical and statistical reasoning.[29]

We first focus on the different available sets of classification criteria. To evaluate their performances, the studies conducted on populations who were not included in the development step of the proposed set of criteria will be emphasized. The evaluations of six different classification criteria (four related to AS and two related to SA) are available. Furthermore, some of these sets of classification criteria have been evaluated in several studies, whereas no diagnostic criteria have been evaluated. The only study available on diagnostic criteria is a development study. Therefore, classification criteria are often used in daily practice as an aid in making the diagnosis, although they were not elaborated for this aim and the psychometric properties might not be appropriate to use these criteria for this purpose.

TABLE 11.1 CLINICAL PRESENTATION OF SPONDYLOARTHRITIS	
Disease Subgroups	Clinical Features
Ankylosing spondylitis	*Rheumatologic manifestations*
Psoriatic arthritis	Axial involvement
Reactive arthritis	Peripheral arthritis
Inflammatory bowel disease related arthritis	Enthesitis
Undifferentiated spondyloarthritis	*Extraarticular features*
	Acute anterior uveitis
	Genetic background
	Family history
	HLA-B27 antigen
	Specific manifestations
	Psoriasis
	Inflammatory bowel disease

Classification Criteria

Ankylosing spondylitis classification criteria
Rome criteria

Definition

The first classification criteria for AS were proposed at the Rome conference in 1963 (Table 11.2).[17] The Rome criteria classified AS as "bilateral sacroiliitis *and* one of the five following clinical criteria present," or "four of five clinical criteria present." The clinical criteria are low back pain and stiffness for more than 3 months, which is not relieved by rest, pain, and stiffness in the thoracic region, limited motion in the lumbar spine, limited chest expansion, and history or evidence of iritis or its sequelae.

TABLE 11.2 ROME CLASSIFICATION CRITERIA FOR ANKYLOSING SPONDYLITIS*

Clinical criteria

1. Low back pain and stiffness for more than 3 months that is not relieved by rest

2. Pain and stiffness in the thoracic region

3. Limited motion in the lumbar spine

4. Limited chest expansion

5. History or evidence of iritis or its sequelae

Radiologic criterion

6. X-ray film showing bilateral sacroiliac changes characteristic of ankylosing spondylitis

*A patient is considered to have ankylosing spondylitis if bilateral sacroiliitis and one of the five clinical criteria are present or if four of the clinical criteria are present. From Kellgren JH, Jeffrey MR, Ball J. The Epidemiology of Chronic Rheumatism. Oxford, England: Blackwell Scientific Publications; 1963;I:326–327.

Evaluation and performances

The performance of the Rome criteria was evaluated in two studies, which are the same studies in which the inflammatory back pain criteria for AS were evaluated[5,30] (Table 11.3). Each individual clinical criterion was evaluated. The performances of two items were very different in the two evaluation studies: these items are low back pain and stiffness for more than 3 months and limited motion of the lumbar spine. The other clinical items, thoracic pain and stiffness, limited chest expansion, and iritis had a high specificity but a low sensitivity in both studies. They were therefore poor epidemiologic discriminators. The radiologic criterion "bilateral sacroiliitis" was evaluated in one study only: it was both sensitive (93%) and specific (91%).

The Rome criteria can be fulfilled in two ways (either with four clinical criteria or with one radiologic and one clinical criterion). These options were compared in one study:[30] there was a clear difference between the performances of the option "four clinical criteria" (sensitivity 27% and specificity 99%) and the option "one clinical criterion with bilateral sacroiliitis" (sensitivity 87% and specificity 95%). This difference emphasizes the importance of the radiologic item in this set of criteria.

Comments and limitations

When four of the five clinical items were present, it was possible for the criteria for AS to be fulfilled without radiologic evidence of the disease. However, bilateral sacroiliitis was recognized as the most important criterion and had a weight three times greater than that for any of the clinical criteria. The weight attributed to this radiologic item has been criticized: because radiologic sacroiliitis appears late in the course of the disease, the

---

TABLE 11.3 COMPARISON OF THE PERFORMANCES OF THE ROME CRITERIA: COMPARING TWO STUDIES

	Sensitivity (%)		Specificity (%)		PPV (%):	NPV (%):
	Study 1[5]	Study 2[30]	Study 1[5]	Study 2[30]	Study 1[5]	Study 2[30]
Low back pain >3 months' duration	38	63	94	95	62	86
Thoracic pain and stiffness	38	43	88	98	44	85
Limited motion of the lumbar spine	52	73	89	72	55	88
Limited chest expansion*	10	43	100	94	100	81
Iritis	10	27	99	99	67	81
Rome bilateral AS sacroiliitis		93		91		
Four clinical criteria		27		99		
Bilateral sacroiliitis + one clinical criterion		87		95		

*The cut-off in these studies was set at 2.5 cm.
AS, ankylosing spondylitis; PPV, positive predictive value; NPV, negative predictive value.

Rome criteria are not going to be useful to classify early AS or mild forms of the disease.

The imprecise labeling of three items of the Rome criteria magnified interobserver variability. This led to some modifications of these items:

- "Limited motion of the lumbar spine" was not clearly defined. To be more precise, the New York criterion measured axial ankylosis in "all three planes."
- The Rome criterion "limited chest expansion" led to the more precise New York criterion "limited chest expansion with a cut-off at 2.5 cm." In fact, in both evaluation studies, a cut-off at 2.5 cm was chosen to measure chest expansion, and, therefore, the Rome criterion, which does not rely on objective measurement, was not really evaluated.
- The item "iritis" was considered by some authors as imprecise and was therefore deleted from the New York criteria.

New York criteria

Definition

The New York criteria were formulated in 1966[27] and were based on the Rome criteria. The New York criteria comprise clinical and radiologic items (Table 11.4).

Clinical criteria are 1) a history or the presence of pain at the dorsolumbar junction or in the lumbar spine; 2) limitation of the motion of the lumbar spine in all three planes: anterior flexion, lateral flexion, and extension; and 3) limitation of chest expansion to 1 inch (2.5 cm) or less, measured at the level of the fourth intercostal space. In the study, the chest expansion was measured in strict conditions: it had to be assessed twice, at the fourth intercostal space, with breathing instructions. The aim was to minimize interobserver variation.

The radiologic criterion is sacroiliitis graded from 1 to 4 on plain x-ray films (grade 0 = normal, grade 1 = suspicious changes, grade 2 = minimum abnormality, small erosion, or sclerosis without alteration in the joint width, grade 3 = unequivocal abnormality, erosion, or sclerosis alteration in the joint width, and grade 4 = several abnormality [total ankylosis]).

A patient is considered to have a definite AS if there is a grade 3 or 4 bilateral sacroiliitis with any clinical criterion or grade 2 bilateral or 3 or 4 unilateral sacroiliitis with either clinical criterion 1 or both clinical criteria 2 and 3.

Evaluation and performances

Table 11.5 summarizes the performances of the New York criteria as evaluated in three studies: two are the studies described earlier[5,30]; the third is an evaluation in 232 relatives with or without sacroiliitis, of 104 probands who had PsA, with 76 spouses as control subjects.[31] In this study it was assumed that sacroiliitis reflected the true diagnostic status, and it was against this parameter that each clinical criterion was evaluated. For each clinical item, although the values of specificity and sensitivity varied, the results showed the same trend, with a medium or low sensitivity and a higher specificity (Table 11.5). The sensitivity of the items relying on measurements ("limitation of the motion of the lumbar spine in all three planes" and "limitation of chest expansion less than 2.5 cm") had high variability (7% to 67% and 10% to 43%, respectively), which is an interesting paradox.

The radiologic criterion was evaluated only in one study[30] and was both sensitive (73%) and specific (98%). The performances of the whole set of New York criteria were evaluated only in one study[30] (using as the definition of AS the clinician's final opinion); sensitivity reached 73% and specificity 98%.

Comments and limitations

- "Limitation of chest expansion < 2.5 cm" had a very low sensitivity (10% to 43%). In one study,[5] the sensitivity of this item improved when the cut-off was 5 cm instead of 2.5 cm, but in this case specificity was much lower (68%). This clinical feature appears late in the disease and might be influenced by treatment and exercises. Moll and Wright[32] showed a physiologically progressive

---

TABLE 11.4 NEW YORK CLASSIFICATION CRITERIA FOR ANKYLOSING SPONDYLITIS

A. Diagnosis

1. Limitation of the motion of the lumbar spine in all three plans: anterior flexion, lateral flexion, and extension

2. History or presence of pain at the dorsolumbar junction or in the lumbar spine

3. Limitation of chest expansion to 2.5 cm or less, measured at the level of the fourth intercostal space

B. Grading

Definite ankylosing spondylitis:

1. Grade 3–4 bilateral sacroiliitis with at least one clinical criterion

2. Grade 3–4 unilateral or grade 2 bilateral sacroiliitis with clinical criterion 1 or with both clinical criteria 2 and 3

Probable ankylosing spondylitis:

Grade 3–4 bilateral sacroiliitis with no clinical criterion

From Bennett PH, Burch TA. Population Studies of the Rheumatic Diseases. Amsterdam, Netherlands: Excerpta Medica; 1968:456–457.

TABLE 11.5 COMPARISON OF THE PERFORMANCES OF THE NEW YORK CRITERIA ACCORDING TO THREE STUDIES

Studies	Sensitivity (%)			Specificity (%)		
	Study 1[5]	Study 2[30]	Study 3[31]	Study 1[5]	Study 2[30]	Study 3[31]
History of (dorso)lumbar pain	62	77	68	43	52	49
Limitation of motion of the lumbar spine in all three planes	38	67	7	96	84	100
Limitation of chest expansion	10	43	15	100	94	93
Grade 3–4 bilateral sacroiliitis		73			78	
New York criteria		73			98	

reduction of chest expansion with age, and in females chest expansion was lower than in males. Therefore, normograms corrected for age and sex should be used.

- The criterion "history or presence of pain at the dorsolumbar junction or in the lumbar spine" had a low discriminating value (sensitivity 68% to 77% and specificity 49% to 52%), whereas the more precise original Rome criterion "low back pain and stiffness for more than 3 months that is not relieved by rest" performed better (sensitivity 38% to 63% and specificity 94% to 95%) and was therefore chosen for the modified New York criteria.
- The New York criterion "limitation of lumbar spine in all three planes" performed better than the Rome criterion "limited motion of the lumbar spine," but its very low sensitivity might lead to many undiagnosed occurrences. Therefore, the choice of a measurement in "two planes" only was made for the modified New York criteria.
- Overall, once again, the major role of radiologic evidence of sacroiliitis and of ankylosis in the New York criteria made these criteria not appropriate for early diagnosis or undifferentiated SA.

Modified New York criteria

Definition

In 1984, the modified New York criteria were formulated based on the comparison of the existing sets of criteria in relatives of patients with AS and in population control subjects, as detailed earlier.[5] The modified New York criteria are similar to the New York criteria, but the New York pain criterion (which was not specific enough) was replaced by a slightly modified Rome pain criterion (Table 11.6).

Clinical criteria are the following:

- Low back pain and stiffness for more than 3 months that improves with exercise, but is not relieved by rest.

- Limitation of motion of the lumbar spine in both the sagittal and the frontal planes.
- Limitation of chest expansion relative to normal values corrected for age and sex.

The radiological criterion is as follows:

- Sacroiliitis grade 2 or higher bilaterally or sacroiliitis grade 3 to 4 unilaterally.

AS is considered definite if the radiologic criterion is associated with at least one clinical criterion and probable if three clinical criteria are present or if the radiologic criterion is present without any signs or symptoms corresponding to the clinical criteria.

TABLE 11.6 MODIFIED NEW YORK CLASSIFICATION CRITERIA FOR ANKYLOSING SPONDYLITIS

A. Diagnosis

1. Clinical criteria

a. Low back pain and stiffness for more than 3 months that improves with exercise, but is not relieved by rest

b. Limitation of motion of the lumbar spine in both the sagittal and the frontal planes

c. Limitation of chest expansion relative to normal values corrected for age and sex

2. Radiologic criterion: sacroiliitis grade ≥ 2 bilaterally or sacroiliitis grade 3–4 unilaterally

B. Grading

1. Definite ankylosing spondylitis if the radiologic criterion is present with at least one clinical criterion

2. Probable ankylosing spondylitis if

a. Three clinical criteria are present

b. The radiologic criterion is present without any signs or symptoms fulfilling the criteria.

From Van der Linden S, Valkenburg HA, Cats A. Evaluation of diagnostic criteria for ankylosing spondylitis. A proposal for modification of the New York criteria. Arthritis Rheum 1984;27:361–368.

Evaluation and performances

The items of the modified New York criteria have not been evaluated separately. In the only evaluation of the whole set of criteria, the Rome low back pain criterion with stiffness was mixed with the New York criterion of three-plane limitation; this evaluation revealed a sensitivity of 80% and a specificity of 81%.[30] In the presence of a positive clinical history screening test, the modified New York criteria performed better than the New York criteria and the Rome criteria in terms of sensitivity.[33]

Comments and limitations

Currently, the modified New York criteria are widely used both in clinical practice and in clinical trials to classify patients with AS. They have been shown to be superior to the New York and Rome criteria, which are now rarely used. The modified New York criteria are also often used as an aid for diagnosis even though they were not designed as such and do not perform well in early disease. A prospective study indicated that the sensitivity of the modified New York criteria increased with the disease duration (sensitivity of 0% for a disease duration of 2 years versus 60.2% for a disease duration of more than 10 years) (Table 11.7).[28] The delay before radiologic evidence of sacroiliitis is seen might explain these results. Although the modified New York criteria are sensitive, they cannot be used to identify mild, undifferentiated, or early forms of the disease. For these purposes, the classification criteria for SA can not be used, and there is an ongoing study to create diagnostic criteria for early disease.

Spondyloarthritis classification criteria

Introduction

As seen in the previous sections, in sets of classification criteria for AS there is an insistence on axial features including sacroiliitis. They are very restrictive in that it is impossible to include and classify either patients with early disease or patients with extraaxial features without axial characteristics. The concept of SA, which considers the spectrum of theses diseases rather than each individual diagnosis and classification (e.g., AS or PsA), (see Table 11.1) led to two different sets of classification criteria: Amor's classification criteria and the ESSG classification criteria.[28,29]

Amor's classification criteria

Definition

The aim of Amor's classification criteria was to be more sensitive to include undifferentiated spondyloarthropathy but without losing too much specificity. The aim was that a patient could fulfill the criteria without a discriminating feature, i.e., there is no "entry criterion." These criteria were developed by Amor in 1990[28] based on personal experience. The Amor criteria comprise 11 clinical and 1 radiologic criteria, all with weighted numbers (Table 11.8).

The clinical criteria are lumbar or dorsal pain at night or morning stiffness of the lumbar or dorsal spine, asymmetrical oligoarthritis; buttock pain; sausage-like toes or digits; heel pain or other well defined enthesiopathic pain; iritis; non-gonococcal urethritis or cervicitis within 1 month before the onset of the disease; acute diarrhea within 1 month before the onset of the arthritis, psoriasis, balanitis, or IBD; the presence of HLA-B27 and/or a family history of AS; PsA or IBD; clear-cut improvement within 48 hours after intake of nonsteroidal anti-inflammatory drugs (NSAIDs) or rapid relapse of the pain after their discontinuation.

The radiologic criterion is sacroiliitis, bilateral grade 2 or unilateral grade 3.

A patient is considered to have an SA if total criteria score is at least 6.

Evaluation and performances

Amor's classification criteria were first evaluated in 1219 patients with SA and 157 control subjects with other rheumatic diseases.[28] Disease was diagnosed according to expert opinion (a senior rheumatologist), and possible SA was excluded. In this study, the specificity of the Amor criteria was 86.6%, and sensitivity reached 90%. Three items had excellent sensitivity: lumbar and buttock pain at night,

TABLE 11.7 SENSITIVITY OF THE MODIFIED NEW YORK CRITERIA AND AMOR'S CLASSIFICATION CRITERIA FOR SPONDYLOARTHRITIS RELATED TO THE DURATION OF THE DISEASE						
Disease duration (years)	<2	< 4	< 6	<10	>10	Total
Number of patients	10	52	25	40	123	250
Sensitivity of New York criteria (%)	0.0	15.4	20.0	25.0	60.2	39.6
Sensitivity of Amor's criteria (%)	80.0	96.2	96.0	97.5	96.7	96.0

Data from Amor B, Dougados M, Mijiyawa M. Criteria of the classification of spondylarthropathies. Rev Rhum Mal Osteoartic 1990;57:85–89.

TABLE 11.8 AMOR'S CLASSIFICATION CRITERIA FOR SPONDYLOARTHRITIS*	
Parameter	Scoring
A. Clinical symptoms or past history of	
1. Lumbar or dorsal pain at night or morning stiffness of lumbar or dorsal spine	1
2. Asymmetrical oligoarthritis	2
3. Buttock pain Or if alternate	1 2
4. Sausage-like toe or digit	2
5. Heel pain or other well defined enthesopathic pain	2
6. Iritis	2
7. Nongonococcal urethritis or cervicitis within 1 month before the onset of the disease	1
8. Acute diarrhea within 1 month before the onset of the arthritis	1
9. Psoriasis, balanitis, or inflammatory bowel disease	2
B. Radiological findings	
10. Sacroiliitis (bilateral grade 2 or unilateral grade 3)	3
C. Genetic background	
11. Presence of HLA-B27 and/or a family history of ankylosing spondylitis, psoriatic arthritis, or inflammatory bowel disease	2
D. Response to treatment	
12. Clear-cut improvement within 48 hours after NSAID intake or rapid relapse of the pain after their discontinuation	1

*A patient is considered to suffer from a spondyloarthritis if the sum is ≥6. From Amor B, Dougados M, Mijiyawa M. Criteria of the classification of spondylarthropathies. Rev Rhum Mal Osteoartic 1990;57:85–89.

morning stiffness, and good response to intake of NSAIDs.

The sensitivity of Amor's criteria was equivalent for AS and undifferentiated SA and varied from 88.9% for Reiter's disease to 98% for AS. Amor's criteria also performed better in early SA than the sets of criteria detailed earlier, classifying patients with a short disease duration; for the whole group of spondylarthropathies, the sensitivities of modified New York criteria versus Amor's criteria were, respectively, 39.6% versus 96% (Table 11.7). In this study,[2] all the patients with AS according to modified New York criteria fulfilled Amor's criteria, but nearly 7% of the patients fulfilling Amor's criteria did not satisfy the modified New York criteria.

In another study in 1995,[34] each individual criterion was evaluated in 124 patients with SA and 1964 control subjects (Table 11.9). The items with the highest sensitivity were spinal pain, HLA-B27 and/or positive family history, and response to NSAIDs. The items with the highest specificity were sacroiliitis, diarrhea, and urethritis for less than 1 month. The items performing well in terms of sensitivity and specificity were spinal pain, sacroiliitis, HLA-B27 and/or positive family history, and response to NSAIDs.

Comments and advantages and limitations
With Amor's classification, a patient with uveitis but with no spinal involvement or oligoarthritis can fulfill the criteria for SA, because there is no specific "entry criterion." This is not the case with the other sets of criteria. Amor pointed out that the three points indicated by the item "sacroiliitis" are needed to confirm the diagnosis in only 10% of spondylarthropathies.[28] However, the criterion "heel pain" is controversial because it might introduce confusion between talalgia and Achilles tendonitis. Furthermore, the associated item "other enthesitis" might be considered too vague and may heighten interobserver variability.

European Spondyloarthropathy Study Group classification criteria

Definition
In 1991, a European Task Force[29] proposed another set of classification criteria for SA, with the same aim as Amor: to encompass patients with undifferentiated disease ignored in epidemiologic studies because of inadequacy of existing criteria. Features of SA were listed, with a detailed description of each feature so that all physicians could agree on reliable ways of recognizing it (Table 11.10). The following classification emerged (Table 11.11): "Inflammatory spinal pain or synovitis (asymmetric or predominant to the lower limbs), together with at least one of the following items: positive family history, psoriasis, inflammatory bowel disease, urethritis or acute diarrhea, alternate buttock pain, enthesiopathy, and sacroiliitis as determined from pelvic radiography."

Evaluation and performances: comparison of Amor's classification criteria and the ESSG classification criteria
A cross-sectional study of 2228 patients was performed to compare the two new sets of classification criteria for SA.[35] A Spanish study was also performed to evaluate the positive and negative predictive values of the two sets of classification criteria[36] in 102 patients with "possible spondyloarthritis," to determine after 5 years whether Amor's criteria or the ESSG criteria could lift this uncertainty.

TABLE 11.9 PERFORMANCE OF ITEMS OF AMOR'S CLASSIFICATION CRITERIA FOR SPONDYLOARTHRITIS EVALUATED IN 2088 PATIENTS WITH RHEUMATIC DISEASES*

Item	Sensitivity	Specificity	PPV	NPV
1. Spinal pain	71.4	77.3	17.7	98.2
2. Oligoarthritis	44.3	94.7	34.6	96.4
3a. Buttock pain	66.9	81.7	18.2	97.5
3b. Alternate buttock pain	38.7	97.6	50.5	96.2
4. Sausage-like digit	26.6	98.6	41.2	95.5
5. Heel pain	51.6	92.2	29.6	96.8
6. Uveitis	13.7	99.6	73.9	94.8
7. Urethritis <1 month	10.5	99.7	72.2	94.6
8. Diarrhea <1 month	14.5	99.2	54.5	94.8
9. Psoriasis/balanitis/inflammatory bowel disease	35.5	97.4	46.8	96.0
10. Sacroiliitis	59.7	99.7	93.7	97.5
11. Genetic feature	71.0	96.5	56.8	98.1
12. Response to NSAIDs	70.0	86.0	22.1	97.3

*Patients included 124 patients considered to have spondyloarthritis and 1964 control patients. All values are given as percentages. PPV, positive predictive value, NPV, negative predictive value.
From Amor B, Dougados M, Listrat V, et al. Are classification criteria for spondylarthropathy useful as diagnostic criteria? Rev Rhum Engl Ed 1995;62:10–15.

TABLE 11.10 SPECIFICATION OF THE VARIABLES OF THE ESSG CRITERIA FOR SPONDYLOARTHRITIS

Variable	Definition
Inflammatory spinal pain	History or present symptoms of spinal pain in back, dorsal, or cervical region, with at least four of the following: a) onset before age 45, b) insidious onset, c) improvement with exercise, d) associated with morning stiffness, or e) at least 3 months duration.
Synovitis	Past or present asymmetric arthritis or arthritis predominantly in the lower limbs
Family history	Presence in first- or second-degree relatives of any of the following: a) ankylosing spondylitis, b) psoriasis, c) acute uveitis, d) reactive arthritis, or e) inflammatory bowel disease
Psoriasis	Past or present psoriasis diagnosed by a physician
Inflammatory bowel disease	Past or present Crohn's disease or ulcerative colitis diagnosed by a physician and confirmed by radiographic examination or endoscopy
Alternating buttock pain	Past or present pain alternating between the right and left gluteal regions
Enthesopathy	Past or present spontaneous pain or tenderness at examination of the site of the insertion of the Achilles tendon or plantar fascia
Acute diarrhea	Episode of diarrhea occurring within 1 month before arthritis
Urethritis	Nongonococcal urethritis or cervicitis occurring within 1 month before arthritis
Sacroiliitis	Bilateral grade 2–4 or unilateral grade 3–4, according to the following radiographic grading system: 0 = normal, 1 = possible, 2 = minimal, 3 = moderate, 4 = ankylosis

From Dougados M, Van der Linden S, Juhlin R, et al., for the European Spondyloarthropathy Study Group. The European Spondylarthropathy Study Group preliminary criteria for the classification of spondylarthropathy. Arthritis Rheum 1991;34:1218–1227.

TABLE 11.11 ESSG CLASSIFICATION CRITERIA FOR SPONDYLOARTHRITIS

Inflammatory spinal pain	*or*	Synovitis: asymmetric or predominantly in lower limbs
	And one or more of the following: Positive family history Psoriasis Inflammatory bowel disease Urethritis, cervicitis, or acute diarrhea within the month before arthritis Buttock pain alternating between right and left gluteal areas Enthesitis Sacroiliitis	

From Dougados M, Van der Linden S, Juhlin R, et al., for the European Spondyloarthropathy Study Group. The European Spondyloarthropathy Study Group preliminary criteria for the classification of spondylarthropathy. Arthritis Rheum 1991;34:1218–1227.

Equivalent performances of both sets were obtained. There was slight superiority for Amor's classification criteria (Table 11.12) with a high specificity (98% for Amor's criteria and 96% for ESSG criteria) and a good sensitivity for the subgroup of "definite spondyloarthritis" (92% for Amor's criteria and 87% for the ESSG criteria).

Nevertheless, sensitivity fell to 62% for Amor's criteria and 63% for ESSG criteria if the whole group of spondylarthropathies was considered. Amor's criteria at baseline had better predictive values especially in the second study (Table 11.12).

The difference in the performances of the two sets of criteria might be explained by the facts that the ESSG criteria require the presence of either spinal or peripheral joint involvement and thus have "entry criteria" or that the ESSG criteria do not include a response to NSAIDs, which is the 12th item of the Amor classification. In fact, because Amor's criteria are based on the weighted sum of 12 variables without any prerequisite, they might be more helpful than the ESSG criteria for making a diagnosis in an individual patient (because the patient can be classified as having SA whatever the target symptom, for example, dactylitis or uveitis). Viewed overall, Amor's criteria performed slightly better than the ESSG criteria in classifying early SA.

Conclusion

Table 11.13 shows a review and comparison of the sensitivity and specificity of all these classification criteria. The New York criteria are the criteria used most often for clinical research in AS. In considering the whole population, SA classification criteria perform much better in terms of sensitivity and specificity than AS classification criteria. SA criteria are used more often in clinical practice. Nevertheless, these two sets of criteria are not diagnostic criteria.

A Set of Diagnostic Criteria for Spondyloarthritis: Wishful Thinking?

In fact, no diagnostic criteria for SA have been evaluated. Early diagnosis is the current challenge, especially because of the new, dramatically powerful drugs available for spondyloarthropathies. However, for the reasons outlined in the first part of this chapter, no diagnostic criteria have been evaluated for SA.

A new and interesting approach, based on a decision tree, was proposed by Rudwaleit et al. in 2004[37] to help the physician in making an early diagnosis in a patient with axial SA (Fig. 11.1). This was a development study, and these criteria have not been evaluated yet.

The aim of the study was to provide data on the probability of early axial SA in patients with chronic

TABLE 11.12 COMPARISON BETWEEN AMOR'S AND ESSG CLASSIFICATION CRITERIA, BASED ON A STUDY OF 2228 PATIENTS (STUDY 1) AND 154 PATIENTS (STUDY 2)

Characteristics	AMOR'S CRITERIA		ESSG CRITERIA	
	Study 1[35]	Study 2[36]	Study 1[35]	Study 2[36]
Sensitivity (%)	91.9		87.1	
Specificity (%)	97.9		96.4	
Positive predictive value (%)	73.1	76	60.3	46
Negative predictive value (%)	99.5	89	99.2	82

TABLE 11.13 COMPARISON OF THE SENSITIVITY AND SPECIFICITY OF EXISTING CLASSIFICATION CRITERIA FOR ANKYLOSING SPONDYLITIS AND SPONDYLOARTHRITIS

	Sensitivity (%)	Specificity (%)
Ankylosing spondylitis		
Rome (radiological criteria + one clinical criterion)	87	95
Rome (four clinical criteria)	27	99
New York	73	98
Modified New York	80	81
Spondyloarthritis		
Amor's	91.9	97.9
ESSG	87.1	96.4

Data were derived from the following studies: Rigby AS, Wood PH. Observations on diagnostic criteria for ankylosing spondylitis. Clin Exp Rheumatol 1993;11:5–12; and Amor B, Dougados M, Listrat V, et al. Evaluation of the Amor criteria for spondylarthropathies and European Spondylarthropathy Study Group (ESSG). A cross-sectional analysis of 2,228 patients. Ann Med Interne (Paris) 1991;142:85–89.

back pain, according to the absence or presence of certain clinical features, laboratory tests, and skeletal imaging. The entry criterion was inflammatory back pain because this symptom is present in a great majority of patients with AS. This study was based on patients with AS or undifferentiated spondyloarthritides, without radiographic sacroiliitis, but with clinically predominant axial involvement.

The result is expressed as a percentage of probability for SA with axial involvement. The rate above which "axial SA" is considered as definite is 90%. If the probability is between 80% and 90%, the diagnosis is considered as highly probable. The probability of having an axial SA reached 90% in the presence of inflammatory back pain and at least three of seven further SA features: family history, heel pain, uveitis, synovitis, dactylitis, good response to NSAIDs, and HLA-B27 positivity. The author calculated a likelihood ratio based on a literature review for each parameter studied. The likelihood ratio expresses the odds that a given level of a diagnostic test result would be expected in a patient with (or without) the target disorder. The likelihood ratio captures both the sensitivity and specificity of a given test parameter. In this study, the presence of inflammatory spinal pain with only two features with a high likelihood ratio (for instance, acute anterior uveitis, HLA-B27 positivity, or MRI evidence) was sufficient to reach a probability of disease greater than 90%. The use of HLA-B27 makes sense as long as it is used in combination with the other parameters; in this study it had a high sensitivity and high specificity, resulting in a high likelihood ratio. HLA-B27 typing does not rely on a patient's memory or physician examination, it is relatively cheap to perform, and it is reliable. MRI also had a high sensitivity and specificity and is useful because it visualizes inflammation directly. However, this test has the disadvantages of high costs and possible interpretation variability.

Rudwaleit et al.[37] propose the following diagnostic algorithm (Fig. 11.1):

- First step: We consider a patient with inflammatory spinal pain according to the Calin criteria, without any change on pelvic radiography. The probability that the patient has axial SA is 14%.
- Second step: The physician checks for the other features of SA.
- If the patient has three or more of the other features, the probability of having the disease is 80% to 95% (probable to definite diagnosis); if the patient has one or two features, the probability varies from 35% to 70%; and if he or she has no other feature, the probability of suffering from the disease stays at 14%.
- Third step: When there are two or fewer other features associated with spinal inflammatory pain and normal radiography, HLA-B27 typing is recommended. At this step:
  - If HLA-B27 typing is positive in a patient with two other features, the probability of suffering from an axial SA is 80% to 90% (probable diagnosis);
  - If the patient has no other features, the probability falls to 59%. In this last case only, MRI is recommended.
  - In both cases, when HLA-B27 is negative, another diagnosis has to be considered.
- Fourth step: If MRI shows signs of sacroiliitis, the probability of the patient having the disease is 80% to 95%. If MRI results are negative, the probability is 10% to 20%, and another diagnosis has to be considered. Because of its cost and reduced availability, this diagnostic algorithm proposes the prescription of MRI as a final diagnostic step.

This decision tree is a new, original, and interesting way to consider making a diagnosis that is usable in daily clinical practice. However, it should be evaluated further before becoming an everyday tool in clinical practice.

CONCLUSION

The several successive proposed sets of classification criteria retrace the history of the spondyloarthritides and of medical and scientific research.

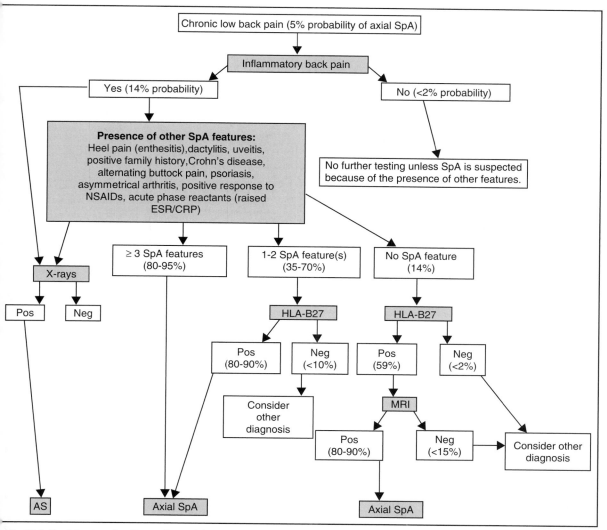

Fig. 11.1 Decision tree for diagnosing axial spondyloarthritis (SA). The starting point is the presence or absence of inflammatory back pain (IBP) in patients presenting with chronic back pain. In general, for making the diagnosis of axial SpA, a disease probability >90% is suggested. If the probability of disease exceeds 90% diagnosis of axial SpA is definite; if the probability is 80% to 90% the diagnosis is probable. AS, ankylosing spondylitis; ESR, erythrocyte sedimentation rate; CRP, C-reactive protein.

Questions that still remain concerning such criteria are the following:

- Should these criteria be proposed for the whole group of spondyloarthritides?
- Should they be proposed as diagnostic criteria?
- Should they be proposed as "potentially severe disease" criteria?

It is clear that such questions have been highlighted by the data recently observed with anti-tumor necrosis factor-α (TNF-α) therapies, suggesting that such treatments, if administered at an early stage of the disease, might prevent further progression.

Therefore, it is the opinion of the authors that further research is needed to recognize patients with a very early stage of disease (diagnostic criteria) but also to identify patients for whom therapies such as anti-TNF-α might be of interest. In this latter case, studies have to be conducted to propose a set of criteria for potentially severe disease. The use of these criteria in daily practice will be interesting because of the availability of new effective treatments.

REFERENCES

1. Dougados M, Hochberg MC. Why is the concept of spondyloarthropathies important? Best Pract Res Clin Rheumatol. 2002;16:495–505.

2. Dougados M. Diagnosis and monitoring of spondyloarthropathy. Compr Ther. 1998;24:590–595.

3. Dougados M. Diagnostic features of ankylosing spondylitis. Br J Rheumatol. 1995;34:301–303.

4. Dougados M. How to diagnose spondylarthropathy? Clin Exp Rheumatol. 1993;11:1–3.

5. Van der Linden S, Valkenburg HA, Cats A. Evaluation of diagnostic criteria for ankylosing spondylitis. A proposal for modification of the New York criteria. Arthritis Rheum. 1984;27:361–368.

6. Calin A, Porta J, Fries JF. Clinical history as a screening test for ankylosing spondylitis. JAMA. 1977;237:2613–2614.

7. Khan MA. Ankylosing spondylitis: clinical features. In Klippel JH, Dieppe PA, eds. Rheumatology. 2nd ed. London: Mosby-Wolfe; 1998;6.16.1–6.16.10.

8. Polley HF, Slocumb CH. Rheumatoid spondylitis: a study of 1035 cases. Ann Intern Med. 1974;26:240–249.

9. Feldtkeller E, Khan MA, van der Heijde D, van der Linden S, Braun J. Age at disease onset and diagnosis delay in HLA B27 negative versus positive patients with ankylosing spondylitis. Rheumatol Int. 2003;23:61–66.

10. Puhakka KB, Jurik AG, Schiottz-Christensen B, et al. MRI abnormalities of sacroiliac joints in early spondylarthropathy: a 1-year follow-up study. Scand J Rheumatol. 2004;33:332–338.

11. Remy M, Bouillet P, Bertin P, et al. Evaluation of magnetic resonance imaging for the detection of sacroiliitis in patients with early seronegative spondylarthropathy. Rev Rheum Engl Ed. 1996;63:577–583.

12. Puhakka KB, Jurik AG, Egund N, et al. Imaging of sacroiliitis in early seronegative spondylarthropathy. Assessment of abnormalities by MRI in comparison with radiography and CT. Acta Radiol 2003;44:218–229.

13. McGonagle D, Gibbon W, Emery P. Classification of inflammatory arthritis by enthesitis. Lancet. 1998;352:1137–1140.

14. Balint PV, Kane D, Wilson H, McInnes IB, Sturrock RD. Ultrasonography of entheseal insertions in the lower limb in spondyloarthropathy. Ann Rheum Dis. 2002;61:905–910.

15. D'Agostino MA, Said-Nahal R, Hacquard-Bouder C, Brasseur JL, Dougados M, Breban M. Assessment of peripheral enthesitis in the spondylarthropathies by ultrasonography combined with power Doppler: a cross-sectional study. Arthritis Rheum. 2003;48:523–533.

16. Kamel M, Eid H, Mansour R. Ultrasound detection of heel enthesitis: a comparison with magnetic resonance imaging. J Rheumatol. 2003;30:774–778.

17. Kellgren JH, Jeffrey MR, Ball J. The Epidemiology of Chronic Rheumatism. Oxford, England: Blackwell Scientific Publications; 1963;I:326–327.

18. Brewerton DA. A reappraisal of rheumatic diseases and immunogenetics. Lancet. 1984;2:799–802.

19. Sadowska-Wroblewska M, Filipowicz A, Garwolinska H, Michalski J, Rusiniak B, Wroblewska T. Clinical signs and symptoms useful in the early diagnostic of ankylosing spondylitis. Clin Rheumatol. 1983;2:37–43.

20. Schlosstein L, Terasaki PI, Bluestone R, Pearson CM. High association of an HL-A antigen, W27, with ankylosing spondylitis. N Engl J Med. 1973;5:704–706.

21. Braun J, Bollow M, Remlinger G, et al. Prevalence of spondylarthropathies in HLA-B27 positive and negative blood donors. Arthritis Rheum. 1998;41:58–67.

22. Hulsmeyer M, Fiorillo MT, Bettosini F, et al. Dual, HLA-B27 subtype-dependent conformation of a self-peptide. J Exp Med. 2004;199:271–281.

23. Bremner RG. Ankylosing spondylitis. Univ Toronto Med J. 1949;27:57–61.

24. Edmunds L, Elswood J, Calin A. New light on uveitis in ankylosing spondylitis. J Rheumatol. 1991;18:50–52.

25. Rosenbaum JT. Acute anterior uveitis and spondyloarthropathies. Rheum Dis Clin North Am. 1992;18:143–151

26. Gofton JP, Lawrence JS, Bennett PH. Sacroillitis in eight populations. Ann Rheum Dis. 1966;25:528–533.

27. Bennett PH, Burch TA. Population Studies of the Rheumatic Diseases. Amsterdam, Netherlands: Excerpta Medica; 1968: 456–457.

28. Amor B, Dougados M, Mijiyawa M. Criteria of the classification of spondylarthropathies. Rev Rhum Mal Osteoartic. 1990;57:85–89.

29. Dougados M, Van der Linden S, Juhlin R, et al., for the European Spondylarthropathy Study Group. The European Spondylarthropathy Study Group preliminary criteria for the classification of spondylarthropathy. Arthritis Rheum. 1991; 34:1218–1227.

30. Rigby AS, Wood PH. Observations on diagnostic criteria for ankylosing spondylitis. Clin Exp Rheumatol. 1993;11:5–12.

31. Moll JM, Wright V. New York clinical criteria for ankylosing spondylitis. A statistical evaluation. Ann Rheum Dis. 1973;3:354–363.

32. Moll JM, Wright V. An objective clinical study of chest expansion. Ann Rheum Dis. 1972;31:1–8.

33. Goie The HS, Steven MM, Van der Linden SM, Cats A. Evaluation of diagnostic criteria for ankylosing spondylitis: a comparison of the Rome, New York and modified New York criteria in patients with a positive clinical history screening test for ankylosing spondylitis. Br J Rheumatol. 1985;24:242–249.

34. Amor B, Dougados M, Listrat V, et al. Are classification criteria for spondylarthropathy useful as diagnostic criteria? Rev Rhum Engl Ed. 1995;62:10–15.

35. Amor B, Dougados M, Listrat V, et al. Evaluation of the Amor criteria for spondylarthropathies and European Spondylarthropathy Study Group (ESSG). A cross-sectional analysis of 2,228 patients. Ann Med Interne (Paris). 1991;142:85–89.

36. Collantes E, Veroz R, Escudero A, et al. Can some cases of 'possible' spondyloarthropathy be classified as 'definite' or 'undifferentiated' spondyloarthropathy? Value of criteria for spondyloarthropathies. Spondyloarthropathy Study Group. Joint Bone Spine. 2000;67:516–520.

37. Rudwaleit M, van der Heijde D, Khan MA, Braun J, Sieper J. How to diagnose axial spondyloarthritis early. Ann Rheum Dis. 2004;63:535–543.

12 Clinical Aspects of Ankylosing Spondylitis

Shirley W. Pang and John C. Davis, Jr.

INTRODUCTION

Ankylosing spondylitis (AS) is a systemic inflammatory disease of unknown etiology characterized by inflammation of the axial skeleton and adjacent structures as well as involvement of multiple organs including the eyes, lungs, and heart. The severity of disease ranges widely, from mild with limited sacroiliac joint involvement to severe with debilitating ankylosis of the spine.

CLINICAL MANIFESTATIONS

Systemic

Most patients with AS experience general constitutional symptoms including low-grade fever, fatigue, malaise, anorexia, and overall reduced quality of life.[1]

Musculoskeletal

Enthesitis is the hallmark feature of AS and is characterized by inflammation at the sites of insertion of ligaments, tendons, or joint capsules to bone.[2] Both enthesitis and synovitis contribute greatly to the axial and peripheral arthritis observed in AS. Along the spine, enthesitis occurs at capsular and ligamentous attachments as well as at discovertebral, costovertebral, and costotransverse joints. The bony attachments of interspinous and paravertebral ligaments may also be involved. Enthesitis is largely responsible for the pain, stiffness, and limitations of the spinal joints and pain. This can result in the eventual fusion of the sacroiliac joints.[3] Enthesitis also involves multiple extra-axial sites. The most commonly affected sites are the insertion of the plantar fascia and Achilles tendon at the calcaneus, producing significant heel pain and decreased mobility. Calcaneal spurs due to plantar fasciitis may be visible radiographically usually within several months. Other extra-axial sites include tibial tubercles, ischial tuberosities, pelvic adductor insertions into the femur, and costochondral junctions.[4]

Symptoms of sacroiliitis typically develop in the late teens up to the third decade of life. Patients usually present with unilateral or bilateral buttock pain. Over time, the pain may become persistent and bilateral, typically aggravated at night and interfering with sleep. Initially, the lower anterior synovial portion of the sacroiliac (SI) joint is affected. Subsequently, associated osteopenia and osteitis develop. Radiographically, SI joints appear widened due to erosions within the joint. Once endochondral ossification caused by osteitis occurs, erosions of the lower aspect of the SI joints appear on radiographs. These may, however, take several years to become evident. With further progression of the disease, capsular enthesitis occurs on both the anterior and posterior part of the joint throughout its length, corresponding to radiographic joint obscuration. Chronic inflammation in long-standing disease may then lead to bony ankylosis of the SI joints.[3]

Approximately 75% of patients present classically with chronic inflammatory low back pain (Table 12.1). Back stiffness subsequently develops and typically is worse after periods of prolonged inactivity. Over time, progressive ankylosing of the spine results in fixed deformities, including flattening of the lumbar spine, causing loss of lumbar lordosis and accentuated dorsal spine kyphosis.[3] Arthritis of "root" joints (the hips and

TABLE 12.1 INFLAMMATORY BACK PAIN FEATURES
1. Younger age at onset of pain (peak 26 years)
2. Pain and early morning stiffness of the spine or buttocks
3. Improvement with exercise/activity
4. Insidious/gradual in onset
5. Symptoms lasting longer than 3 months
6. Restriction of spinal mobility and deep breathing
7. Radiographic evidence of sacroiliitis or ankylosis
8. Difficulty sleeping due to pain

145

shoulders) is seen in about one third of patients.[3] With advanced disease, patients may develop a flexion contracture of the hip resulting in severe postural changes. Advanced hip joint disease often requires total hip arthroplasty.[4]

Peripheral joint involvement can occur in up to 50% of patients and become chronic in 25% of patients.[1] Peripheral joint synovitis can occur at any stage of the disease and typically involves the lower extremities such as the hips, knees, ankles, and metatarsophalangeal joints in an asymmetric fashion. Upper extremity involvement is rare, except in cases of concurrent psoriasis or inflammatory bowel disease (IBD). The synovitis is characteristically oligoarticular, asymmetric, and episodic. Peripheral arthritis is often thought to reflect more severe disease activity.[5] Temporomandibular joints may also be affected, resulting in symptoms of discomfort with mastication and reduction in oral aperture. Dactylitis (sausage-like digits) can also occur in one or more digits with symptoms lasting for months. However, this may resolve spontaneously.[4] Several studies have indicated that the incidence of peripheral joint involvement was significantly higher in women.[6–8] Studies of female patients with AS have shown a prevalence of peripheral arthritis ranging between 23% and 75%.[9,10] In a study of 412 Korean patients with AS, hand joint involvement was also found to be more common in women.[11]

Lastly, osteoporosis may be a significant feature of AS. Osteoporosis, observed in more than one third of patients, is related to disease activity and may become evident within the first few years of disease, especially in patients with very active disease. Osteoporosis can result in an increased cumulative risk for vertebral fractures.[12–15] Vertebral fractures not only adversely affect quality of life, but also increase mortality. In fact, patients with AS have higher morbidity and mortality associated with vertebral fractures than with hip fractures.[15] Osteoporosis in patients with AS can be difficult to identify. As seen on posterior-anterior dual-energy x-ray absorptiometry (DEXA) scans, patients with early AS demonstrate decreased vertebral column bone mineral density (BMD). However, with the progression of disease, the vertebral column BMD paradoxically increases. The increase in BMD is as a result of nontrabecular, cancellous bone expansions through syndesmophyte formation and ligamentous thickening and calcification. Because the increased BMD reflects nontrabecular bone expansion, the bone laid down is of poor structural integrity and more susceptible to fractures.[16]

Ophthalmologic

Acute anterior uveitis (AAU) is the most common extraarticular manifestation of AS, occurring in 25% to 40% of patients.[17] AAU is characterized by inflammation of the iris and ciliary body. Patients commonly present with an abrupt onset of ocular pain, photophobia, redness, lacrimation, and blurring of vision. The activity and severity of ocular complications are not associated with articular disease. However, patients who develop peripheral arthritis are more likely to develop AAU.[18]

In patients with AS, AAU is typically characterized by frequent recurrence of acute alternating unilateral attacks, with each attack separated by varying intervals of time.[19] Recurrence is usually described as occurring randomly in either eye; however, results in one case series of 175 patients with HLA-B27–associated uveitis suggested that recurrence in the same eye was more common than recurrence in the other eye, postulating that breakdown of the blood-aqueous barrier may be responsible for this phenomenon.[20] The frequency of attacks appears to decrease over the course of disease. In one study of 148 patients with HLA-B27+–associated uveitis, the median duration of an AAU attack was 6 weeks, and the median number of recurrences with more than 12 months of follow-up was three.[21] In addition, the first episode of uveitis is typically preceded by rheumatologic symptoms. However, some reports in the literature indicate that in 0% to 11.4% of patients, uveitis was the first manifestation of spondyloarthropathy.[22,23]

Prompt treatment consists of topical administration of steroids and a mydriatic agent, with resolution within several weeks. If HLA-B27–associated uveitis is identified early, the overall prognosis is generally favorable, and permanent visual impairment is a rare complication. In one case series only 6.9% of patients showed significant impairment in visual acuity.[20] However, if not promptly treated, inflammation progresses with debris subsequently accumulating in the anterior chamber causing papillary and lens dysfunction. In rare patients, the posterior chamber can become involved, often due to anterior chamber inflammation (frequency between 0% and 21%).[19,21,24–26] Posterior chamber inflammation may cause macular edema with visual compromise. Macular edema has been demonstrated to be the key factor determining visual outcomes in uveitis.[27] Formation of synechiae (scarring and pinning down of the iris) occurs in the setting of nonaggressive and delayed treatment. Cataracts can also occur and are associated with synechiae.[21]

Cardiovascular Disease

Cardiac complications due to AS usually occur in patients after many years of disease. There appears to be no association with skeletal disease activity, and rarely does cardiac involvement precede axial symptoms.[28] Common manifestations of cardiac involvement may include valvular dysfunction (aortic and mitral regurgitation), variable degrees of conduction system disturbances, and left ventricular dysfunction.[29,30] Interestingly, in one case report a patient with mitral stenosis in addition to mitral regurgitation and aortic regurgitation was described.[31] However, except for this case report, there has been no previous reported association of mitral stenosis with AS.

The prevalence of valve dysfunction increases with age and disease duration, with reports of 2% after 10 years of disease and 12% after 30 years of disease.[32,33] The overall prevalence for cardiac complications ranges from 24% to 100% in postmortem series and from 8% to 31% by transthoracic echocardiography.[34-36] Transesophageal echocardiograms reveal an even higher incidence of valvular abnormalities of approximately 80% but most appear not to be hemodynamically significant.[28] In aortic regurgitation, three factors contribute: 1) aortic root thickening and dilation, 2) aortic cusp thickening and retraction, and 3) inward rolling of the edges of the cusps. Aortic regurgitation is diagnosed in 2% to 10% of patients with AS.[37,38] Mitral regurgitation is less common and may be the result of subaortic fibrosis of the anterior leaflet with impaired mobility or may be due to left ventricular dilation from aortic regurgitation.[39] Valvular dysfunction is associated with cardiovascular morbidity.[32] The presence of an audible aortic regurgitation murmur signals a progression of disease to eventual heart failure, usually over the course of several years. With significant valvular dysfunction, the treatment of choice is valvular replacement.

Multiple types of atrioventricular conduction blocks have been reported in patients with AS.[40] After examining electrocardiograms of 190 patients with AS, Bernstein and Broch[40] found that 29 (15%) patients had first-degree and 3 (1.6%) patients had complete heart block. A longitudinal follow-up of these patients revealed that up to one third exhibited cardiac conduction abnormalities including atrioventricular and intraventricular blocks. The blocks were intermittent in nature, suggesting that the underlying process involves reversible inflammation and not fibrosis.[41,42] Third-degree heart block has been identified in 1% to 9% of patients with AS.[37,40,41,43,44] The block occurs primarily at the atrioventricular node itself, as demonstrated by electrophysiologic studies.[45,46] Heart block can progress to a subsequent need for pacemaker placement. The prognosis is considered to be good and generally does not affect longevity.[47] Arrhythmias have also been reported, including bradycardia or pauses due to sinus node dysfunction.[45,46]

Left ventricular dysfunction with systolic and diastolic abnormalities are not uncommon manifestation in patients with AS. In one study, 17% of patients with AS without valvular abnormalities had subclinical systolic dysfunction.[48] Diastolic filling abnormalities were documented echographically.[34,49,50] These abnormalities do not appear to be associated with age, disease duration, or severity of peripheral joint disease.[49]

Other rarer cardiac manifestations include aneurysm of the ascending aorta, amyloidosis, pericarditis, and pericardial effusion. Based on both clinical features and on histopathologic examination, pericarditis is a rare feature that has been recognized in 1% or less of patients.[48]

The vast majority of patients with cardiac involvement are HLA-B27 positive. Subsequently, the concept of HLA-B27-related cardiac syndrome has been proposed, consisting of the combination of aortic root disease and conduction system abnormalities. This concept is supported by immunogenetic, histopathologic, clinical, and electrophysiologic studies.[51] It has been noted that as many as 15% to 20% of male patients with permanent pacemakers may have an HLA-B27–associated disease as the cause of their bradycardia.[52-54] In addition, the syndrome of severe conduction system abnormalities plus aortic regurgitation is strongly associated with HLA-B27, which is found in 67% to 88% of patients with these two concomitant conditions.[55,56] Histopathologically, the pathologic lesions noted in cardiac and aortic tissues are similar to those found in affected joints.[29,51] In HLA-B27–associated disease, high-degree atrioventricular blocks are relatively selective and are typically located in the atrioventricular node, even in patients with concomitant fascicular or bundle-branch blocks.[45,46]

Pulmonary

The exact prevalence of pulmonary disease is rare and remains to be fully studied. Pulmonary involvement is typically asymptomatic, consisting of abnormalities of the thoracic cage and lung parenchyma. Rarely the cricoarytenoid joint is affected, with patients developing symptoms of hoarseness. If pulmonary involvement is severe, upper airway obstruction and acute respiratory failure can occur.[57] The cause of pulmonary involvement remains controversial, but it is postulated that it develops in patients with severe bone changes.

Restriction in thoracic expansion occurs as a result of ankylosing of the thoracic spine and inflammation of costovertebral and costosternal joints. In the study of Fournie et al.,[58] 50% of the patients exhibited enthesopathy of the manubriosternal symphysis and sternoclavicular joints. The decreased chest expansion can contribute to restrictive ventilatory impairment and loss of respiratory function.[59] Abnormalities noted are usually mild on pulmonary function testing. In a series of 32 patients with AS, the mean vital capacity (VC) was 88% of the predicted values.[60] This reduction in VC is due to decreased thoracic cage compliance from chest wall fixation rather than parenchymal disease because diffusion capacity was normal.[61] To preserve normal lung functions, chest wall fixation is counterbalanced by several factors: thorax fixation at greater lung volumes, increased ventilatory contribution by the diaphragm, and maintenance of chest wall symmetry and vertical axis of rib excursion.[59,62,63] The degree of pulmonary function abnormalities is correlated with the mobility of the thoracic cage and disease duration.[60]

The association of AS and pleuropulmonary disease was first reported in 1941 by Dunham and Kautz[64] and in 1949 by Hamilton.[65] The most common pleuropulmonary manifestation of the disease is believed to be bilateral upper lobe fibrotic changes.[66] The fibrocystic apical process has been reported to occur in from 1.3% to 30% of patients.[66–68] In a study of 2080 patients with AS, 25 patients were noted to exhibit apical fibrobullous changes, and 2 had pleural effusions. Wolson and Rohwedder[69] found two occurrences of apical lung fibrosis after a record review of 52 patients with AS.

Apical fibrocystic disease typically presents in adulthood with the duration between onset of rheumatologic manifestations and onset of pulmonary lesions varying from 6 to 35 years with a mean of 15 years or more.[70,71] However, there have been rare case reports of patients who had bilateral apical pulmonary fibrosis before any rheumatologic symptoms appeared.[72] Apical fibrocystic disease predominantly occurs in men with a male-to-female ratio of 50:1.[73] The fibrosis is typically asymptomatic.[59,62] Patients become symptomatic in situations of secondary superinfection of cavities by bacteria or fungi. Superinfections of the cavities can be seen in up to one third of patients, with *Aspergillus* being identified in some of these patients.[74,75] The cause of apical fibrocavitary disease is unknown; however, several hypotheses has been put forth including diminished upper lobe ventilation caused by chest wall rigidity, altered apical mechanical stresses, recurrent pulmonary infections, repeated aspiration pneumonitis due to esophageal muscle dysfunction, and airway inflammation.[63,64,76,77]

Radiographic changes in early disease consist of small apical nodular or linear infiltrates and pleural thickening. Infiltrates rarely involve the lower half of the lung fields.[68,71] Unilateral involvement presents more often in the right upper zone than in the left.[70] This process may initially be unilateral but usually evolves to become bilateral.[71] The disease typically progresses with subsequent coalescence of the nodules into larger opacities. No treatment has been shown to alter the natural course of this disease.[68,69] In advanced disease, cysts, cavities, and fibrosis of the parenchyma and pleura can be seen.[71] These radiographic findings may mimic those of chronic tuberculosis with apical fibrocavitary changes and cyst formation. Fibrosis can be severe to produce

upper lobe bronchiectasis and upward retraction of the hila.[63,68] In one study of 26 patients with AS, high-resolution computed tomography (CT) scanning showed abnormalities in 19 (70%) patients. Abnormal findings included interstitial lung disease (4 patients), bronchiectasis (6 patients), emphysema (4 patients), apical fibrosis (2 patients), mycetoma (1 patient), and nonspecific interstitial lung disease (12 patients). Interestingly, plain radiographs revealed abnormalities in only 4 patients.[78] Additional abnormalities noted on CT scans include tracheobronchomegaly, mediastinal lymphadenopathy, bronchial wall thickening, and bronchiolitis obliterans organizing pneumonia. Paraseptal emphysema has been documented in a series of patients with AS, some of whom were smokers.[75,79] Smoking is associated with worse long-term clinical, functional, and radiographic outcome.[80] In 53 patients with AS with median disease duration of 20 years, significant differences were noted between smokers and nonsmokers in the following tests: the Schober test, occiput-wall distance, stiffness, spine radiographic scores, total spine movement, and functional index.[80]

Renal

The most common renal manifestation in AS is secondary amyloidosis (62%).[81] Secondary amyloidosis is uncommon, reported in 1% to 3% of patients with long-standing active disease. It has been more commonly reported in Europe than in the United States. Patients typically present with proteinuria, often in the nephrotic range, that can progress to renal failure. With renal failure, the prognosis is poor. Gratacos et al.[82] reported that 10 (13.7%) of 137 patients with AS had positive results on abdominal fat pad biopsies for amyloid. However, upon follow-up of 2 to 10 years, only 5 (6.9%) patients were symptomatic.

Immunoglobulin (Ig) A nephropathy, another renal manifestation of ankylosing spondylitis (30%), is also uncommon. This disease should be considered in patients presenting with hematuria and proteinuria, with or without mild renal impairment. At presentation, these patients also have an elevated serum IgA level (93%) and renal insufficiency (27%).[83] In up to 35% of patients, microscopic hematuria and proteinuria can be seen. The prognostic significance these findings for a subsequent decline in renal function is unclear.[82]

Patients can also present with analgesic abuse nephropathy resulting from therapy with nonsteroidal anti-inflammatory drugs and traditional disease-modifying antirheumatic drugs such as sulfasalazine.[8] Other common renal manifestations include mesangioproliferative glomerulonephritis (55%) with rare involvement including membranous nephropathy (1%), focal segmental glomerulosclerosis (1%), and focal proliferative glomerulomenephritis.[81]

Genitourinary

There appears to be an increased prevalence of varicocele in men with AS on the basis of a small study of 21 Turkish patients and 25 control subjects.[85] By physical examination and ultrasonography, unilateral or bilateral varicoceles were noted in a majority of patients but were only seen in one fifth of control subjects. In another recent study of 65 men erectile dysfunction (ED) in patients with AS was evaluated.[86] These patients experienced significantly lower erectile function, orgasmic function, intercourse satisfaction, and overall satisfaction scores on the International Index of Erectile Function. The ED appears to be associated with morning stiffness. The pathogenesis of ED is thought to be multifactorial—from the accelerated atherosclerosis due to inflammation and medications such as glucocorticoid or methotrexate, to severe disturbances of body image, to limited mobility causing physical dysactivity.[86–89] Interestingly, this finding of limited sexual activities in male patients with AS was not found in another study of sexual function in patients with AS.[90] However, the different results could be explained by cultural differences in the study populations as well as in methodology.[86]

Neurologic

Neurologic complications can occur in the setting of several spinal diseases. Spinal fractures are not a rare complication in patients with advanced AS. Fractures can be classified into two basic categories.[91]

The first category consists of fractures of ankylosed spines caused by even minor trauma. Cooper et al.[15] reported vertebral fracture rates peaking two to three decades after diagnosis, and a cumulative incidence of 15% in patients with AS compared with an incidence of 2% to 3% in the control group. In a study of 111 patients with AS, Ralston et al.[92] reported a 16% prevalence of vertebral fractures. The most common sites are the C5–C6 and C6–C7 interspaces. Lower dorsal lumbar spine fractures are rare. In most patients, fractures are three column, involving both anterior and posterior elements. They are typically unstable and can cause devastating consequences when they occur at the cervical level because of the associated cord trauma.[93,94] In one study, the mortality rate was found to be 35%, which is twice the rate seen with similar fractures involving normal spines.[95] Fractures initially may be nondisplaced and presentation can be subtle, easily missed on plain radiographs. In one study of 300 patients, Bohlman[96] found that only 50% of acute cervical spine fractures were diagnosed in the emergency room by physical examination and cervical spine radiographs. Of these 300 patients, 80% became paralyzed and 50% died of complications of the cervical spine fracture. Computed tomography (CT) and magnetic resonance imaging

(MRI) can be used to detect occult fractures. Because of the instability of these fractures, patients must be immobilized to allow for healing to prevent ensuing damage to the spinal cord.[93]

The second category consists of stress fracture, typically occurring near the cervicothoracic and thoracolumbar junction. Patients with long-standing disease usually present with new pain or increased spinal range of motion. Radiographic findings on initial presentation may be subtle; on later presentation, a pseudoarthritis can develop at the site of the stress fracture, appearing radiographically as vertebral end-plate erosion or destruction.[97]

Spontaneous atlantoaxial-axial joint subluxation, atlanto-occipital subluxation, and upward subluxation of the axis are recognized complications of AS, similar to rheumatoid arthritis. Without stabilization, spinal cord compression can result. In a study of 103 patients, Ramos-Remus et al.[98] noted anterior subluxation in 21% of patients and posterior subluxation in 2%. In a 2-year follow-up study, anterior subluxation was noted to progress in 50% of patients. Spontaneous anterior subluxation was reported to be more common in patients with peripheral arthritis than in those with exclusively axial involvement.[98]

In patients with long-standing disease, slowly progressive cauda equina due to arachnoiditis is a rare but serious reported complication. Symptoms are secondary lumbosacral nerve root damage from arachonoiditis.[99,100] Patients may present with sensory loss and motor function loss. Less often, patients may have lower extremity weakness and pain, loss of ankle reflex, impotence, and urinary and fecal incontinence. Motor symptoms are typically mild if present. MRI and CT are key to diagnosing this complication.

There have been published case reports of a possible increased association between multiple sclerosis (MS) and AS. Most of these case reports describe patients with AS who have a neurologic finding consistent with an MS-like syndrome, such as monophasic myelopathy or transverse myelitis.[101,102] However, only four occurrences of MS-like clinical and cerebral magnetic resonance lesions in patients with long-standing AS have been reported to date. One of these case reports describes the possible coexistence of MS-like symptoms corroborated with MRI findings in a black patient, which is interesting because many of the reports suggesting a possible association between AS and MS were found in Caucasian patients.[98,103–105] In addition, the incidence of both AS and MS is higher than expected when individual prevalences of each disease are compared. In one study of 420 patients with MS, Hanrahan et al.[106] found that the prevalence of HLA-B27 was 10.2%. With further clinical and radiographic evaluation for AS, 5 of the 20 HLA-B27–positive patients met the criteria for AS. The prevalence rates of HLA-B27 positivity in MS patients are between 12% and 25%, whereas in the normal population, the prevalence rates are between 1% and 2%.[106] Also, there appears to be a role for immunogenetic predisposition factors in both diseases. There is a very strong association between HLA-B27 and AS; likewise, there is an observation of increased HLA-A3, B7, DR3, and Dw2 haplotypes in patients with MS.[107,108] In both diseases, T-lymphocyte activations appear to play an important role. In addition, environmental factors seem to be involved in the expression of both diseases based on the lack of concordance of disease expression in monozygotic twin studies.[109] However, there is no conclusive evidence to establish an association between MS and AS.[98,103]

Gastrointestinal

Macroscopic and microscopic subclinical intestinal inflammation has been seen in up to 60% of patients with AS by ileocolonoscopy.[110–113] The intestinal inflammation usually involves the ileum; however, microscopic colitis has also been reported.[113,114] A close relationship appears to exist between the subclinical intestinal inflammation and the inflammation in Crohn's disease, with the ileal biopsy findings of giant cells, granulomas, and fissures being almost identical in both AS and Crohn's disease.[114] In one study, it was reported that 26% of 123 patients with chronic AS have ileocolonoscopic findings of inflammation resembling Crohn's disease.[113]

For the vast majority of these patients with AS, the subclinical mucosal ulcerations do not become symptomatic. However, a small portion of these patients do eventually develop overt IBD, usually Crohn's disease.[110,115] The 123 patients previously studied with ileocolonoscopy were then prospectively studied with a follow-up period of 2 to 9 years. The findings from this study demonstrated that 6.5% of patients who initially presented with subclinical inflammatory gut lesions developed clinically overt Crohn's disease. In addition, all of these patients developed AS, often with persistent peripheral arthritis.[116] Interestingly, in a minority of patients with colitis and peripheral arthritis, peripheral joint disease may become quiescent after total colectomy.[4] However, many patients complain of a fibromyalgia-like disorder with widespread discomfort, even after colectomy.[4] In other studies, 10% of patients with the initial diagnosis of AS associated with subclinical ileitis had developed overt IBD when they were restudied several years later.[116,117]

Risk factors found to be associated with evolution of IBD include chronic inflammatory gut lesions, persistently elevated levels of inflammatory serum markers, and HLA-B27 negativity in the presence of sacroiliitis.[118] Also, no direct link appears to exist between AS and IBD because the inflammatory activity of each disease appears to occur independently of each other.[4]

The significance of these mucosal changes is not known, but studies to address the nature and importance of intestinal inflammation in AS are currently being conducted.[114] One suggestion was that intestinal inflammation in AS may represent subclinical Crohn's disease. Another was that intestinal inflammation may play a pathogenic role in the arthropathy of AS. It is hypothesized that through increased intestinal permeability to human antigens and or bacteria, there is an HLA-B27–dependent immune response to elements of fibrocartilage, thereby resulting in the arthropathy.[114]

DIAGNOSIS OF ANKYLOSING SPONDYLITIS

To establish a definite diagnosis of AS, the modified New York criteria (Table 12.2) have been developed. With these criteria the diagnosis of AS depend on unilateral or grade 2 or greater bilateral radiographic demonstration of grade 3 or 4 sacroiliitis based on the Stoke Ankylosing Spondylitis Spine Score. In addition, one or more clinical symptoms or signs must be present. A definite diagnosis cannot be established if sacroiliitis occurs alone, although this may an early sign or mild form of AS.[119]

ASSESSMENT OF DISEASE ACTIVITY

Various domains can be evaluated to assess disease activity. These domains include physical function, pain, spinal mobility, stiffness, peripheral joint involvement, enthesopathy, laboratory parameters (acute-phase reactants), and structural damage identified with radiography.

TABLE 12.2 MODIFIED NEW YORK CRITERIA FOR DEFINITIVE AS*
Clinical symptoms and signs
1. Low-back pain of ≥3 months' duration that is improved by exercise and not relieved by rest
2. Limitation of lumbar spine in sagittal and frontal plans
3. Chest expansion decreased relative to normal values for age and sex
Radiography†
Bilateral sacroiliitis, grade 2–4
Unilateral sacroiliitis, grade 3–4

*The diagnosis of AS is definite if unilateral grade 3 or 4 or bilateral grade 2 to 4 sacroiliitis and any clinical criteria are present.
†Grading of radiographs: 0 = normal, 1 = suggestive; 2 = minimal sacroiliitis; 3 = moderate sacroiliitis; 4 = complete ankylosis.
From Van der Linden S, Valkenburg HA, Cats A. Evaluation of diagnostic criteria for ankylosing spondylitis. A proposal for modification of the New York criteria. Arthritis Rheum. 1984;27:361–367.

Various composite indexes have been developed to evaluate disease activity, including the Bath Ankylosing Spondylitis Disease Activity Index (BASDAI). The BASDAI includes the domains of fatigue, axial pain, peripheral pain, stiffness, and enthesopathy on a visual analog scale.[120,121] More recently, the Assessment in Ankylosing Spondylitis (ASAS) Working Group developed a composite index for the criteria for both responder and partial remission. These criteria include the core domains of pain, functional impairment, patient's global assessment, and inflammation (assessed by morning stiffness).[122] With the ASAS response criteria, there must be a 20% improvement and a minimum of a 10-point absolute change on a zero to 100 point scale in each of the three domains, with no worsening of the fourth domain.

REFERENCES

1. Yu DT, Wisenhutter CW. Clinical manifestation of ankylosing spondylitis. UpToDate. 2004;12.1.
2. Granfors K, Marker-Hermann E, de Keyser F, Khan MA, Veys EM, Yu DT. The cutting edge of spondylarthropathy research in the millennium. Arthritis Rheum. 2002;46:606–613.
3. Khan MA. Clinical features of ankylosing spondylitis. In: Hochberg M, Silman A, Smolen JS, eds. Rheumatology. 3rd ed. St. Louis, Mosby; 2003;2:1161–1181.
4. Klippel JH, Crofford LJ, Stone JH, Weyland CM. Seronegative spondyloarthropathies. In: Klippel JH, ed. Primer on the Rheumatic Diseases. 12th ed. Atlanta, GA: Arthritis Foundation; 2001:251–252.
5. Heuft-Dorenbosch L, van Tubergen A, Spoorenberg A, et al. The influence of peripheral arthritis on disease activity in ankylosing spondylitis patients as measured with the Bath Ankylosing Spondylitis Disease Activity Index. Arthritis Rheum. 2004;51:154–159.
6. Goodman CE, Lange RK, Waxman J, Weiss TE. Ankylosing spondylitis in women. Arch Phys Med Rehabil. 1980;61:167–170.
7. Kidd B, Mullee M, Frank A, Cawley M. Disease expression of ankylosing spondylitis in males and females. J Rheumatol. 1988;15:1407–1409.
8. Marks SH, Barnett M, Calin A. Ankylosing spondylitis in women and men: a case-control study. J Rheumatol. 1983;10:624–628.
9. Jimenez-Balderas F, Mintz G. Ankylosing spondylitis: clinical course in women and men. J Rheumatol. 1993;20:2069–2072.
10. Gran JT, Ostensen M, Husby G. A clinical comparison between males and females with ankylosing spondylitis. J Rheumatol. 1985;12:126–129.
11. Lee JH, Jun JB, Jung S, et al. Higher prevalence of peripheral arthritis among ankylosing spondylitis patients. J Korean Med Sci. 2002;17:669–673.
12. Gratacos J, Collado A, Pons F, et al. Significant loss of bone mass in patients with early, active ankylosing spondylitis: a followup study. Arthritis Rheum. 1999;42:2319–2324.
13. El Maghraoui A, Bordene D, Cherruau B, et al. Osteoporosis, body composition, and bone turnover in ankylosing spondylitis. J Rheumatol. 1999;26:2205–2209.
14. Maillefert JF, Aho LS, El Maghaoui A, Dougados M, Roux C. Changes in bone density in patients with ankylosing spondylitis: a two-year follow-up study. Osteoporos Int. 2001;12:605–609.
15. Cooper C, Carbone L, Michet CJ, Atkinson EJ, O'Fallon WM, Melton LJ. Fracture risk in patients with ankylosing spondylitis: a population based study. J Rheumatol. 1994;21:1877–1882.
16. Meirelles ES, Borelli A, Camargo OP. Influence of disease activity and chronicity on ankylosing spondylitis bone mass loss. Clin Rheumatol. 1999;18:364–368.
17. Wakefield D, Montanaro A, McCluskey P. Acute anterior uveitis and HLA-B27. Surv Ophthalmol. 1991;36:223–232.
18. Maksymowych WP, Chou CT, Russell AS. Matching prevalence of peripheral arthritis and acute anterior uveitis in individuals with ankylosing spondylitis. Ann Rheum Dis. 1995;54:128–130.
19. Rothova A, van Veenedaal WG, Linssen A, Glasius E, Kijlstra A, de Jong PT. Clinical features of acute anterior uveitis. Am J Ophthalmol. 1987;103:137–145.
20. Monnet D, Breban M, Hudry C, Dougados M, Brezin AP. Ophthalmic findings and frequency of extraocular manifestations in patients with HLA-B27 uveitis: a study of 175 cases. Ophthalmology. 2004;111:802–809.
21. Tay-Kearney ML, Schwam BL, Lowder C, et al. Clinical features and associated systemic diseases of HLA-B27 uveitis. Am J Ophthalmol. 1996;121:47–56.
22. Hantzschel H, Otto W, Romhild N, et al. Characteristics of the early phase of ankylosing spondylitis. Z Gesamte Inn Med. 1981;36:189–192.
23. Amor B, Santos RS, Nahal R, Listat V, Dougados M. Predictive factors for the longterm outcome of spondyloarthropathies. J Rheumatol. 1994;21:1883–1887.
24. Rothova A, Suttorp-van Schulten MS, Frits Treffers W, Kiljstra A. Causes and frequency of blindness in patients with intraocular inflammatory disease. Br J Ophthalmol. 1996;80:332–336.
25. Rodriguez A, Akova YA, Pedroza-Seres M, Foster CS. Posterior segment ocular manifestations in patients with HLA-B27-associated uveitis. Ophthalmology. 1994;101:1267–1274.
26. Dodds EM, Lowder CY, Meisler DM. Posterior segment inflammation in HLA-B27+ acute anterior uveitis: clinical characteristics. Ocul Immunol Inflamm. 1999;7:85–92.
27. Rothova A. Comment on 'Posterior segment inflammation in HLA-B27+ acute anterior uveitis: clinical characteristics.' Ocul Immunol Inflamm. 2000;8:73–75.
28. Roldan CA. Valvular disease associated with systemic illness. Cardiol Clin. 1998;16:531–550.
29. Bulkley BH, Roberts WC. Ankylosing spondylitis and aortic regurgitation. Description of the characteristic cardiovascular lesion from study of eight necropsy patients. Circulation. 1973;48:1014–1027.
30. Davidson P, Baggenstoss AH, Slocumb CH, Daugherty GW. Cardiac and aortic lesions in rheumatoid spondylitis. Mayo Clin Proc. 1963;38:427–435.
31. Gupta BK, Panwar RB, Kabra PK, Kaushik AN, Meena GL, Chadda VS. Ankylosing spondylitis in association with mitral stenosis, mitral regurgitation, and aortic regurgitation: a case report and review of the literature. Echocardiography. 2003;20:275–277.
32. Roldan CA, Chavez J, Weist PW, Qualls CR, Crawford MH. Aortic root disease and valve disease associated with ankylosing spondylitis. J Am Coll Cardiol. 1998;32:1397–1404.
33. Graham DC, Smythe HA. The carditis and aortitis of ankylosing spondylitis. Bull Rheum Dis. 1958;9:171–174.
34. O'Neill TW, King G, Graham IM, Molony J, Bresnihan B. Echocardiographic abnormalities in ankylosing spondylitis. Ann Rheum Dis. 1992;51:652–654.
35. Alves MG, Espirito-Santo J, Queiroz MV, Madeira H, Macieira-Coelho E. Cardiac alterations in ankylosing spondylitis. Angiology. 1988;39(7 Pt 1):567–571.
36. Tucker CR, Fowles RE, Calin A, Popp RL. Aortitis in ankylosing spondylitis: early detection of aortic root abnormalities with two dimensional echocardiography. Am J Cardiol. 1982;49:680–686.
37. Kinsella T, Johnson LG, Ian R. Cardiovascular manifestations of ankylosing spondylitis. Can Med Assoc J. 1974;111:1309–1311.
38. Bachmann F, Hartl W, Veress M, Frind W. Cardiovascular complications of ankylosing spondylitis (Bechterew's disease). Med Welt. 1976;27:2149–2150.
39. Porciello PI, Capella G, Aralda D, Rossi P. Mitral and aortic regurgitation: a rare association in ankylosing spondylitis (author's transl). G Ital Cardiol. 1978;8:564–567.
40. Berstein L, Broch O. Cardiac complications in spondylarthritis ankylopoietica. Acta Med Scand. 1949;135:185–194.

41. Bergfeldt L, Edhag O, Vallin H. Cardiac conduction disturbances, an underestimated manifestation in ankylosing spondylitis. A 25-year follow-up study of 68 patients. Acta Med Scand. 1982; 212:217–223.

42. Cass RM, Richeson JF, Akiyama T. Reversible complete heart block. Hosp Pract (Off Ed). 1991;26:51.

43. Sukenik S, Pras A, Buskila D, Katz A, Snir Y, Horowitz J. Cardiovascular manifestations of ankylosing spondylitis. Clin Rheumatol. 1987;6:588–592.

44. Weed CL, Kulander BG, Massarella JA, Decker JL. Heart block in ankylosing spondylitis. Arch Intern Med. 1966;117:800–806.

45. Bergfeldt L, Vallin H, Edhag O. Complete heart block in HLA-B27 associated disease. Electrophysiological and clinical characteristics. Br Heart J. 1984;51:184–188.

46. Nitter-Hauge S, Otterstad JE. Characteristics of atrioventricular conduction disturbances in ankylosing spondylitis (Mb. Bechterew). Acta Med Scand. 1981;210:197–200.

47. Bergfeldt L, Allebeck P, Edhag O. Mortality in pacemaker-treated patients. A follow-up study of the impact of HLA-B27 and associated rheumatic disorders. Acta Med Scand. 1987;222: 293–299.

48. Nagyhegyi G, Nadas I, Banyai F, et al. Cardiac and cardiopulmonary disorders in patients with ankylosing spondylitis and rheumatoid arthritis. Clin Exp Rheumatol. 1988;6:17–26.

49. Crowley JJ, Donnelly SM, Tobin M, et al. Doppler echocardiographic evidence of left ventricular diastolic dysfunction in ankylosing spondylitis. Am J Cardiol. 1993;71:1337–1340.

50. Sun JP, Khan MA, Farhat AZ, Bahler RC. Alterations in cardiac diastolic function in patients with ankylosing spondylitis. Int J Cardiol. 1992;37:65–72.

51. Bergfeldt L, Edhag O, Rajs J. HLA-B27-associated heart disease. Clinicopathologic study of three cases. Am J Med. 1984;77: 961–967.

52. Bergfeldt L. HLA-B27–associated cardiac disease. Ann Intern Med. 1997;127(8 Pt 1):621–629.

53. Bergfeldt L. HLA-B27-associated rheumatic diseases with severe cardiac bradyarrhythmias. Clinical features and prevalence in 223 men with permanent pacemakers. Am J Med. 1983;75: 210–215.

54. Bergfeldt L, Edhag O, Vedin L, Vallin H. Ankylosing spondylitis: an important cause of severe disturbances of the cardiac conduction system. Prevalence among 223 pacemaker-treated men. Am J Med. 1982;73:187–191.

55. Bergfeldt L, Insulander P, Lindblom D, Moller E, Edhag O. HLA-B27: an important genetic risk factor for lone aortic regurgitation and severe conduction system abnormalities. Am J Med. 1988;85:12–18.

56. Qaiyumi S, Hassan ZU, Toone E. Seronegative spondyloarthropathies in lone aortic insufficiency. Arch Intern Med. 1985;145:822–824.

57. Libby DM, Schley WS, Smith JP. Cricoarytenoid arthritis in ankylosing spondylitis. A cause of acute respiratory failure and cor pulmonale. Chest. 1981;80:641–642.

58. Fournie B, Boutes A, Dromer C, et al. Prospective study of anterior chest wall involvement in ankylosing spondylitis and psoriatic arthritis. Rev Rhum Engl Ed. 1997;64:22–25.

59. Wiedemann HP, Matthay RA. Pulmonary manifestations of the collagen vascular diseases. Clin Chest Med. 1989;10:677–722.

60. Feltelius N, Hedenstrom H, Hillerdal G, Hallgren R. Pulmonary involvement in ankylosing spondylitis. Ann Rheum Dis. 1986;45:736–740.

61. Franssen MJ, van Herwaarden CL, van de Putte LB, Gribnau FW. Lung function in patients with ankylosing spondylitis. A study of the influence of disease activity and treatment with nonsteroidal antiinflammatory drugs. J Rheumatol. 1986;13:936–940.

62. Hunninghake GW, Fauci AS. Pulmonary involvement in the collagen vascular diseases. Am Rev Respir Dis. 1979;119: 471–503.

63. Tanoue LT. Pulmonary involvement in collagen vascular disease: a review of the pulmonary manifestations of the Marfan syndrome, ankylosing spondylitis, Sjögren's syndrome, and relapsing polychondritis. J Thorac Imaging. 1992;7:62–77.

64. Dunham CL, Kautz F. Spondylarthritis ankylopoietica: a review and report of twenty cases. Am J Med Sci. 1941;201:232–250.

65. Hamilton K. Pulmonary disease manifestations of ankylosing spondylarthritis. Ann Intern Med. 1949;31:216–227.

66. Rosenow E, Strimlan CV, Muhm JR, Ferguson RH. Pleuropulmonary manifestations of ankylosing spondylitis. Mayo Clin Proc. 1977;52:641–649.

67. Thai D, Ratani RS, Salame S, Steiner RM. Upper lobe fibrocavitary disease in a patient with back pain and stiffness. Chest. 2000;118:1814–1816.

68. Lee-Chiong TL Jr. Pulmonary manifestations of ankylosing spondylitis and relapsing polychondritis. Clin Chest Med. 1998;19:747–757, ix.

69. Wolson AH, Rohwedder JJ. Upper lobe fibrosis in ankylosing spondylitis. Am J Roentgenol Radium Ther Nucl Med. 1975; 124:466–471.

70. Gupta SM, Johnston WH. Apical pulmonary disease in ankylosing spondylitis. NZ Med J. 1978;88:186–188.

71. Rumancik WM, Firooznia H, Davis MS Jr, et al. Fibrobullous disease of the upper lobes: an extraskeletal manifestation of ankylosing spondylitis. J Comput Tomogr. 1984;8:225–229.

72. Ferdoutsis M, Bouros D, Meletis G, Patsourakis G, Siafakas NM. Diffuse interstitial lung disease as an early manifestation of ankylosing spondylitis. Respiration. 1995;62:286–289.

73. Boulware DW, Weissman DN, Doll NJ. Pulmonary manifestations of the rheumatic diseases. Clin Rev Allergy. 1985;3:249–267.

74. Campbell AH, Macdonald CB. Upper lobe fibrosis associated with ankylosing spondylitis. Br J Dis Chest. 1965;59:90–101.

75. Fenlon HM, Casserly I, Sant SM, Breatnach E. Plain radiographs and thoracic high-resolution CT in patients with ankylosing spondylitis. AJR Am J Roentgenol. 1997;168:1067–1072.

76. Stewart RM, Ridyard JB, Pearson JD. Regional lung function in ankylosing spondylitis. Thorax. 1976;31:433–437.

77. Scobie BA. Disturbed oesophageal manometric responses in patients with ankylosing spondylitis and pulmonary aspergilloma. Australas Ann Med. 1970;19:131–134.

78. Casserly IP, Fenlon HM, Breatnach E, Sant SM. Lung findings on high-resolution computed tomography in idiopathic ankylosing spondylitis—correlation with clinical findings, pulmonary function testing and plain radiography. Br J Rheumatol. 1997;36: 677–682.

79. Primack SL, Muller NL. Radiologic manifestations of the systemic autoimmune diseases. Clin Chest Med. 1998;19:573–586, vii.

80. Averns HL, Oxtoby J, Taylor HG, Jones PW, Dziedzic K, Dawes PT. Smoking and outcome in ankylosing spondylitis. Scand J Rheumatol. 1996;25:138–142.

81. Strobel ES, Fritschka E. Renal diseases in ankylosing spondylitis: review of the literature illustrated by case reports. Clin Rheumatol. 1998;17:524–530.

82. Gratacos J, Orellana C, Sanmarti R, et al. Secondary amyloidosis in ankylosing spondylitis. A systematic survey of 137 patients using abdominal fat aspiration. J Rheumatol. 1997;24:912–915.

83. Lai KN, Li PK, Hawkins B, Lai FM. IgA nephropathy associated with ankylosing spondylitis: occurrence in women as well as in men. Ann Rheum Dis. 1989;48:435–437.

84. Vilar MJ, Cury SE, Ferraz MB, Sesso R, Atra E. Renal abnormalities in ankylosing spondylitis. Scand J Rheumatol. 1997;26:19–23.

85. Ozgocmen S, Kocakoc E, Kiris A, Ardicoglu A, Ardicoglu O. Incidence of varicoceles in patients with ankylosing spondylitis evaluated by physical examination and color duplex sonography. Urology. 2002;59:919–922.

86. Pirildar T, Muezzinoglu T, Pirildar S. Sexual function in ankylosing spondylitis: a study of 65 men. J Urol. 2004;171:1598–1600.

87. Torzewski J, Torzewski M, Bowyer DE, et al. C-reactive protein frequently colocalizes with the terminal complement complex in the intima of early atherosclerotic lesions of human coronary arteries. Arterioscler Thromb Vasc Biol. 1998;18:1386–1392.

88. Haagsma CJ, Blom HJ, van Riel PL, et al. Influence of sulphasalazine, methotrexate, and the combination of both on plasma homocysteine concentrations in patients with rheumatoid arthritis. Ann Rheum Dis. 1999;58:79–84.

89. Fisher S. Body Images and Personality. 2nd ed. New York, NY: Dover Publications; 1968:375–363.

90. Elst P, Sybesma T, van der Stadt RJ, Prins AP, Muller WH, den Butter A. Sexual problems in rheumatoid arthritis and ankylosing spondylitis. Arthritis Rheum. 1984;27:217–220.

91. Karasick D, Schweitzer ME, Abidi NA, Cotler JM. Fractures of the vertebrae with spinal cord injuries in patients with ankylosing spondylitis: imaging findings. AJR Am J Roentgenol. 1995;165:1205–1208.

92. Ralston SH, Urquhart GD, Brzeski M, Sturrock RD. Prevalence of vertebral compression fractures due to osteoporosis in ankylosing spondylitis. BMJ. 1990;300:563–565.

93. Taggard DA, Traynelis VC. Management of cervical spinal fractures in ankylosing spondylitis with posterior fixation. Spine. 2000;25:2035–2039.

94. Weinstein PR, Karpman RR, Gall EP, Pitt M. Spinal cord injury, spinal fracture, and spinal stenosis in ankylosing spondylitis. J Neurosurg. 1982;57:609–616.

95. Murray GC, Persellin RH. Cervical fracture complicating ankylosing spondylitis: a report of eight cases and review of the literature. Am J Med. 1981;70:1033–1041.

96. Bohlmann H. Acute fractures and dislocations of the cervical spine: an analysis of 300 hospitalized patients and review of the literature. J Bone Joint Surg Am. 1979;61:1119–1142.

97. Bennett DL, Ohashi K, El-Khoury GY. Spondyloarthropathies: ankylosing spondylitis and psoriatic arthritis. Radiol Clin North Am. 2004;42:121–134.

98. Ramos-Remus C, Gomez-Vargas A, Hernandez-Chavez A, et al. Two year followup of anterior and vertical atlantoaxial subluxation in ankylosing spondylitis. J Rheumatol. 1997;24:507–510.

99. Bartleson JD, Cohen MD, Harrington TM, Goldstein NP, Ginsburg WW. Cauda equina syndrome secondary to long-standing ankylosing spondylitis. Ann Neurol. 1983;14:662–669.

100. Sant, SM, O'Connell D. Cauda equina syndrome in ankylosing spondylitis: a case report and review of the literature. Clin Rheumatol. 1995;14:224–226.

101. Libbrecht N, De Bleecker J. Ankylosing spondylitis and multiple sclerosis. Acta Clin Belg. 1999;54:30–32.

102. Oh D, Jun JB, Kim HT, Lee SW, Jung SS, Lee IH, Kim SY. Transverse myelitis in a patient with long-standing ankylosing spondylitis. Clin Exp Rheumatol. 2001;19:195–197.

103. Cellerini M, Gabbrielli S, Bongi SM. Cerebral magnetic resonance imaging in a patient with ankylosing spondylitis and multiple sclerosis-like syndrome. Neuroradiology. 2001;43:1067–1069.

104. Thompson AJ, Miller D, Youl B, et al. Serial gadolinium-enhanced MRI in relapsing/remitting multiple sclerosis of varying disease duration. Neurology. 1992;42:60–63.

105. Whitman GJ, Khan MA. Unusual occurrence of ankylosing spondylitis and multiple sclerosis in a black patient. Cleve Clin J Med. 1989;56:819–822.

106. Hanrahan PS, Russell AS, McLean DR. Ankylosing spondylitis and multiple sclerosis: an apparent association? J Rheumatol. 1988;15:1512–1514.

107. Thomson G. HLA disease associations: models for the study of complex human genetic disorders. Crit Rev Clin Lab Sci. 1995;32:183–219.

108. Benjamin R, Parham P. Guilt by association: HLA-B27 and ankylosing spondylitis. Immunol Today. 1990;11:137–142.

109. Ebers GC, Bulman DE, Sadovnick AD, et al. A population-based study of multiple sclerosis in twins. N Engl J Med. 1986;315:1638–1642.

110. Mielants H, Veys EM, Cuvelier C, De Vos M. Course of gut inflammation in spondylarthropathies and therapeutic consequences. Baillieres Clin Rheumatol. 1996;10:147–164.

111. Mielants H, Veys EM, Goemaere S, Goethals K, Cuvelier C, De Vos M. Gut inflammation in the spondyloarthropathies: clinical, radiologic, biologic and genetic features in relation to the type of histology. A prospective study. J Rheumatol. 1991;18:1542–1551.

112. Mielants H, Veys EM, Joos R, Cuvelier C, De Vos M. Repeat ileocolonoscopy in reactive arthritis. J Rheumatol. 1987;14:456–458.

113. Leirisalo-Repo M, Turunen U, Stenman S, Helenius P, Seppala K. High frequency of silent inflammatory bowel disease in spondylarthropathy. Arthritis Rheum. 1994;37:23–31.

114. Smale S, Natt RS, Orchard TR, Russell AS, Bjarnason I. Inflammatory bowel disease and spondylarthropathy. Arthritis Rheum. 2001;44:2728–2736.

115. De Keyser F, Elewaut D, De Vos M, et al. Bowel inflammation and the spondyloarthropathies. Rheum Dis Clin North Am. 1998;24:785–813, ix–x.

116. Mielants H, Veys EM, Cuvelier C, et al. The evolution of spondyloarthropathies in relation to gut histology. III. Relation between gut and joint. J Rheumatol. 1995;22:2279–2284.

117. De Vos M, Cuvelier C, Mielants H, Veys E, Barbier F, Elewaut A. Ileocolonoscopy in seronegative spondylarthropathy. Gastroenterology. 1989;96(2 Pt 1):339–444.

118. De Keyser F, Mielants H. The gut in ankylosing spondylitis and other spondyloarthropathies: inflammation beneath the surface. J Rheumatol. 1998;30:2306–2307.

119. van der Linden S, Valkenburg HA, Cats A. Evaluation of diagnostic criteria for ankylosing spondylitis. A proposal for modification of the New York criteria. Arthritis Rheum. 1984;27:361–368.

120. Garrett S, Jenkinson T, Kennedy LG, Whitelock H, Gaisford P, Calin A. A new approach to defining disease status in ankylosing spondylitis: the Bath Ankylosing Spondylitis Disease Activity Index. J Rheumatol. 1994;21:2286–2291.

121. Calin A, Nakache JP, Gueguen A, Zeidler H, Mielants H, Dougados M. Defining disease activity in ankylosing spondylitis: is a combination of variables (Bath Ankylosing Spondylitis Disease Activity Index) an appropriate instrument? Rheumatology (Oxford). 1999;38:878–882.

122. Dougados M, van der Heijde D. Ankylosing spondylitis: how should the disease be assessed? Best Pract Res Clin Rheumatol. 2002;16:605–618.

13 Treatment

Walter P. Maksymowych

INTRODUCTION

Ankylosing spondylitis (AS) is among the most common of the chronic inflammatory joint disorders. Despite this, the pace of therapeutic development has been rather slow in comparison to that for other inflammatory joint disorders such as rheumatoid arthritis (RA). Despite the obvious phenotypic and etiologic differences between these disorders, the rationale for using therapeutics in AS has been based almost entirely on their ability to ameliorate inflammation in RA. Factors that have hampered therapeutic development and appropriate management of patients with AS have included the long delay between onset of symptoms and diagnosis, the lack of availability of standardized and validated outcome instruments with which to assess the effectiveness of therapy, the lack of diagnostic tools that demonstrate sufficient sensitivity and specificity in early disease, a lack of understanding of the pathogenesis of disease (particularly events occurring at disease onset), and the assessment of new therapeutics in patients with long-standing disease. For these various reasons, the effects of therapeutics developed for and most commonly used in the management of AS are largely symptomatic, although there has been considerable progress in addressing these impediments to therapeutic development and there is now increasing evidence that recently introduced therapies may be disease modifying. The primary objectives in the management of AS are to reduce symptoms of pain and stiffness, to improve and/or maintain function and mobility, to prevent disability, to improve quality of life, and to prevent structural damage. In this chapter we will discuss the current state of knowledge regarding the treatment of AS, recognizing that this is a disease that requires decades of management for most patients and a comprehensive treatment plan that may include educational, physical, medical, and surgical treatment modalities. Each treatment approach is outlined with respect to the evidence-based medical literature and discussed with respect to the implications for management in routine clinical practice. Consensus approaches to treatment based on an overall assessment of the medical literature and key issues that remain to be resolved are highlighted later in the chapter.

OUTCOME ASSESSMENT

Two developments have transformed the approach to developing new therapeutics for AS and their use in routine clinical practice. The first has been the development of a research agenda, achievement of consensus on relevant outcomes, and their validation and international standardization by an international body of experts in AS, the Assessments in Ankylosing Spondylitis (ASAS) Working Group. The work of this group and others has led to the development of a variety of disease-specific instruments that measure disease activity, function, mobility, quality of life, and structural damage on plain radiography that are outlined in detail in Chapter 15. A major advance has been the development of a composite response measure that can discriminate patients receiving active therapy from control subjects based on both relative (20%) and absolute improvement in pain, patient global assessment, function, and inflammation that has been designated the ASAS20 response criterion.[1] This response now constitutes the most widely used primary outcome in clinical trials of therapeutics for AS. ASAS50 and ASAS70 composite response measures have also been assessed in clinical trials of therapeutics for AS.

A second development has been the finding that magnetic resonance imaging (MRI) demonstrates abnormalities in the spine and sacroiliac joints before the appearance of plain radiographic abnormalities. In particular, the introduction of fat suppression sequences has allowed the visualization of lesions within subarticular bone marrow that may be obscured on conventional MRI by marrow fat. This has led not only to a more sensitive diagnostic method but also to the development of MRI-based outcome tools that measure disease activity in the spine and sacroiliac joints. These tools are discussed in detail in Chapter 14.

PATIENT EDUCATION

Overview

There is a widespread view that patient education is a generic approach that should be used to limit disability in rheumatic disease and achieve improvement in quality of life. In particular, level of education attained is a strong independent predictor of outcome in many chronic diseases. In a recent survey of members of the ASAS group, 73% indicated that there were educational programs available for patients with AS which included individual (60%) as well as group (48%) programs.

The objectives of patient education are to improve patient behaviors leading to 1) increased regular exercise; 2) appropriate use of non-pharmacologic pain management techniques, relaxation, and cognitive distraction; 3) appropriate use of aids and devices; and 4) development of action plans ultimately leading to improved health status and long term outcomes.

These objectives formed the conceptual framework for the development of the Arthritis Self-Management Program, and there are now several reports documenting its effectiveness in arthritis.[2] A major factor thought to account for the program's effectiveness is the improvement in personal perceived self-efficacy, defined as the confidence of patients in their ability to manage the consequences of their arthritis and thereby actively seek and implement solutions.

Evidence-Based Literature

A literature review revealed only six studies that were focused on the evaluation of a patient-education intervention in AS (Table 13.1). One study indicated that patients who participated in educational support groups acquired significantly increased knowledge about their disease and its treatment so that there was a trend toward compliance with prescribed exercise programs.[3] However, this approach did not enhance the patients' ability to cope with their disease. The application of a cognitive behavioral treatment program in a group setting format with components of relaxation, cognitive restructuring, and the promotion of well-being was described in two reports.[4,5] Both studies demonstrated a beneficial effect in measures of pain severity, anxiety, depression, psychophysiologic complaints, and sleep disturbance at 6 months in patients with AS that persisted at the 12-month follow-up compared with patients who served as waiting-list control subjects. In a further study of this intervention, patients with AS were compared with patients who had alternative diagnoses such as low back pain, tension headache, and RA.[6] Pain reduction was least in patients with AS.

TABLE 13.1 STUDIES OF EDUCATION INTERVENTIONS IN PATIENTS WITH AS			
Study	Intervention	Main Endpoint(s)	Main Conclusion
Gross and Brandt. 1981[3]	Educational support group	Compliance with exercise program, knowledge of disease, coping	Improved knowledge but not exercise compliance or coping
Rehfisch and Basler. 1989[4]	Cognitive-behavioral group program for pain management	Pain diary, anxiety, depression, psychophysiological complaints, sleep	Improvement in most outcomes at 6 months maintained at 1 year
Basler and Rehfisch. 1991[5]	Cognitive-behavioral group program for pain control	Pain severity, anxiety, depression, psychophysiological complaints, sleep disturbance	Improvement in most outcomes at 6 months maintained at 1 year
Basler. 1993[6]	Group cognitive-behavioral program for pain management	Pain severity, anxiety, depression, sleep disturbance	Pain reduction greatest in nonspecific and least in AS back pain
Barlow and Barefoot. 1996[7]	Group patient education (self-management course for AS) over 3 weeks	Self-efficacy, depression, psychological well-being, home exercise activity	Improvement at 3 weeks with sustained trend at 6 months
Sweeney et al. 2002[8]	Mailed exercise video, educational booklet, exercise wall chart/reminder stickers	BASDAI, BASFI, BASGI, Stanford self-efficacy scale, exercise self-efficacy, self-reported mobility and aerobic exercise	Improvement only for exercise self-efficacy and self-reported mobility/aerobic exercise

AS, ankylosing spondylitis; BASDAI, Bath Ankylosing Spondylitis Disease Activity Index; BASFI, Bath Ankylosing Spondylitis Functional Index; BASGI, Bath Ankylosing Spondylitis General Index.

In one study the effectiveness of group patient education administered as a self-management course was examined.[7] Improvements in depression, self-efficacy, and psychologic well-being were evident at 3 weeks and persisted up to 6 months. Although a beneficial effect on home exercise activity was noted at 3 weeks, this was not maintained at 6 months.

In a controlled study researchers examined an educational intervention delivered by mail that consisted of an exercise/educational video focusing on the benefits and barriers to exercise, an educational booklet, an exercise progress wall chart, and exercise reminder stickers.[8] Of 200 patients randomly selected from a database of 4569 members of an AS patient society and hospital outpatients, 155 completed the study, and at 6 months there was no significant difference between the groups in disease activity (Bath Ankylosing Spondylitis Disease Activity Index [BASDAI]), function (Bath Ankylosing Spondylitis Functional Index [BASFI]), and patient global assessment (Bath Ankylosing Spondylitis General Index [BASGI]). Self-efficacy for exercise and self-reported AS mobility and aerobic exercise showed a significant improvement in the intervention group. The modest benefits demonstrated in this study should be weighed against the fact that most of the recruited patients belonged to a patient organization and thus were already motivated to exercise. On the other hand, the long disease duration (greater than 20 years) of patients may have limited the potential for improvement in function.

Conclusions

Few conclusions can be drawn regarding the possible effectiveness of patient-education programs, which appear to vary widely in content and application. There appears to be general agreement that patient education is important to promote change in behavior, which may lead to mild improvement in symptoms, facilitates adjustment to new social and economic circumstances, and promotes coping with the emotional consequences of disease diagnosis and participation in decisions concerning treatment. It is also difficult to evaluate the contribution of concomitant therapies such as physiotherapy.

Management Issues in Clinical Practice

Patient support groups such as the Spondylitis Association of America (www.spondylitis.org) provide extensive resources that help patients manage their disease. This support is particularly valuable for physicians serving in relatively remote areas and in countries that lack educational resources. Many physiotherapy departments affiliated with rheumatic disease units in referral hospitals also conduct educational activities as an integral component of the physiotherapy program.

Finally, patients should be encouraged to participate in self-management programs to promote coping skills and self-efficacy in pain management.

PHYSICAL MODALITIES

Overview

The importance of physiotherapy in the management of patients with AS was first recognized in the 1940s when it was observed that military recruits who exercised had less severe symptoms and improved mobility. Since then, physiotherapy has become established in the treatment of this disease. Various forms of physiotherapy have been used including massage, manual therapy, electrotherapy, and exercises. The specific modality of treatment used in any particular center usually depends more on the experience and preconceived notions of effectiveness on the part of physiotherapists and rheumatologists rather than on the weight of evidence-based medicine. Physiotherapy is usually focused on maintaining and improving mobility of the spine and peripheral joints, strengthening the axial and proximal musculature, improving general fitness, and improving the patient's overall understanding of the necessity and appropriateness of regular exercise. Most physiotherapy therefore incorporates a patient-education program, and many centers have instituted multidisciplinary programs that not only incorporate instruction on appropriate exercise but also promote techniques that facilitate relaxation, the adoption of appropriate sporting activities, knowledge about the disease and its treatment, and the adoption of healthy lifestyles.

Although there is no evidence to support a standard protocol of specific exercises, several different types of exercise regimens have been described in the literature:

1. Unsupervised individual exercises include both exercises prescribed by a physiotherapist according to a predefined protocol of instruction and recreational exercises that have been adopted as part of a regular daily routine.
2. Supervised individual exercises may be performed at home and/or in a physiotherapy center. This approach is often chosen early after diagnosis when there is a necessity to educate patients on appropriate exercise, recreational activity, and posture. This approach is also aimed to improve exercise self-efficacy so that eventually a patient can pursue a regular program of unsupervised exercise at home.
3. Supervised group physical therapy is offered by many physiotherapy centers in recognition of the fact that many patients find it difficult to comply with an unsupervised program of regular exercise.

The primary aim of this program is to motivate patients to continue exercising in an environment where they have social contact with other patients who are also exercising.

4. In-patient physiotherapy typically consists of a 2- to 4-week program of more intensive exercise focused on correcting posture, improving flexibility, and motivating patients to pursue regular exercise when they leave the program. Many programs also include hydrotherapy and other treatment modalities with the aim of relieving symptoms. Some programs incorporate education about the disease and include attendance by diverse allied health professionals who provide advice on appropriate appliances for patients with arthritis, information on insurance reimbursement for new therapies, and information on support networks through patient societies.

5. Spa therapy for rheumatic disease has a long tradition, particularly in some European countries. It incorporates a variety of treatment modalities including exercises, hydrotherapy, massage, and, of course, rest and relaxation.

Until recently there was no consensus or standardized approach to the evaluation of these various modalities of physical therapy. There has since been agreement among experts in the ASAS Working Group that a core set of domains should be included in the assessment of the efficacy of physiotherapeutic interventions. These include physical function, pain, stiffness, patient global assessment, and spinal mobility. The studies described in the following are therefore described in light of these recommendations.

Evidence-Based Medical Literature
(Table 13.2)

Unsupervised, self-administered, or individual exercises

In a longitudinal study researchers examined the effects of unsupervised recreational exercise and back exercises on patient-reported pain severity, stiffness severity, and functional disability as recorded by the Health Assessment Questionnaire (HAQ) in a prospective cohort of 220 patients with AS followed for a median of 4.5 years.[9] Two primary analyses were performed: the first showed that neither exercise duration nor the frequency of back exercises was associated with short-term (6-month) changes in pain, stiffness, or HAQ disability in the patient group as a whole. However, among those who had AS for 15 years or less, pain severity and stiffness severity scores did improve significantly during periods when exercise was performed for more than 200 minutes per week compared with periods when exercise was performed for 30 minutes per week or less. The second analysis showed that progression of functional disability over time was least in those who reported a consistently high frequency of back exercise in the subgroup of patients with disease duration of more than 15 years. The important conclusion of this study is that consistent back exercise for years may help stabilize or decrease the rate of progression of functional disability in AS.

A cross-sectional study included a survey of 4282 patients who completed a self-administered questionnaire regarding physical exercise to determine the relationship between exercise and demographic and clinical variables.[10] Most patients reported either 2 to 4 hours of exercise per week or no exercise at all. The group who performed a moderate level of exercise (2 to 4 hours/wk) had improved function and lower disease activity whereas the group who performed intensive exercise (10 or more hours/wk) had improved function but no difference in disease activity. Adherence to a regular exercise regimen was associated with rheumatologist follow up, beliefs in the benefits of exercise, and a higher educational level. The conclusion was that consistency rather than quantity was most important in relation to improvement in health status measures and reinforced the importance of patient education.

Supervised individual exercises

The effectiveness of supervised individual physical therapy has been evaluated in only two reports. One open-label study included 144 patients who received 12 supervised individual treatments of 30 minutes in a 6-week course.[11] Of the various mobility measures examined, only cervical rotation showed significant improvement at the 6-week end point. Significant, although relatively modest, improvement was also noted in fitness (4%), functioning (14%), and patient global assessment (22%). There was no association between disease duration and changes in outcome variables.

In the second study, patients were randomly allocated to either physiotherapy and patient education administered by specially trained physiotherapists ($n = 26$) or no therapy ($n = 27$).[12] The physiotherapy intervention included administration of heat or cold modalities, demonstration of correct posture, and application of therapeutic exercise to increase mobility, muscle strength, and endurance. This was augmented by self-administered daily exercise programs. At 4 months, there was significant improvement in fingertip-to-floor distance (42%) and function (23%) between treatment groups. There was no improvement in degree of pain or stiffness. In a follow-up study,[13] patients in the control group were offered the active intervention and patients in the active group were maintained on a follow-up program as needed. There was no improvement in mobility in control patients who switched to active therapy.

TABLE 13.2 RANDOMIZED, CONTROLLED STUDIES OF PHYSIOTHERAPEUTIC INTERVENTIONS FOR ANKYLOSING SPONDYLITIS

Study/Patient No.	Intervention/ Duration	ASAS Outcome Domains							Main Conclusions
		Pain	Global	Function	Stiffness	CE	OWD	Sch	
Kraag et al. 1990[12] 26 active 27 control	Individual supervised physiotherapy and education 4 months	↑	nd	↑	↑	↑	↑	↑	Improvement in mobility (FFD) (42%) and function (23%) over control group.
	Other endpoints: FFD (↑), sleep (→)								
Hidding et al. 1993[17] 68 active 76 control	Weekly group physiotherapy 9 months	↑	↑	↑	↑	↑	nd	nd	Minor improvement in mobility (TLF, TLE) (7%), fitness (5%), patient global (28%), over control group.
	Other endpoints: TLF (↑), TLE (↑), CR (→), fitness (↑)								
Hidding et al. 1994[18] 34 active 34 control	Weekly group physiotherapy 9 months	↑	↑	↑	↑	↑	nd	nd	Improvement in time for exercises at home (58%), patient global (28%), function (HAQ-S) (32%), over control group.
	Other endpoints: TLF (→), TLE (→), CR (→), fitness (→)								
Analay et al. 2003[19] 27 active 24 control	Out-patient group physiotherapy 3 × week 6 weeks	↑	nd	↑	↑	↑	nd	↑	Improvement in all parameters except pain at 6 weeks and 3 months after treatment compared to control group.
	Other endpoints: FFD (↑), TTW (↑), IMD (↑), depression (↑), fitness (↑)								
Helliwell et al. 1996[31] 15 active Group I 15 active Group II 14 control	Group I: 3 weeks intensive in-patient physiotherapy Group II: 2 × week hydrotherapy plus home exercise 5 × week 6 weeks	↑	nd	nd	↑	↑	nd	↑	Significant improvement in active groups at 6 weeks. No group differences at 6 months after treatment.
	Other endpoints: CR (↑)								
Van Tubergen et al. 2001[32] 40 spa group I 40 spa group II 40 control	Spa therapy for 3 weeks (2 different sites). 40 weeks	↑	↑	↑	↑	nd	nd	nd	Spa exercise is superior to weekly group therapy alone over 40 weeks but not at 40 weeks.

CE, chest expansion; CR, cervical rotation; FFD, finger-to-floor distance; HAQ-S, health assessment questionnaire for the spondyloarthopathies; IMD, intermalleolar distance; OWD, occiput-to-wall distance; Sch, Schober's test; TLE, thoraco-lumbar extension; TLF, thoraco-lumbar flexion; TTW, tragus-to-wall distance.

Supervised group physical therapy

The effectiveness of group physical therapy has been addressed in very small open-label studies. These generally have shown small improvements in spinal mobility immediately after treatment that did not persist for more than a few months.[14–16]

The effectiveness of weekly supervised group physical therapy in addition to unsupervised exercises was examined in three randomized, controlled trials. In the first study, 144 patients were randomly assigned to exercises at home ($n = 76$) or to the same plus weekly group physical therapy ($n = 68$) for 9 months.[17] Both groups had received 6 weeks of supervised individual therapy before randomization. Active treatment led to a 28% improvement in global health compared with the control intervention but had no impact on patient's symptoms (pain, stiffness, or function) and was only marginally more effective for mobility. In a follow-up study, patients who received the active intervention were randomly assigned for another 9 months to unsupervised daily exercises at home (discontinuation group) or continuation of weekly sessions of supervised group physical therapy (continuation group).[18] A significant increase in global health of 28% was found in the continuation group compared with the discontinuation group, although function did not change and mobility deteriorated.

In a third study 51 patients were randomly assigned to either an intensive group therapy program given 3 days a week at 50 minutes a day or a home physiotherapy program.[19] All patients had a 1-hour training program at entry and were given information about the disease and the purpose of physical exercises. The exercise program included stretching, mobilization, axial strengthening exercises, aerobic exercises on a static bike, and postural and respiratory exercises. At the end of the 6-week treatment, significant improvement was noted in function (24%), all measures of spinal mobility, duration of morning stiffness, physical fitness, and degree of depression, but there was no improvement in pain. These benefits were maintained 3 months after treatment with the exception of the depression score.

In-patient physiotherapy

Several researchers have examined a short course (2–3 weeks) of intensive in-patient physical therapy not only for its effectiveness but also for the development of outcome instruments. These validation studies demonstrated a 16% improvement in disease activity (BASDAI),[20] a 20% improvement in function (BASFI),[21] a 29% improvement in patient global assessment (BASGI),[22] and a 30% improvement in mobility (Bath Ankylosing Spondylitis Metrology Index [BASMI]).[23] A subsequent study of 236 patients who received a 3-week course of intensive in-patient physiotherapy at various times over 18 months confirmed improvement of 18% to 27% in these outcome instruments,[24] although a further study showed no improvement in function compared with waiting list control subjects.[25]

Several researchers have also examined in-patient physiotherapy to determine which axial mobility measurements are most responsive to change and whether improvement in mobility is sustained in the long-term.[26–28] Although effects on mobility were generally short lived, detectable improvement in fingertip-to-floor distance was sustained beyond 1 year after a single 3-week course of treatment.

The value of physiotherapy given specifically to improve mobility of the neck and hip has been addressed in two controlled, although nonrandomized, studies. In one study of 35 patients and 35 matched control subjects 25 patients showed a significant improvement in all cervical measurements after 3 weeks of intensive in-patient physiotherapy, and this improvement was maintained in 11 patients at 3 months.[29] In the second study 29 patients and 12 control subjects were recruited, and the effects of daily passive stretching of the hip joints during a 3-week in-patient physiotherapy course were examined.[30] Significant improvement in the range of all movements, except for flexion, was noted immediately after treatment and was maintained at the 6-month follow-up in 7 patients.

The effects of in-patient physiotherapy have been reported in only one randomized, controlled study.[31] Forty-four patients were randomly assigned to three groups: group A ($n = 15$) received 3 weeks of intensive in-patient physiotherapy, group B ($n = 15$) received hydrotherapy twice weekly and performed home exercises twice daily, and group C ($n = 14$) performed home exercises only. At 6 weeks, significant improvement was noted in pain, stiffness, and cervical rotation in the two intervention groups although at 6 months these differences were no longer present.

Spa therapy

The efficacy of 3 weeks of combined spa-exercise therapy as an adjunct to standard treatment with drugs and weekly group physical therapy were reported in one randomized, controlled trial.[32] Two groups of 40 patients each were randomly allocated to treatment at two different spas (one in Austria and the other in the Netherlands). A control group of 40 patients stayed at home and received weekly physiotherapy for 40 weeks. The spa therapy consisted of physical exercises, walking, postural correction, hydrotherapy, sports, and bathing in thermal water or a sauna. After the spa intervention, all patients continued weekly group physical therapy for another 37 weeks. The primary outcome was a pooled index of change based on the preliminary ASAS core set for physical therapy and included function (BASFI), patient global assessment, pain intensity, and morning stiffness. By 4 weeks, significant improvement was evident in the spa group compared with the control group. A significant benefit over control subjects was evident until 28 weeks but lost significance by 40 weeks. The maximum difference between the groups was 30% for pain, 24% for function, and 33% for patient global assessment.

Systematic Reviews

A Cochrane review and a subsequent modification have been completed in an attempt to summarize available evidence on the effectiveness of physiotherapeutic interventions in AS.[33,34] Of 43 studies that were considered for inclusion in this review, only 6 trials met the criteria for inclusion. A total of 561 participants were included in the updated review of whom 241 had been discussed in the original version. Two trials comparing individualized home exercise programs with no intervention were considered to provide low-quality evidence for effects on spinal mobility and physical function in favor of the home exercise program.[12,13] Three trials comparing supervised group physiotherapy to an individualized home exercise program were considered to provide moderate-quality evidence for small differences in spinal mobility and patient global assessment in favor of supervised group exercise.[17–19] A spa therapy clinical trial was considered to provide moderate-quality evidence for effects on pain, physical function, and patient global assessment in favor of the combined spa and exercise therapy.[32]

Several limitations were highlighted in these reports, including the often heterogeneous nature of the intervention among studies, lack of consistency in the approach to measurement of spinal mobility, lack of concealment of allocation, inadequate reporting of co-interventions, high loss to follow-up, lack of use of independent blinded assessors, and poorly described interventions. It was also concluded that patients who participated in group physiotherapy may have shown improvement owing to the contribution of nonphysical factors such as mutual motivation and exchange of experience with similarly affected participants.

Conclusions

Findings in these studies are generally consistent in demonstrating that neither home physiotherapy nor group physical therapy benefit symptoms but do lead to modest improvement in spinal mobility, function, and global-health status. Limited data also support a role for in-patient physiotherapy in improving function and mobility. Both in-patient and spa physiotherapy may also provide limited relief of symptoms. Effects on mobility may be maintained over the long term, although it appears that the intervention may need to be maintained to preserve the benefit.

Management Issues in Clinical Practice

It is consistently recommended that physiotherapy be considered part of the overall management plan for patients with AS, despite the limited data on effectiveness, which is largely confined to exercise interventions. Furthermore, in-patient physiotherapy for patients with rheumatic diseases is increasingly an unrealistic option in the context of limited hospital budgets. An outpatient group physiotherapy program at the time of diagnosis and perhaps during disease exacerbations is probably the most pragmatic and cost-beneficial approach, as is a prescription for 30 minutes of back exercises per day 5 days a week and encouragement of recreational exercise. Such physiotherapy programs for patients with AS are often available at regional referral centers for patients with rheumatic diseases and incorporate essential elements of patient education, motivation, and development of self-efficacy, which have been associated with long-term health benefits.

MEDICAL MODALITIES

Symptom-Modifying Antirheumatic Drugs

For the past several decades, pharmacologic approaches to management have relied on the use of symptom-modifying antirheumatic drugs (SMARDs). These drugs have been defined by the ASAS Working Group as agents that improve symptoms and clinical features of inflammatory manifestations of disease. The ASAS group has proposed that the same outcome domains be used for the assessment of SMARDs as for physical therapy, namely, physical function, pain, stiffness, mobility, and patient global assessment. By definition, these agents are not disease modifying in terms of their ability to prevent the development of erosions, syndesmophytes, and spinal ankylosis. Two categories of drugs have been used for their symptom-modifying properties: nonsteroidal anti-inflammatory agents (NSAIDs), and adjuvant therapies such as analgesics and antidepressants.

Nonsteroidal Anti-Inflammatory Drugs
Overview

These agents have been the cornerstone of pharmacologic intervention for AS since their introduction in the 1950s. A survey of NSAID use in 1331 patients with AS from the United Kingdom indicated that 86% of these patients are taking NSAIDs.[35] Numerous studies have shown that these agents rapidly reduce signs and symptoms in patients with AS followed by rebound of symptoms within a few days (5 or 6 half-lives after discontinuation). There is as yet little evidence that NSAIDs influence laboratory markers of disease, although preliminary data suggest that they may have a role in preventing structural damage evident on x-ray films. Several NSAIDs are available with differences in chemical structure, dosage, pharmacology, half-life, and adverse effects. The relatively recent introduction of cyclooxygenase (COX)-2 selective agents has added to this diversity.

Rationale

It is now well established that the mechanism of action of these agents centers on their ability to suppress the production of pro-inflammatory prostaglandins through their inhibition of COX. However, these agents have also been shown to suppress neutrophil functions such as generation of free oxygen radicals and superoxide, adhesion to endothelium, and chemotaxis.[36] COX has recently been shown to constitute a superfamily of prostaglandin synthase genes that encode a constitutively expressed COX-1, the enzyme believed to be responsible for the physiologic production of cytoprotective prostaglandins in the gastric mucosa, highly regulated COX-2, which is increased in inflammatory tissues, and a COX-3 isoform that appears to be preferentially expressed in the central nervous system and constitutes the primary site of activity of acetaminophen and related compounds.[37] Although COX-2 is highly regulated and expressed primarily at the onset of inflammation, constitutive expression has been observed in the kidneys, spleen, and osteoblasts. COX-2 also plays a role in vascular homeostasis by sustaining vascular prostacyclin production.[38,39] These enzymes differ in their sensitivity to inhibition by NSAIDs, which depends not only on the agent itself but also on the assay used to measure inhibition.[40] The introduction of highly selective COX-2 inhibitors such as celecoxib into clinical practice has not only expanded the range of therapeutic possibilities for AS but also the possibility of suppressing symptoms with a lower risk of gastrointestinal (GI) side effects. The relatively low potency of aspirin and salicylates in inhibiting COX-2 might account for their relative lack of efficacy in patients with AS.

Evidence-based literature

A large number of clinical trials of NSAID therapy in patients with AS have been conducted but most have used different study designs to compare the efficacy and tolerability of two or more NSAIDs. The first NSAID to be widely used for AS and still considered to be the most effective is phenylbutazone. One retrospective analysis showed that this agent might also prevent radiologic progression of disease.[41] Unfortunately, patient tolerance was poor, and the risk of severe hematologic adverse events such as agranulocytosis has led to restrictions or an outright ban on its use in most countries.

Placebo-controlled trials

NSAID treatment has been compared with placebo in six randomized, controlled trials although one has been reported in abstract form only (Table 13.3). The first was a 2-week study of piroxicam 20 mg daily in 80 patients judged to have active disease after withdrawal of maintenance NSAID therapy for 3 days.[42] Patients receiving piroxicam had significantly greater improvement in pain, function, and fingertip-to-floor distance but not in morning stiffness, frequency of nocturnal awakening, chest expansion, or the Schober test.

The second was a crossover study of a propionic acid derivative, ximoprofen 50 mg twice daily.[43] After a 3-day washout from maintenance NSAIDs, 36 patients meeting prespecified criteria for disease flare received either ximoprofen or placebo for 1 week. There was then a crossover to alternative therapy for a second 1-week period. Of the 36 patients, 28 considered ximoprofen to be more effective compared with 4 who received a placebo. A significant difference was noted in favor of ximoprofen for pain severity, analgesic consumption, morning stiffness, frequency of nocturnal awakening, function, and mobility (fingertip-to-floor distance). The study drug was well tolerated with no discontinuations because of side effects, which were comparable to those seen in patients receiving placebos.

A third trial was a dose-ranging study of 2 weeks' duration evaluating 5, 10, 20, and 30 mg daily versus placebo.[44] A total of 285 patients meeting prespecified criteria for disease flare after a 2-day washout from maintenance NSAIDs were recruited, although those with peripheral arthritis were excluded. A responder was defined as a patient in whom a decrease of at least 50% was noted in the pain visual analog scale (VAS) (0 to 100 mm). Significantly higher percentages of responders were noted in all the ximoprofen groups (54%, 41%, 53%, and 56%, respectively) compared with patients receiving placebos (21%). A significant improvement was also noted in duration of morning stiffness, frequency of nocturnal awakening, function, mobility, and analgesic consumption in patients who received ximoprofen. Adverse events were similar in all groups.

In a fourth study the aim was to examine the efficacy and tolerability of two NSAIDs, piroxicam and meloxicam, over both the short term (6 weeks) and the long term (1 year).[45] The study included 473 patients meeting prespecified criteria for disease flare after withdrawal of maintenance NSAIDs for 2 to 15 days although patients with peripheral articular disease were excluded. Patients were randomly assigned to receive piroxicam 20 mg, meloxicam 15 mg or 22.5 mg, or placebo. At 6 weeks, the percentage of patients who achieved at least a 50% reduction in pain score were 49% in the piroxicam group, 53% in the meloxicam 15 mg group,

TABLE 13.3 RELATIVE PERCENTAGE IMPROVEMENT OVER PLACEBO IN ASAS OUTCOME DOMAINS IN PATIENTS RECEIVING ACTIVE NSAID THERAPY (ABSOLUTE BENEFIT/BASELINE MEAN IN CONTROL GROUP) IN DOUBLE-BLIND PLACEBO-CONTROLLED TRIALS

Study	Patient No	Disease Duration	Study Duration	ASAS Outcome Domains						
				Pain	Stiffness	Function	Global	CE	OWD	Sch
Dougados et al. 1988[42]	Piroxicam (20 mg) = 38 Placebo = 42	NS	2 weeks	26.2*	22.9	13.3*	na	0.6.	na	37.9
Dougados et al. 1989[43]	Ximoprofen (30 mg) = 18 Placebo = 18	10 years 8 years	2 weeks†	50.5*	37.1*	27.8*	na	−2.5	na	3.8
Dougados et al. 1994[44]	Ximoprofen (30 mg) = 50 Ximoprofen (20 mg) = 45 Ximoprofen (10 mg) = 49 Ximoprofen (5 mg) = 46 Placebo = 95	10 years 8 years 8 years 10 years 10 years	2 weeks	37.3 26.9 20.9 26.9	93.2* 52.5 66.1* 44.1	32.6* 34.7* 27.1* 20.1*	na	na	na	0.0 0.0 0.0 3.1
Dougados et al. 1999[45]	Meloxicam (22.5 mg) = 124 Meloxicam (15 mg) = 120 Piroxicam (20 mg) = 108 Placebo = 121	12 years 13 years 12 years 12 years	6 weeks‡ 6–52 weeks	26.4* 23.6* 23.6*	35.2* 22.7* 18.2	25.0* 23.1* 18.8*	35.5* 37.1* 37.1*	23.7 13.1 13.1	na	2.3 1.6 1.6
Dougados et al. 2001[46]	Celecoxib (200 mg) = 80 Ketoprofen (200 mg) = 90 Placebo = 76	11 years 11 years 11 years	6 weeks	20.0* 11.4	40.7 39.5	31.4* 17.4*	23.8 12.0	8.9 8.2	na	2.5 2.7
Van der Heijde et al. 2005[47]	Etoricoxib (120 mg) = 92 Etoricoxib (90 mg) = 103 Naproxen (1000 mg) = 99 Placebo = 93	NS	6 weeks§ 6–52 weeks	53.9* 53.1* 43.6*	na	35.3* 35.8* 27.0*	41.4* 43.4* 32.5*	na	na	na

*statistically significant improvement over placebo.

†cross-over design with each treatment period of 1 week.

‡6-week trial with 6–52 weeks double-blind extension phase. Outcome data is presented for the 6-week phase.

§6-week placebo-controlled trial with 6–52 week active comparator extension. Outcome data is presented for the 6-week phase.

ASAS, Assessments in Ankylosing Spondylitis; CE, chest expansion; na, not available; NS, not stated; NSAID, nonsteroidal anti-inflammatory drug; OWD, occiput-to-wall distance; Sch, Schober's test.

and 49% in the meloxicam 22.5 mg group versus 22% of patients taking placebo. Significant improvement was also noted in function although not in spinal mobility. At 1 year, the percentage of responders was similar in the various treatment groups although when discontinuation of therapy for any reason was examined over the course of 1 year, more patients discontinued piroxicam (53%) and lower dose meloxicam (53%) than higher dose meloxicam (37%). A significant increase in withdrawal due to epigastric and intestinal disorders was also noted in piroxicam patients (32%) over the course of 1 year compared with placebo (13%) and the two meloxicam (15 mg [18%]; 22.5 mg [20%]) groups. Furthermore, all the gastroduodenal ulcers recorded in patients receiving piroxicam occurred during the 6- to 52-week period. Thus, beyond the readily apparent benefits demonstrable over 6 weeks, survival analysis also showed significant differences between active treatment arms in favor of meloxicam 22.5 mg, indicating that a long-term study is a more appropriate trial design to detect both efficacy and safety differences between NSAIDs and different dosages of a given NSAID than the conventional short-term parallel group design.

In a fifth study a selective COX-2 inhibitor, celecoxib, at 100 mg twice daily was compared with ketoprofen 100 mg twice daily and placebo.[46] The same entry criteria for active disease were used as in the preceding trial, and patients with peripheral articular disease were again excluded. A significantly higher percentage of patients in the celecoxib (48%) and ketoprofen (36%) groups experienced a reduction of at least 50% in pain severity score compared with those receiving placebo (19.7%). Significant improvement was also noted in function and mobility in actively treated patients compared with the placebo group. Both the incidence of adverse events and withdrawal from the study because of adverse events were greater in the active treatment groups, particularly for epigastric pain and diarrhea, and there was no difference between celecoxib and ketoprofen in these respects. In a second study of a COX-2 selective agent, eterocoxib, 387 patients were recruited and randomly assigned to receive eterocoxib 90 or 120 mg daily, naproxen 1000 mg daily, or placebo for 6 weeks followed by an active comparator extension phase to week 52, whereby placebo patients were randomly allocated to one of the active therapy groups.[47] More patients in the placebo (47.3%) and naproxen (22.2%) groups than in the etoricoxib (7.8% and 9.8%) groups discontinued treatment because of lack of efficacy. Discontinuation for adverse events was similar across groups. Severity of pain score, patient global assessment, and function improved significantly in patients receiving etoricoxib versus those receiving placebo or naproxen. Five serious cardiovascular thrombotic events occurred in the extension phase, all in etoricoxib-treated patients. Three patients receiving etoricoxib and 4 receiving naproxen experienced peptic ulcer bleeds.

Active-comparator trials

The efficacy and tolerability of two or more NSAIDs were compared in a large number of studies.[48] Most studies showed no significant differences in either efficacy or safety among different NSAIDs. In one study continuous therapy with celecoxib 200 mg daily was compared with on-demand therapy with the same agent in 214 patients for 2 years.[49] Dose escalation was permitted to 200 mg twice daily if symptoms were poorly controlled although the scheme of administration did not change. Patients developing adverse events requiring discontinuation of celecoxib were allowed to use an alternative NSAID but, again, the scheme of administration was preserved. X-ray films of the cervical and lumbar spine were performed at baseline and 2 years. Radiologic progression was significantly less evident in the continuous therapy arm though the difference between the two groups was small. However, there was no significant difference in disease activity over the course of 2 years.

NSAID toxicity

Because the onset of AS is relatively early in life with the potential of continuous therapy being required for several decades, the toxicity of NSAID therapy is a major consideration. Between 10% and 60% of patients receiving NSAIDs experience minor GI symptoms such as nausea, dyspepsia, epigastric pain, and diarrhea, whereas more serious effects in the form of symptomatic ulcers, upper GI bleeding, and perforation occur in approximately 1% to 2% of patients using NSAIDs for 3 months and 2% to 4% of patients using NSAIDs for 12 months.[50,51] A prospective survey of AS patients in the United Kingdom indicated that between 8% and 15% of patients taking indomethacin, naproxen, piroxicam, or diclofenac at study entry had discontinued these medications due to toxicity after 2 years.[34] On the other hand, another prospective longitudinal study of 241 patients with AS followed for a median of 4.5 years showed that although the median duration of use of ibuprofen, indomethacin, diclofenac, piroxicam, and nabumetone was 6 months or less, discontinuation was usually not due to toxicity.[52] Overall more patients discontinued piroxicam due to toxicity (23.5%) compared with celecoxib (8.0%), indomethacin (10%), or naproxen (12.3%). The factors that potentiate the risk for an NSAID-associated serious GI event include previous peptic ulcer or GI bleeding, increasing age, use of multiple NSAIDs, combined use of NSAIDs and corticosteroids, and comorbid medical diseases.[53] An additional consideration is the concomitant presence of inflammatory bowel disease (IBD) in 5% to 10% of patients with AS in whom NSAID use is associated with exacerbation of bowel inflammation.

COX-2 selective agents (celecoxib and rofecoxib) are associated with significantly decreased risk of major GI side effects although rates of less serious and more common GI symptoms (dyspepsia, abdominal pain, nausea, flatulence, and diarrhea) are not significantly reduced.[54] The majority of patients with AS develop their disease relatively early in life and tend to fall into a group with a fairly low risk for serious GI complications so that the absolute and relative risk reduction in serious GI events associated with the use of COX-2 selective agents in patients with AS is likely to be quite small. Moreover, a recent controlled trial, together with several longitudinal studies, has shown that rofecoxib is associated with an increased risk for significant cardiovascular events.[55,56]

Both groups of NSAIDs are associated with the development and/or exacerbation of hypertension, peripheral edema, and congestive heart failure. They may also compromise renal function in patients who already have or are at risk of developing renal dysfunction.

Conclusions

Both nonselective and COX-2–selective NSAIDs are effective in relieving symptoms of pain and stiffness and improving function in patients with AS. When given for prolonged periods of up to 1 year, there also appears to be improvement in spinal mobility and acute-phase reactants. Preliminary data from a single long-term randomized trial suggest that continuous administration of NSAIDs may also prevent structural damage.

Management Issues in Clinical Practice

NSAIDs are the mainstay of the pharmacologic management of AS. The choice of the NSAID should be governed by the clinician's experience with specific NSAIDs and the patient's risk of developing serious adverse events. It is appropriate to use a nonselective NSAID for the majority of patients with AS who tend to be relatively young and without comorbid conditions. COX-2–selective agents can be reserved for patients older than age 65, particularly those with prior peptic ulceration or other GI adverse events. They should be used with extreme caution, if at all, in patients with a history of cardiovascular or renal disease. Surveys show that a sizable proportion of patients use these agents intermittently even when they are prescribed for continuous use. Approximately 60% to 70% of patients with AS have symptoms that appear to be well controlled with NSAIDs and physical modalities of therapy.[57] Of the 241 new courses of NSAIDs that were stopped for any reason during one longitudinal study,[52] 34% were followed immediately by treatment with another NSAID.

In contrast, 69 courses (29%) were followed by a delay of 6 months or more before another NSAID was taken, suggesting decreased need for these medications in a substantial minority of patients and perhaps a more rational approach whereby NSAID therapy is only taken at the time of disease flare. For these patients, intermittent use may be appropriate. Some patients are reluctant to take prescribed NSAID therapy for fear of side effects even though symptoms may be inadequately controlled. Such patients should be encouraged to take adequate NSAID therapy to ensure symptomatic relief, especially in view of preliminary findings that NSAIDs might ameliorate structural damage. Compliance could be further improved by using agents requiring once-daily administration.

The rapid-acting and substantial symptomatic effect of NSAIDs has also been suggested as a potential tool to facilitate diagnosis of this disease. Substantial improvement of back pain within 48 hours of NSAID administration and/or rapid relapse upon withdrawal of the drug is listed as one of the diagnostic criteria for spondyloarthropathy (SpA) proposed by Amor et al.[58] In a cross-sectional, multicenter study, SpA was diagnosed in 69 of 741 patients who had back pain.[59] All of these patients received at least one NSAID for their clinical symptoms. This treatment was considered effective by 53 patients with SpA (77%), but only 102 patients with mechanical back pain found it effective (15%). NSAID efficacy therefore had sensitivity of 77%, specificity of 85%, positive predictive value of 34%, and negative predictive value of 97%. In clinical practice, this can be interpreted as indicating that a patient with back pain who has no significant symptomatic response to an NSAID is highly unlikely to have AS.

For patients who report an inadequate symptomatic response to a new NSAID prescription, it would be important to confirm that the patient is receiving the optimal dosage. Dosing is often inadequate for ibuprofen, which should be administered in doses of ≥ 2.4 g/day if tolerated. It is also advantageous to administer NSAIDs, particularly those with a short half life, late in the evening to alleviate pain and stiffness that is often maximal in the morning. Clinical trials have also shown that up to 2 weeks may be required to demonstrate maximum symptomatic benefit from an NSAID. If these strategies have been used and the symptomatic benefit is still inadequate, a switch to a second NSAID, preferably from a structurally unrelated class of compound, is recommended.

Management of Nonsteroidal Anti-Inflammatory Drug Therapy in the Setting of Comorbid Conditions

It is not uncommon for patients to develop hypertension during the course of AS. Aside from the reappraisal of NSAID dosing to the minimum required to control symptoms, it is also important to note that calcium channel blocker therapy is the most effective approach to managing hypertension in patients receiving concomitant NSAID therapy.[60]

NSAIDs have been associated with onset or exacerbation of IBD and are listed in the practice guidelines of the American College of Gastroenterology among factors recognized to exacerbate Crohn's disease.[61] This possibility is particularly relevant for the 5% to 10% of patients with AS who have concomitant Crohn's disease. Should NSAIDs be used at all in these patients and do COX-2–selective agents offer any advantages over nonselective agents? In one retrospective case review study 27 patients who had received COX-2 inhibitors through the IBD clinic were identified.[62] Over a median follow-up of 9 months, 2 patients were felt to have had an exacerbation of their IBD. In one prospective open-label study the safety and efficacy of a 20-day regimen of rofecoxib 12.5 to 25 mg/day were examined in 32 patients with IBD and concomitant arthritis.[63] Rofecoxib had to be withdrawn in 3 patients (9%) after a few days due to GI complaints, which ceased immediately after drug discontinuation. In a second prospective open-label trial rofecoxib 12.5 mg/day was examined in 45 patients with inactive IBD, and a control group of 30 patients with dyspepsia was also included.[64] Drug withdrawal was necessary in 9 (20%) patients with IBD due to disease relapse compared with only 1 control patient. Although induction of the COX-2 enzyme has been documented in inflamed bowel mucosa, there is also evidence that the COX-2 enzyme becomes activated in an effort to repair damaged tissue. All NSAIDs should therefore be avoided in patients with active symptoms of IBD and/or moderate to severe disease. Patients with ulcerative colitis appear to have a risk similar to those with Crohn's disease. NSAIDs could be cautiously introduced at low doses only in those patients with mild, inactive disease and the dosage cautiously escalated after 1 month if there has been no exacerbation of IBD.

Adjuvant Symptom-Modifying Drugs
Simple analgesics and opioids

It is readily apparent that patients with AS take a variety of over-the-counter medications including simple analgesics such as acetaminophen, low-dose ibuprofen, and naproxen as well as a variety of alternative therapies. A survey of patients with AS conducted in the late 1980s revealed that a substantial proportion (34%) took simple analgesics and 15% purchased over-the-counter drugs.[65] More than half of the patients (57%) considered pain relief as their first priority for drug treatment. It is therefore not surprising that many patients and practitioners also use opiate strategies either alone or in combination with acetaminophen for control of pain. A retrospective study examined

opiate use in a cohort of 644 rheumatology clinic patients.[66] Opioid prescriptions were found for 290 (45%) patients of whom 137 (21%) had used opioids, primarily codeine and oxycodone, for at least 3 months. Opioids significantly reduced rheumatic disease pain severity scores, and side effects were mild, consisting of nausea, dyspepsia, constipation, and sedation. Doses were stable for prolonged periods with escalations of opioid doses almost always related to worsening of the painful condition or a complication thereof rather than the development of tolerance.

Antidepressants

Patients have identified fatigue and sleep disturbance as major symptoms in AS. Low-dose amitriptyline has been used to decrease pain and fatigue and improve sleep in patients with fibromyalgia. In one placebo-controlled study 100 patients were randomly assigned to either low-dose amitriptyline 30 mg nightly or placebo for 2 weeks.[67] Compared with those taking a placebo, patients taking amitriptyline showed significantly greater improvement in restful sleep and disease activity scores although there was no effect on pain, fatigue, morning stiffness, or function scores.

Disease-Controlling Antirheumatic Therapies

Prospective follow-up of patients with AS recruited from both academic and community-based centers reporting new treatment courses of NSAIDs that were stopped for any reason showed that approximately one third were followed immediately by treatment with another NSAID, implying inadequate effectiveness of the first treatment.[52] Data from a placebo-controlled trial of two NSAIDs, celecoxib and ketoprofen, showed that approximately 50% of patients reported greater than 50% reduction in pain severity.[46] Consequently, there is a substantial need for additional therapies in up to half of all patients with AS. The obvious candidates are the disease-modifying agents used for the treatment of RA. The ASAS Working Group has defined a disease-controlling therapy as any agent that decreases inflammatory manifestations of disease and sustains or improves function. It must also be shown to prevent or decrease the rate of progression of structural damage. These are concepts that have been well developed in RA from the perspective of both appropriate outcome assessment and clinical trial design so that there is now conclusive data that MTX (MTX), salazopyrine (SSPN), leflunomide, and several biologic therapies are disease controlling. Several of these agents have also been examined on a limited basis in AS although most of the studies predated the development and validation of appropriate outcome instruments. Appropriate radiologic instruments have only recently been developed for the assessment of structural damage in AS (see Chapter 15). The ASAS group has recommended a core set of nine outcome domains that should be included in the assessment of disease-controlling therapies. In addition to the five domains included in the core set for symptom-modifying therapies (pain, stiffness, patient global assessment, function, and mobility), these domains include fatigue, peripheral joint inflammation/enthesitis, acute-phase reactants, and plain radiographs. Each of the therapies described below will be discussed in light of these recommendations.

Salazopyrine and related compounds

Overview

SSPN was first synthesized in the 1930s and was one of the first agents to be developed on the principle of rational drug design. At that time it was thought that RA was caused by a group B streptococcal intestinal infection and so it was considered appropriate to combine salicylic acid with the antibacterial sulfapyridine. This combination was then shown to be useful for both RA and IBD. The use of SSPN for the treatment of AS was first suggested by Amor et al. in 1984,[68] particularly in those patients who had peripheral arthritis. The rationale for this approach was based on the well-documented association between AS and IBD, the demonstration of inflammatory lesions in the intestine of patients with AS, the success of SSPN in the management of IBD, and its potential antimicrobial properties on intestinal bacteria thought to be involved in the pathogenesis of AS. Since that time, the findings of 10 double-blind, placebo-controlled trials have been published. There are few reports, however, that have assessed the scope of use of SSPN for AS. A prospective longitudinal study of 241 patients with AS followed for a median of 4.5 years reported 49 new treatment courses in 42 (17.4%) patients at a median dose of 2 g/day.[52] Median duration of drug use was 12 months. Baseline information for patients with AS recruited to phase III clinical trials of anti–tumor necrosis factor (TNF)-α therapy showed that 20% of patients had been using this agent.[69,70]

Rationale

SSPN is administered orally and cleaved in the colon to 5-aminosalicylic acid (5-ASA) and sulfapyridine (SP). The latter is well absorbed and may exert systemic anti-inflammatory effects whereas the former remains in the colon and may exert a local anti-inflammatory effect. However, the parent molecule also has immunomodulating properties. Several modes of action have been proposed, including inhibition of leukocyte mobility and chemotaxis, inhibition of the generation of reactive oxygen species and pro-inflammatory prostaglandins, and modification of bacterial bowel flora.[71] More recent work has shown that SSPN inhibits 5-aminoimidazole-carboxamide-ribonucleotide (AICAR) transformylase,

an enzyme involved in de novo purine biosynthesis.[72] This in turn leads to the accumulation of AICAR and its metabolites, which have a direct inhibitory effect on at least two additional key enzymes, adenosine deaminase and adenosine monophosphatase deaminase. The end result is increased concentrations of adenosine and adenine nucleotides. Adenosine has a variety of anti-inflammatory effects on different cell types. In neutrophils, these include inhibition of oxygen radical formation and elastase expression, inhibition of adherence to endothelium, and inhibition of phagocytosis.[73] In macrophages, adenosine inhibits phagocytosis, generation of superoxide anions, and generation of various pro-inflammatory cytokines, including TNF-α.[74] Other work has shown that SSPN but not 5-ASA or SP induced apoptosis of T cells through inhibition of phosphorylation of nuclear factor (NF)-κB, which is a key transcriptional factor involved in the regulation of apoptosis.[75]

Evidence-based literature

Open-label studies

SSPN was first evaluated in an open-label study of 8 patients with peripheral arthritis. The drug was effective in 6 patients.[68] It was then evaluated in 48 patients with reactive arthritis of whom 16 fulfilled the criteria for AS with ileocolonoscopic follow-up of 3 to 24 months.[76] Approximately half showed clinical remission. In a further prospective study from this group, 123 patients meeting the European Spondyloarthropathy Study Group (ESSG) criteria for spondyloarthritis who had ileal colonoscopy were reviewed after 2 to 9 years.[77] AS was diagnosed in 52 patients, and 49 had a second ileocolonoscopy at follow up. The prevalence of clinical remission of joint disease during SSPN treatment was significantly higher in patients with inflammatory gut lesions at the first ileal colonoscopy than in patients who presented with normal gut histology.

Controlled studies (Table 13.4)

The first controlled study evaluated SSPN 2 g/day over a 6-month period in 60 patients.[78] An intent-to-treat analysis was used to evaluate eight clinical parameters. More SSPN (50%)-treated than placebo (20%)-treated patients considered themselves responders according to a global rating score. Changes in individual parameters were only reported for those who completed the study and demonstrated significant group differences for only two clinical parameters, NSAID usage and function. In a second study 37 patients were randomly assigned to receive SSPN 3 g/day or a placebo for a period of 12 weeks.[79] Of the 10 clinical and 3 laboratory variables studied, only sleep disturbance and acute-phase reactants (serum haptoglobin and orosomucoid) showed significant improvement in the active

TABLE 13.4 RANDOMIZED, CONTROLLED STUDIES OF SALAZOPYRIN FOR AS

Study	Patient No./ Study Duration	Disease Duration	Pain	Stiffness	Function	Global	Mobility	ESR/CRP	Main Conclusions
			ASAS Outcome Domains						
Dougados et al. 1986[78]	SSPN (2 g) = 30 Placebo = 30 6 months	10 years 10 years	↑	↑	↑	↑	↑	↑	Overall efficacy greater in SSPN (50%) than in placebo (20%) patients. SSPN superior to placebo for function (15%) and NSAID use (31%) from 3 months onwards.
	Other end points: sleep disturbance, serum haptoglobin and awakening								
Feltelius et al. 1986[79]	SSPN (3 g) = 18 Placebo = 19 12 weeks	12 years 10 years	↑	↑	nd	↑	↑	↑	SSPN superior to placebo only for sleep disturbance, serum haptoglobin and orosomucoid.
	Other end points: sleep disturbance, serum haptoglobin and orosomucoid								
Nissala et al. 1988[80]	SSPN (3 g) = 43 Placebo = 42 26 weeks	4 years 5 years	↑	↑	nd	↑	↑	↑	SSSPN superior to placebo for morning stiffness (34%), chest expansion (19%), ESR (36%). No difference between axial and peripheral subgroups of AS.
	Other end points: tender and swollen joints, serum immunoglobulins								
Davis et al. 1989[81]	SSPN (2 g) = 15 Placebo = 13 3 months	9 years 8 years	?	?	nd	nd	?	?	Between group comparisons were not performed.
	Other end points: sleep disturbance, serum orosomucoid, serum IgA								
Corkill et al. 1990[82]	SSPN (2 g) = 32 Placebo = 30 48 weeks	12 years 16 years	↑	↑	nd	nd	↑	↑	SSPN superior to placebo only for peripheral joint pain at week 4.
	Other end points: peripheral joint pain, tender and swollen joints, serum immunoglobulins								
Taylor et al. 1991[83]	SSPN (2 g) = 20 Placebo = 20 12 months	11 years 11 years	↑	↑	nd	↑	↑	↑	SSPN superior to placebo only for pain (39%).
	Other end points: radiological progression, sleep disturbance, forced vital capacity, swollen joints, NSAID requirement, serum orosomucoid and IgA								
Kirwan et al. 1993[84]	SSPN (2 g) = 44 Placebo = 45 3 years	19 years 22 years	↑	↑	↑	↑	↑	↑	Fewer episodes of peripheral joint symptoms in SSPN group.
	Other end points: NSAID use, sleep disturbance, episodes of peripheral arthritis, episodes of uveitis, flares in AS symptoms, episodes of heel pain								
Dougados et al. 1995[85]	SSPN (3 g) = 134 Placebo = 172 6 months	11 years 9 years	↑	↑	↑	↑	↑	↑	Analyses primarily based on patients who completed the trial.
	Other end points: swollen joints, new episodes of uveitis, physician global								
Clegg et al. 1996[86]	SSPN (2 g) = 131 Placebo = 133 36 weeks	18 years 19 years	↑	↑	↑	↑	↑	↑	SSPN superior to placebo only for ESR. Response to SSPN greater in peripheral arthritis subgroup of patients.
	Other end points: nocturnal pain, swollen and tender joints, dactylitis score, enthesopathy index, physician global								

AS, ankylosing spondylitis; ASAS, Assessments in Ankylosing Spondylitis; CRP, C-reactive peptide; ESR, erythrocyte sedimentation rate; IgA, immunoglobulin A; nd, not done; NSAID, nonsteroidal anti-inflammatory drug; SSPN, salazopyrin.
↑ = significant improvement; → = no change; comparison of active intervention(s) versus controls

treatment group. In a third controlled trial, 85 patients with a relatively short duration of disease (5.4 years in the placebo group and 3.8 years in the SSPN group) were recruited into a 6-month trial of SSPN 3 gdaily.[80] In contrast with the former two studies, almost two thirds of patients had peripheral joint inflammation. Of nine clinical and five laboratory parameters assessed, significant improvement in SSPN-treated patients was only evident in the severity of morning stiffness, chest expansion, erythrocyte sedimentation rate (ESR), and serum immunoglobulin (Ig) levels. Stratification of outcome according to axial and peripheral subtypes of AS revealed no significant differences. In a fourth study, 28 patients were randomly assigned to receive either SSPN 2 g/day or a placebo over a period of 3 months.[81] Of five clinical and five laboratory parameters assessed, two clinical (duration of stiffness and occiput to wall distance) and three laboratory (ESR, C-reactive peptide [CRP] level, and IgA level) showed improvement.

Three long-term controlled trials have been reported. In a 48-week study 62 patients who were randomly assigned to receive either SSPN 2 g daily or placebo were evaluated.[82] There was no significant improvement in severity of spinal pain, spinal stiffness, peripheral joint pain, or measures of spinal mobility compared with the placebo group. In another 1-year trial, 40 patients were randomly assigned to receive either SSPN 2 g daily or placebo.[83] At 1 year, only one of eight clinical parameters assessed, severity of pain score, improved significantly in SSPN-treated patients. Radiologic progression was noted in both treatment groups. In a further long-term study 89 patients with relatively long disease duration (20 years) received either SSPN 2 g daily or a placebo over a 3-year period.[84] The primary outcome variables were measures of spinal mobility. There was no benefit for SSPN over placebo.

Two large, multicenter, randomized, placebo-controlled, double-blind studies of SSPN in the treatment of AS have been reported. The first was a 6-month study of SSPN 3 g daily in which patients fulfilling the classification criteria of the ESSG were enrolled.[85] Of 351 recruited patients 134 had AS. For the entire group, analysis of primary efficacy variables (VAS pain, patient/physician global assessment, and duration of morning stiffness) showed that there was a significant difference in favor of SSPN only for patient global assessment. Analysis of the AS subgroup was confined to those who completed the study and showed no benefit for SSPN. Significant benefits were observed primarily in patients with psoriatic arthritis (PsA) and polyarticular involvement. In a second placebo-controlled study 264 patients with AS were given SSPN in a dose of 2 g daily for 36 weeks.[86] Responder status was determined according to predefined changes in patient/physician global assessment, duration of morning stiffness, and

severity of back pain. No treatment group differences were noted in either percentage of responders or in any of the individual outcome measures used to define treatment response. Analysis by subgroup showed significant benefits only in those with combined axial and peripheral involvement as compared with those with axial disease alone.

In all trials tolerability has been good with the most common adverse events affecting the GI and central nervous systems, including nausea, vomiting, abdominal pain, dizziness, irritability, and headaches. Serious hematologic, hepatic, and mucocutaneous reactions were rarely reported. Withdrawal due to side effects has varied from 5% to 16%.

Systematic reviews and meta-analyses

Researchers conducting a meta-analysis of SSPN in AS selected five of these trials on the basis of standardized methodologic assessments and concluded that four clinical outcomes reached levels of statistical significance in the pooled analysis of clinical benefit.[87] There was a reduction of 28.2% for duration of morning stiffness, 30.6% for severity of morning stiffness, 7.1% for general well-being, and 26.7% in severity of pain.

Conclusions

The small, controlled studies of both short and long duration demonstrated minimal clinical benefit for SSPN over placebo, which was confirmed in the two large multicenter studies. The latter studies were also consistent in the conclusion that SSPN is not efficacious in those with purely axial disease but may have modest beneficial effects in those with concomitant peripheral synovitis. There is essentially no evidence pointing to a disease-modifying effect of such treatment. A significant limitation in most of these studies was the long disease duration (>10 years) of recruited patients together with a lack of standard inclusion criteria and approach to outcome assessment.

5-Aminosalicylic acid

5-ASA has also been evaluated in open studies in view of its ability to reduce gut inflammation in IBD. Pentasa is a formulation of 5-ASA that is delivered to both large and small bowel and has been examined in 26 patients with AS in a 16-week study using a dose of 1500 mg daily.[88] Dose escalation to 2 g day was permitted from week 8. Significant improvement was noted in outcome parameters measuring symptoms, function, peripheral joint count, ESR, and CRP but not spinal mobility. In a second report, two open analyses were conducted evaluating 2 g daily in 20 patients with inadequate response or adverse events associated with SSPN and in 19 patients without previous exposure to SSPN over a period of 36 weeks.[89] Beneficial effects were primarily noted for physician but not patient global assessment. In contrast, a third formulation of 5-ASA, Salofalk, given at a higher dose of 3 to 4 g daily in a 24-week study of 20 patients demonstrated little efficacy and a high incidence of adverse events was reported.[90]

A 26-week randomized, controlled trial comparing a 5-ASA formulation, Asacol, with SP 1.25 g daily and SSPN 2 g daily in 90 patients with active AS failed to show any clinical improvement in Asacol-treated patients.[91] Furthermore, SSPN- and SP-treated patients did significantly better than those taking Asacol. Consequently, the weight of evidence does not support the use of 5-ASA in the treatment of AS.

Management issues in clinical practice

The primary indication for SSPN in routine practice is for the patient who has concomitant peripheral arthritis and has had an inadequate response to NSAIDs and physical modalities. Gradual introduction of therapy in 500 mg per week increments is recommended to avoid GI side effects. A dose of up to 3 g daily for 6 months represents an adequate trial of therapy although treatment is often discontinued if clinical improvement is not perceptible by 3 to 4 months. A 2 g daily dose represents a relatively safe maintenance dose. Prospective follow-up of patients in routine practice starting new treatment courses of SSPN for AS has shown that 22% report side effects during therapy, mostly diarrhea and upper abdominal pain, although most patients discontinue therapy for lack of efficacy.[52]

Methotrexate

Overview

MTX is a disease-modifying agent that has been in widespread use for the treatment of RA and PsA for the past three decades. It is widely regarded by clinicians as front-rank therapy for RA, and it constitutes the primary benchmark in the development of new therapies for RA. It is therefore not altogether surprising that it has also been used in clinical practice for the treatment of AS, although treatment has been largely empiric with respect to dosing and administration that is entirely based on its experience in RA. There are few reports in which the scope of its use for AS has been assessed. In a prospective longitudinal study of 241 patients with AS followed for a median of 4.5 years 19 new treatment courses for MTX in 14 patients at a median dose of 15 mg/wk were reported.[52] Median duration of drug use was 10 months. Baseline characteristics of patients with AS recruited to phase III clinical trials of anti–TNF-α therapy indicated that between 10% and 15% of patients had been using this agent.[69,70]

Rationale

MTX is a folic acid analog that interferes with the synthesis of DNA and RNA by inhibiting the enzyme dihydrofolate reductase and therefore the production of reduced folate analogs that are required for de novo synthesis of DNA and RNA precursors, such as purines and pyrimidines. This in turn leads to inhibition of cell proliferation, especially in rapidly dividing cells, and accounts for the toxicity observed in the bone marrow and GI tract. The therapeutic effects of this agent have been ascribed to inhibition of lymphocyte proliferation, induction of lymphocyte apoptosis, and impairment of T-cell function.[92,93] However, coadministration of folic acid reverses the effects of MTX on lymphocyte proliferation and apoptosis without reversing its anti-inflammatory effects. In addition, folic acid prevents much of the toxicity of this agent without interfering with its anti-inflammatory efficacy, arguing for an additional mechanism(s) of action.[94]

MTX undergoes cellular uptake through the reduced folate carrier and is then converted into polyglutamates. These polyglutamates constitute the active moiety and induce inhibition of AICAR transformylase, a folate-dependent enzyme, at pharmacologically relevant concentrations of MTX.[95] As for SSPN, this leads to increased concentrations of adenosine and adenine nucleotides. The relevance to in vivo administration is highlighted by the observation that oral MTX therapy leads to a marked increase in adenosine release from whole blood of patients.[96] That adenosine mediates the anti-inflammatory effects of MTX in animal models of acute inflammation is also demonstrated by the absence of an anti-inflammatory effect in adenosine receptor knockout mice.[97] Adenosine has a variety of anti-inflammatory effects on different cell types which include suppression of pro-inflammatory cytokine generation in macrophages, including TNF-α, indicating that at least on theoretical grounds MTX should display anti-inflammatory properties in AS.[98]

Evidence-based literature

Open-label studies (Table 13.5)

There have been several case reports and open analyses, mostly reported in abstract form, on the use of MTX in limited numbers of patients for periods of 6 months to 3 years, at doses from 7.5 to 15 mg/weekly. In the first open-label study, 11 patients with active disease received MTX at an initial dose of 7.5 mg followed by dose escalation to 15 mg at week 12.[99] Efficacy was judged as "good" in 5 patients as defined by improvement of 50% or greater in the majority of outcome variables and the decision to continue treatment beyond 24 weeks based on patient global assessment. Of the patients, 3 experienced disease flares

TABLE 13.5 OPEN LABEL STUDIES EVALUATING METHOTREXATE IN PATIENTS WITH AS

Study	Patient/Disease Duration	Dose/Duration	Main Endpoint(s)	Main Conclusions
Creemers et al. 1995[99]	N = 11 14 years	7.5–15 mg PO per week 24 weeks	Pain, patient global, stiffness, fatigue, enthesitis, function, mobility, swollen joints, ESR/CRP	Good response in 5 patients. Mild side-effects in 7 patients.
Clavaguera et al. 1989[100]	N = 12 ns	7.5 mg PO per week 6 months	Physician's global, swollen joints, mobility,	Improvement in all measures except swollen joints. Mild side-effects in 2 patients.
Ostendorf et al. 1998[102]	N = 10 each for AS, RA, PsA 11 years	10–15 mg PO per week 1 year	Pain, stiffness, mobility, function, patient global, ESR, CRP	No benefit in any AS patient compared to improvement in RA and PsA patients.
Biasi et al. 2000[102]	N = 17 5 years	7.5–10 mg PO per week 3 years	Pain, patient global, mobility, swollen joints, ESR, CRP, X-rays spine/sacroiliac joints, NSAID use	No radiographic progression. Improvement starting from 6 months in all parameters except for swollen joints.
Sampaio-Barros et al. 2000[103]	N = 34 11 years	12.5 mg IM per week 1 year	Stiffness, mobility, swollen joints, ESR, CRP	Improvement in symptoms in 53% and peripheral arthritis in 62% but not mobility.

AS, ankylosing spondylitis; CRP, C-reactive peptide; ESR, erythrocyte sedimentation rate; ns, not stated; NSAID, nonsteroidal anti-inflammatory drug; PsA, psoriatic arthritis; RA, rheumatoid arthritis.

during treatment and 4 experienced flares after treatment discontinuation.

In a second open analysis, 12 patients, a majority of whom had peripheral arthritis, received MTX 7.5 mg/wk for 6 months.[100] Significant improvement was noted in spinal symptomatology and mobility but not in swollen/tender joint count. In one study responses to MTX 10 to 15 mg weekly were compared in 10 patients with AS, 10 with RA, and 10 with PsA over 1 year.[101] No significant response was observed in patients with AS compared with the patients with RA and PsA. In one long-term study the use of MTX (7.5 to 10 mg/wk) was examined over 3 years in 17 patients with relatively early disease (mean duration 4.8 years) who were nonresponders to SSPN.[102] From 6 months onward, significant improvement was noted in severity of pain, patient global assessment, spinal mobility, ESR, and CRP level but not in swollen or tender joint count.

Instead of oral MTX, which has variable bioavailability, one group examined parenteral MTX 12.5 mg/wk in 26 patients over 1 year.[103] A clinical improvement permitting NSAID dose reduction of at least 50% was recorded in 18 (53%) patients and improvement in peripheral arthritis was observed in 16 (61.5%). There was no improvement in spinal mobility. Mild side effects were noted in 68% of patients.

Controlled studies (Table 13.6)
There have been three randomized, controlled studies of MTX in AS. In a 1-year, randomized, although non-blinded, study of 51 patients with AS, oral MTX 7.5 mg weekly plus naproxen 1000 mg daily was compared to naproxen alone.[104] A significant difference between groups was only noted for physician global assessment but not for severity of pain, morning stiffness, patient global assessment, spinal mobility, or acute-phase reactants. Treatment was well tolerated with no withdrawals for adverse events. A second study was a 24-week placebo-controlled trial of MTX 10 mg weekly in 30 patients, of whom 28 completed the study.[105] No improvement in disease activity (BASDAI) or metrology (BASMI) was evident. In a third study 35 patients were randomly assigned to receive either MTX 7.5 mg weekly or a placebo for 24 weeks.[106] Of the patients, 60% had active peripheral arthritis at baseline. Response was defined as at least 20% improvement in at least five of seven measures that included morning stiffness duration, patient global assessment, disease activity (BASDAI), function (BASFI and HAQ-S), physician global assessment, physical well-being and no deterioration (>20%) in any of these domains. Intention-to-treat analysis at 24 weeks showed a significant difference in response rate of 53% in the MTX group and 17% in the placebo group. Analysis of earlier time points showed no significant differences. No comparisons between groups were presented for the individual outcome measures. Peripheral arthritis resolved in 81% and 80% of MTX and placebo patients, respectively. Treatment was well tolerated with no withdrawals due to side effects.

Systematic reviews and meta-analyses
A Cochrane review of the use of MTX in AS was published in May 2003. Only two controlled trials met the inclusion criteria for the review (references 104 and 105).[107] The reviewers concluded that there was no evidence for efficacy and that higher-quality trials

TABLE 13.6 RANDOMIZED, CONTROLLED, TRIALS EVALUATING METHOTREXATE IN PATIENTS WITH AS				
Study	Patient/Disease Duration	Dose/ Duration	Main Endpoint(s)	Main Conclusions
Altan et al. 2001[104*]	MTX plus Naproten = 26 Naproten = 25 10 years	MTX 7.5 mg PO per week Naproxen 1000 mg daily 1 year	Stiffness, pain, patient global, physician global, function, mobility, entheses, ESR, CRP	MTX superior to placebo only in physician global.
Roychowdhury et al. 2001[105]	MTX =16 Placebo = 12 17 years	10 mg PO per week 24 weeks	Disease activity (BASDAI), mobility (BASMI), ESR, CRP	No group differences.
Gonzalez-Lopez et al. 2004[106]	MTX = 17 Placebo = 18 10 years for MTX group 6 years for placebo group	7.5 mg PO per week 24 weeks	Stiffness, physical well-being, patient global, physician global, diease activity (BASDAI), function (BASFI)	53% response in MTX group vs. 17% in placebo group.

*non-blinded study

AS, ankylosing spondylitis; BASDAI, Bath Ankylosing Spondylitis Disease Activity Index; BASFI, Bath Ankylosing Spondylitis Functional Index; BASMI, Bath Ankylosing Spondylitis Metrology Index; CRP, C-reactive peptide; ESR, erythrocyte sedimentation rate; MTX, methotrexate.

of larger sample size and longer duration with a higher dosage of MTX were necessary before any definitive conclusions could be drawn.

Conclusions

Aside from the obvious lack of controlled trial data, most researchers have used doses of MTX that would be regarded as inadequate in the management of RA. Standardized outcome measures have been used in only a few studies, and, as yet, the internationally accepted ASAS20 response criterion has not been used. There is presently little evidence to support the use of MTX in patients with AS.

Management issues in clinical practice

Although the evidence-based literature does not support the use of MTX in clinical practice, there is a need to recognize that many formularies across different countries have severely restricted access to proven therapies, specifically anti–TNF-α agents, or have simply made these agents unavailable for the treatment of AS. Clinicians may therefore have to consider empiric use of this agent when AS fails to respond to conservative therapy with NSAIDs, physical modalities, and even SSPN. In that circumstance, dosing should resemble that used in clinical practice for the management of RA, that is, 15 to 20 mg over a course of at least 4 months. Patient management should include monitoring of disease activity and function using standardized outcome measures (the BASDAI and BASFI) so that clinical perceptions of benefit can be documented in a validated manner.

Anti–TNF-α–Directed Therapies

Overview

The introduction of anti–TNF-α–directed therapies for the treatment of AS marks a significant milestone in the development of new therapies for this disease. However, this therapy was primarily based on circumstantial evidence implicating TNF-α in the pathogenesis of disease and followed their successful development for the treatment of RA. Three agents are currently available for the treatment of RA, two of which are now also approved in some countries for the treatment of AS. The first agent reported to be beneficial for AS was the chimeric monoclonal IgG1, infliximab. Shortly thereafter, a second agent, etanercept, was reported to be beneficial. This is a recombinant 75-kDa TNF receptor IgG1 fusion protein. The third agent, adalimumab, is a humanized monoclonal antibody to TNF-α although experience in AS is presently limited.

Rationale

Speculation that this approach would be useful in the treatment of AS was initially prompted by the observation that targeting TNF-α was effective in Crohn's disease as well as in RA. Intestinal inflammation is common in

AS and may resemble that seen in Crohn's disease. The significance of this cytokine to the pathogenesis of AS is also highlighted in the phenotype of a transgenic mouse model in which overexpression of this cytokine occurs as a consequence of a deletion in the 3′ regulatory region of a TNF-α transgene.[108] The excess TNF-α produced is associated with the development of sacroiliitis, cartilage destruction, and bone erosions that is substantially reduced in animals that receive infliximab.[109] In human studies, dense mononuclear infiltrates invading cartilage together with staining for TNF-α messenger RNA (mRNA) have been described in both sacroiliac joints and entheses.[110,111]

Evidence-based literature

Infliximab

Open-label studies

At least 222 patients with AS have been studied in open trials of infliximab conducted in both Europe and North America. The first report describing the evaluation of infliximab in AS was an open-label trial in 11 patients with AS who had a disease duration of 5 years.[112] The dosing regimen that had become established for Crohn's disease was used, that is, 5 mg/kg at 0, 2, and 6 weeks. Highly significant improvements in all clinical and laboratory parameters of disease activity (BASDAI, ESR, and CRP level) as well as indices of function (BASFI) and spinal mobility (BASMI) were evident as soon as 2 weeks. Almost all patients met the primary end point, an improvement of at least 50% in disease activity, by 12 weeks. In a 1-year follow-up analysis, additional infusions were given whenever disease activity approached greater than 60% of baseline values, which defined relapse.[113] Most patients required repeat infusions at 6- to 8-week intervals.

In a Belgian study, 21 patients with SpAs, of whom 10 had AS, 9 had PsA, and 2 had undifferentiated SpA, were examined in a 12-week trial using the same dosing regimen as that for Crohn's disease.[114] Disease duration was 17 years, and most patients had peripheral arthritis. Significant improvement in various symptomatic measures, acute-phase reactants, and swollen joint count occurred as early as day 3 whereas spinal mobility improved by day 15. Infliximab was subsequently given at intervals of 14 weeks although evaluation of data at 1 year showed that this regimen was inadequate, with most patients experiencing recurrence of symptoms before retreatment.[115] Histologic analysis of synovial biopsy specimens obtained at weeks 0, 2, and 12 revealed decreased infiltration with neutrophils and macrophages accompanied by a reduction in synovial lining layer thickness and decreased vascularity but an increase in B cells and plasma cells.[116]

An open-label study of 21 patients from Canada also showed substantial clinical improvement, which was more apparent in those patients with shorter disease duration and less extensive spinal ankylosis on plain x-ray films.[117] MRI was performed at baseline and 2 days after the first, second, and third infusions of 5 mg/kg infliximab and showed that resolution of subchondral bone marrow inflammation within the sacroiliac joints could be demonstrated by 48 hours after the first infusion. In a second Canadian study the dosing regimen typically used for the treatment of RA, (i.e., 3 mg/kg at 0, 2, and 6 weeks and then every 8 weeks thereafter) was evaluated.[118] Almost 60% of 21 patients demonstrated a reduction in disease activity of at least 50% by week 14 together with significant improvement in function. The severity of inflammation in peripheral joints was also quantified using dynamic MRI with gadolinium augmentation and shown to be significantly reduced at 14 weeks compared with baseline. Changes in serologic markers of articular cartilage degradation and/or turnover, namely, metalloproteinases 1 and 3 and human cartilage glycoprotein-39, were shown to correlate significantly with changes in disease activity. Further follow-up has shown that about half of patients receiving this regimen experience sustained efficacy.

In a French study 50 patients with AS and axial disease alone, who all had elevated CRP levels, were enrolled. Almost 100% of patients were designated as responders by 8 weeks as defined by a reduction in pain score of ≥20%.[119] Substudies demonstrated resolution of enthesitis as detected by ultrasound and improvement in bone mineral density of the spine and hip.

Controlled studies (Table 13.7)
Three controlled studies of this agent in AS have been conducted. The first was a multicenter trial in which 70 patients with AS that was refractory to NSAIDs were randomly assigned to either three infusions of infliximab 5 mg/kg at 0, 2, and 6 weeks or placebo.[120] The primary outcome criterion was an improvement of at least 50% in disease activity (BASDAI), and this was achieved at 12 weeks by 53% of patients receiving infliximab versus 9% of those receiving a placebo. Of infliximab-treated patients, 80% met the ASAS20 response criterion compared with 30% of control subjects. Significant improvement in function (BASFI), spinal mobility (BASMI), quality of life (36-item Short-Form Health Survey [SF-36]), CRP level, and ESR was also apparent in infliximab-treated patients. A substudy of 20 patients who had MRI examination of the spine showed improvement in disease activity that correlated with changes in clinical and laboratory parameters of disease activity.[121] After 12 weeks all patients received open-label therapy with infliximab at 5 mg/kg every 6 weeks. After 3 years, 43 (61.4%) were still being treated with infliximab.[122] Withdrawal of treatment led to disease relapse within 4 months in the majority of patients.[123]

In a second study data were reported from a 12-week single-center placebo-controlled trial enrolling 40 patients with SpA according to the ESSG criteria of whom 19 had AS.[124] Infliximab 5 mg/kg was again given at 0, 2, and 6 weeks. Significant improvement in all variables of disease activity as well as in acute-phase reactants was demonstrable as early as week 2, although no improvement in spinal mobility was evident, probably reflecting the short duration of this study and the lack of responsiveness of the metrology index.

In a pivotal phase III placebo-controlled study of infliximab in AS, 279 patients were recruited of whom 2001 received infliximab 5 mg/kg at 0, 2, and 6 weeks, followed by every 6 weeks thereafter for 2 years.[125] Placebo-treated patients received open-label infliximab after 24 weeks. An ASAS20 response was observed in 61.2% of infliximab-treated patients compared with 19.2% of placebo-treated patients by 24 weeks. Significant improvement was also noted in measures of function (BASFI), mobility (BASMI), quality of life (SF-36), and acute-phase reactants (ESR and CRP level). By week 24, 45 patients in the infliximab group (22.4%) achieved ASAS partial remission compared with one patient in the placebo group (1.3%). Clinical benefit was observed in infliximab-treated patients as soon as two weeks. At week 24, 22.4% in the infliximab group achieved ASAS partial remission compared with 1.3% in the placebo group. Responses were higher in patients with high baseline CRP levels. Treatment was well-tolerated with similar proportions of serious adverse events, infusion reactions, and serious infections.

Etanercept
Open-label studies
A single open-label study of etanercept in AS included semiquantitative MRI assessment of 44 entheseal sites in the sacroiliac joints, lumbar and cervical spine, and peripheral joints of 10 patients with SpA of whom 7 had AS, 2 had Crohn's spondylitis, and 1 had undifferentiated spondyloarthritis.[126] Etanercept 25 mg was given twice-weekly for 6 months. Clinical and quality-of-life outcome parameters improved significantly in all patients. Enthesitis resolved completely in 7 patients and improved in 2 other patients. Complete resolution or improvement was noted in 86% of lesions documented by MRI. Positive clinical responses were sustained for a median of 12 weeks after discontinuation of therapy.

Controlled studies (Table 13.7)
Four controlled evaluations of etanercept 25 mg twice weekly have been conducted. In the first study 40 AS patients were randomly assigned to receive either placebo or active therapy for 4 months.[69] Patients had active disease despite treatment with NSAIDs and second-line agents such as MTX and SSPN. Of patients

TABLE 13.7 RANDOMIZED, PLACEBO-CONTROLLED TRIALS OF ANTI-TNFα AGENTS WITH AS

Study	Patient No.	Disease Duration	Primary Endpoint	Primary Endpoint		Secondary Endpoints	Secondary Endpoints	
				Active	Placebo		Active	Placebo
Braun et al. 2002[120]	Infliximabo= 34 Placebo = 35	16 years 15 years	>50% decrease in BASDAI by 12 weeks	53%	9%	BASFI Patient global CRP	−38.2% −52.2% −75%	−2.0% −8.7% −16.7%
Van den Bosch et al. 2002 [123]	Infliximab= 20* Placebo = 20	10 years† 17 years	A. Patient global B. Physician global at, 12 weeks	−73.1% −75.6%	+29.0% +8.3%	BASDAI BASFI CRP	−54.8% −41.1% −100%	+4.9% +22.1% +0.0%
Gorman et al. 2002[69]	Etanercept = 20 Placebo = 20	15 years 12 years	Composite treatment response by 4 months§	80%	30%	Enthesitis score‡ Chest expansion CRP	−100% 34.6% −65%	−50% −6.5% +33.3%
Davis et al. 2003[70]	Etanercept = 138 Placebo = 139	10 years 10 years	ASAS 20 response at 12 weeks	59%	28%	BASDAI ASAS 50 CRP	−40.6% 43% −68.4%	−7.6% 8% −5%
Brandt et al. 2003[126]	Etanercept = 14 Placebo = 16	15 years 11 years	≥50% decrease in BASDAI by 6 weeks	57%	6%	ASAS 20 BASFI BASMI	78.6% −30.6% −36.6%	25% −3.8% −7.9%
Calin et al. 2004[130]	Etanercept = 45 Placebo = 39	15 years 10 years	ASAS 20 response at 12 weeks	60%	23.1%	ASAS 50 BASDAI Schober's test	48.9% −43.6% +36%	10.3% −13.6% −1.3%
Van der Heijde et al. 2005[124]	Infliximab = 201 Placebo = 78	8 years 13 years	ASAS 20 response at 24 weeks	61.2%	19.2%	ASAS 40 ASAS partial remission ASAS 5/6 BASDAI BASFI	47% 22.4% 49% −43.9% −29.8%	12% 1.3% 8.0% −6.2% 0%

*19 had AS, 18 had psoriatic arthritis, 3 had undifferentiated spondyloarthritis

†AS patients only

‡ modified Newcastle Enthesis Index

§ ≥20% improvement in 3 of 5 measures (morning stiffness, nocturnal spinal pain, BASFI, patient global, swollen joint score) with no worsening in remaining measures.

AS, ankylosing spondylitis; ASAS, Assessments in Ankylosing Spondylitis; BASDAI, Bath Ankylosing Spondylitis Disease Activity Index; BASFI, Bath Ankylosing Spondylitis Functional Index; BASMI, Bath Ankylosing Spondylitis Metrology Index; CRP, C-reactive peptide.

receiving etanercept, 80% achieved a response compared with 30% of the placebo group. Significant improvement was observed in various measures of disease activity, function, quality of life, enthesitis, and acute-phase reactants. Placebo-treated patients experienced a similar response to etanercept in the open-label extension phase over the ensuing 6 months.

In a second trial 30 patients with AS that was refractory to NSAID therapy were recruited. An improvement in disease activity (BASDAI) of at least 50% in 57% of etanercept-treated patients compared with only 6% of placebo-treated patients was reported at 6 weeks.[126] After the placebo-treated patients switched to etanercept at 6 weeks, 56% had improved by week 12. Similarly, pain, function, mobility (BASMI), quality of life, and mean CRP levels improved significantly with etanercept but not with placebo at week 6. Disease relapse occurred a mean of 6.2 ± 3 weeks after discontinuation of etanercept. Twenty-six patients then received long-term open-label therapy. At 2 years, 21 (81%) were still receiving therapy with persistent improvement in disease activity, function, mobility, quality of life, and acute-phase reactants.[128]

In a pivotal phase III multinational study, 277 patients were randomly assigned to receive either etanercept ($n = 138$) or placebo ($n = 139$) for 24 weeks.[70] Patients had active disease despite treatment with NSAIDs and second-line agents such as MTX and SSPN. An ASAS20 response was observed in 57% of etanercept-treated patients compared with 22% of placebo-treated patients. Differences between the two groups were already apparent by 2 weeks. All individual ASAS components, acute-phase reactant levels, and spinal mobility measures were also significantly improved. A substudy also revealed improvement in MRI features of inflammation.[129] In the open-label phase, placebo-treated patients who were switched to etanercept began to show improvement as early as week 4 with a gradual increase in the percentage achieving an ASAS20 response that reached 75% by week 48.[130] Partial remission as defined by the ASAS response was evident in 34% at week 48. A subsequent analysis of placebo patients from this study and the 40 patients recruited to an earlier trial[69] compared these AS patients with those with other medical conditions for health-related quality of life (HRQOL) as measured by the SF36. Patients with AS had the lowest scores in the physical domains—physical functioning, role physical, and bodily pain. Impairments in SF-36 scores for psychosocial domains, such as Social Functioning, Role Emotional, and Mental Health, were somewhat less pronounced. Treatment with etanercept significantly improved the HRQOL of patients with AS on all eight SF-36 scales, especially in the same physical domains that showed the greatest impairments prior to treatment.[131]

In a fourth multicenter study 84 patients who had active disease despite NSAID and second-line therapies were recruited.[132] Significantly more etanercept-treated patients than placebo-treated patients (60% vs. 23.1%) were ASAS20 responders at week 12, the primary efficacy end point. The primary end point was not significantly affected by the concomitant use of disease-modifying antirheumatic drugs (DMARDs), nor was there an interaction effect between DMARDs and etanercept on the ASAS20 response at week 12. Significant improvements in the etanercept group were evident by week 2, the earliest assessment point, and were sustained thereafter. Scores of etanercept-treated patients improved 43% on both the spinal inflammation and back pain measures, 37% on patient global assessment of disease activity, and 35% on the functional impairment index (compared with 16%, 6%, 13%, and 3% improvements, respectively, for placebo-treated patients). Etanercept-treated patients also had significantly greater improvements in acute-phase reactants and spinal flexion.

Adalimumab
There has been a single open-label trial of adalimumab in AS.[133] Fourteen patients with AS that was refractory to NSAIDs received adalimumab 40 mg on alternate weeks over 12 weeks. An ASAS20 response was seen in 70% with 50% reporting a substantial response (ASAS50). Significant improvement was also noted in function, nocturnal pain, and patient global assessment. A further increase in the percentage of ASAS20 responders to 86% was noted at week 20 after an increase in dosage to weekly therapy. This was accompanied by a reduction in sacroiliac joint and spinal inflammation observed on MRI.[134]

Controlled studies
Preliminary data from two controlled trials of adalimumab in AS are now available. In a Canadian study, 44 patients were randomized to placebo and 38 to adalimumab 40 mg on alternate weeks in a 24-week trial.[135] After the week 12 assessment, patients not achieving an ASAS20 response were eligible for early escape therapy with adalimumab. At week 12, the ASAS20 response was higher in adalimumab (47%) versus placebo (27%) patients and differences between treatment groups were already statistically significant by week 2. The second trial was a multinational study that recruited 315 patients and randomized 208 to adalimumab 40 mg on alternate weeks and 107 to placebo for 24 weeks.[136] Patients were allowed to remain on stable second line therapy and were offered the early escape option as for the Canadian study. The number of patients meeting ASAS partial remission criteria was significantly higher amongst adalimumab-treated patients (21.6%) than placebo-treated patients (6.5%)

at 24 weeks. ASAS 5/6 responses were also significantly more common in patients that received adalimumab (44.2%) than placebo (13.1%). Treatment was generally well tolerated in both trials.

Side effects of anti–TNF-α therapies

Reported side effects have been similar for all currently available anti–TNF-α agents and similar to those observed in trials of patients with RA and Crohn's disease. They can generally be summarized into seven categories:

1. Sepsis and tuberculosis. Tuberculosis is often atypical with extrapulmonary manifestations and a failure to form granulomas. One group from Belgium described an observational cohort of 107 patients treated with infliximab for a total of 191.5 patient years and reported eight severe infections, including two of reactivated tuberculosis and three retropharyngeal abscesses.[137] However, a recent study from Spain, describing 1578 courses of treatment with infliximab (86%) and etanercept (14%) primarily in patients with RA, has shown that the incidence of tuberculosis can be substantially minimized with appropriate pretreatment screening procedures.[138]

2. Malignancies. A 2002 report from the Food and Drug Administration MedWatch reported 26 cases of lymphoproliferative disorders with regression being observed in two patients after discontinuation of anti–TNF-α therapy.[139] Most malignancies were non-Hodgkin's lymphoma. The recurrence rate of solid organ malignancies, however, may be less in patients receiving these therapies.[140]

3. Hematologic disorders. Pancytopenia and neutropenia have been described in several case reports, some being associated with a fatal outcome in patients receiving infliximab.[141]

4. Demyelinating disorders. Although uncommon, neurologic events have been reported, primarily in patients receiving etanercept, that were temporally related to anti–TNF-α therapy and that resolved partially or completely on treatment discontinuation.[142] There have also been case reports of central nervous system vasculitis during postmarketing surveillance.

5. Congestive heart failure. Case reports of new-onset heart failure, with no identifiable risk factors in 50% of patients, have been published.[143] Exacerbation of heart failure was also been described in both case reports and in a phase II trial of high-dose infliximab (10 mg/kg) in patients with stable heart failure.[144] However, in a large observational study a decreased prevalence of heart failure was reported in patients receiving anti–TNF-α therapy.[145]

6. Development of autoantibodies/autoimmunity. One report described the development of antinuclear antibodies (ANAs) in the majority of patients with AS treated with infliximab and de novo development of anti-double-stranded (ds) DNA antibodies in 20% although no patient experienced lupus symptoms.[146] The frequency of ANAs in different studies depends on the assay method used and the cut-off chosen for designating a positive result. Anti-dsDNA antibodies are of the IgM and IgA class and have been rarely associated with lupus symptoms although not with major organ involvement.[147] The incidence of ANAs and anti-dsDNA has been much less with etanercept. There have also been several case reports of vasculitis.[148]

7. Infusion and hypersensitivity reactions. The incidence of infusion reactions with infliximab has been reported to be 5% to 10% of infusions affecting 5% to 10% of patients.[149,150] Severe reactions have been noted in 1% of patients. Re-infusion has been possible with the use of a prophylaxis protocol in those patients with mild to moderate reactions. It was anticipated that this would be a concern with the use of infliximab in AS because these patients do not receive concomitant therapy with MTX, as is recommended for RA, which may reduce the development of human anti-chimeric antibodies. However, administration of infliximab without MTX in patients with AS has not been associated with an increased incidence of infusion reactions.[125] Injection site reactions have been noted with etanercept, but this does not usually result in discontinuation of therapy.

Conclusions

There can be little doubt that the anti–TNF-α agents, infliximab and etanercept, are effective in the majority of patients with AS, including those with long-standing disease and severe functional impairment. Furthermore, they are well tolerated, and efficacy is sustained at least over 3 years. Maintenance of efficacy requires ongoing treatment with most patients having a relapse within a few months of treatment discontinuation. For infliximab, optimal disease control requires infusions every 6 to 8 weeks. Although circumstantial data indicate that anti–TNF-α agents may be disease controlling, there is as yet no data demonstrating prevention of structural damage on plain x-ray films.

Management issues in clinical practice

Both infliximab and etanercept are indicated for patients when treatment with NSAIDs and physical modalities has failed. Patients with peripheral arthritis should also have had a trial of SSPN. Preference for a specific anti–TNF-α agent is largely dictated by patient preference with respect to mode and regimen of administration because both infliximab and etanercept appear to be equally efficacious. It would be prudent to initiate infliximab therapy at a dose of 3 mg/kg because at least half of all patients will experience a satisfactory response. Dose escalation to 5 mg/kg can be reserved for those who have an inadequate response. Although predictors of response, such as baseline function, disease activity, ESR, CRP levels, and disease duration, have been identified in a pooled analysis of patients from clinical trials of infliximab and etanercept, these lack sufficient predictive value to assist clinicians in selecting appropriate patients for therapy.[151] In contrast to current practice in RA, combination therapy with MTX is not indicated because there is no evidence that this agent is efficacious in AS. Although this combination is superior to monotherapy in RA, such evidence is lacking in AS. Furthermore, monotherapy with infliximab has not been associated with an increased risk of infusion reactions in AS compared with those in RA despite evidence that MTX may suppress the development of anti-chimeric antibodies. All patients should be screened for active or latent tuberculosis by purified protein derivative testing before therapy. Patients who experience mild or moderate infusion reactions with infliximab can continue to receive further infusions with the use of prophylactic protocols that employ acetaminophen and antihistamines. Patients should be followed in routine practice using standardized and validated outcome instruments such as the BASDAI, BASFI, pain VAS, and patient global VAS, which can be completed in a few minutes.

Miscellaneous Therapies

Glucocorticoids

Overview
Glucocorticoids have been typically used in patients undergoing disease flares although few studies have examined their effectiveness in this disease. Several modes of administration have been used including oral therapy, pulse intravenous therapy, and injection therapy into joints and around painful entheses.

Rationale
Evidence has accumulated that glucocorticoids exert their effects through both genomic and nongenomic mechanisms, the latter being more relevant at higher doses. The most important anti-inflammatory effects are mediated by genomic mechanisms. Glucocorticoid binding to their cytoplasmic receptor is followed by translocation to the nucleus where the complex binds to specific DNA sites, the glucocorticoid response elements that are found within many target genes.[152] Depending on the target gene this binding may then lead to either decreased or increased gene activation. This complex also binds to and inhibits the function of several key transcription factors, such as activator protein 1 (AP-1), NF-κB, and nuclear factor of activated T cells (NF-AT), that activate the expression of various pro-inflammatory cytokines such as TNF-α and interleukin (IL)-1.[153]

Nongenomic actions include the inhibition of cytosolic phospholipase A_2 and a consequent reduction in the release of arachidonic acid. At very high doses such as those used in pulse intravenous therapy, the cytoplasmic receptor is saturated, leading to nonspecific interactions of free glucocorticoid molecules with biologic membranes. These interactions may alter cell functions by interfering with ion transport, which leads to rapid immunosuppression and a reduction in the inflammatory process. Intra-articular injections also result in high glucocorticoid concentrations in the vicinity of inflammatory cells.

Evidence-based literature
Most studies have been open label, examining the effects of either pulse intravenous glucocorticoids or intraarticular injections given into the sacroiliac joints.

Pulse intravenous steroids
In the first report the effects of up to four consecutive daily pulses of 1 g of methylprednisolone were described.[154] An immediate benefit was noted in pain severity, morning stiffness, and spinal mobility that persisted for up to 1 year in those patients who received at least three consecutive daily pulses, allowing them to return to their regular work. An immunologic study in eight patients receiving three daily pulses of 1 g of methylprednisolone revealed an early anti-inflammatory effect with a significant reduction in morning stiffness that was evident for 1 month, and pain and acute-phase reactants improved for 3 months.[155] In a third open-label study seven patients received 1 g of methylprednisolone daily for 3 days; reduced pain severity for up to 6 weeks and in fingertip-to-floor distance for up to 6 months were reported.[156] In a randomized, double-blind dose-response study three consecutive daily intravenous infusions of 1 g and 375 mg of methylprednisolone were compared in 17 patients with AS who were then followed for 6 months.[157] There were no significant differences in pain relief or spinal mobility although pretreatment pain levels were reached in 347 days in the high-dose group compared with 253 days in the low-dose group. Most studies indicated that treatment was well tolerated with only a minority of patients reporting difficulty sleeping, a metallic taste, mood disorder, and flushing.

Intramuscular adrenocorticotropic hormone
In one placebo-controlled study daily injections of adrenocorticotropic hormone (20 IU for 7 days and 10 IU for 5 days) were evaluated in 21 patients with AS

Controlled studies

There has been one controlled dose-response (60 versus 10 mg) evaluation of pamidronate in AS; the frequent occurrence of postinfusion reactions precluded the use of a placebo.[182] Eighty-four patients were recruited, and 72 completed 6 months of therapy. Treatment was well tolerated despite the high incidence of postinfusion reactions after the first exposure to pamidronate with only 1 patient withdrawing for adverse events. Significant efficacy was not observed at 3 months, but significant reductions in disease activity (BASDAI) and improvement in function (BASFI), patient global (BASGI), and mobility (BASMI) were evident by 6 months in the 60-mg group: 63% percent of patients had at least a 25% reduction in disease activity compared with only 30.2% of patients who received the 10-mg dose. There were, however, no significant differences in acute-phase reactants or the degree of peripheral synovitis, which could reflect the short half-life (~1 hour) of the drug in peripheral blood.

Conclusions

There is preliminary evidence that pamidronate given intravenously is effective in AS, particularly axial disease, although treatment has a slow onset of action, requiring at least 3 months of therapy. Treatment appears to be well tolerated. There is as yet no controlled data demonstrating improvement in bone density in patients with AS who are receiving bisphosphonates.

Management issues in clinical practice

Although most clinicians would prefer to administer bisphosphonates by the oral route there is as yet no evidence that such treatment is effective for the symptoms of AS. Furthermore, intravenous administration of bisphosphonate induces immunomodulating effects not observed with oral administration that may be relevant to its mechanism of action.[183] Nevertheless, it would be appropriate to consider screening with bone densitometry for patients with persistent, active, long-standing (>15 years) disease and instituting oral bisphosphonate therapy if concomitant osteoporosis is present. Intravenous pamidronate is a therapeutic option for patients in whom NSAID therapy has failed, particularly if anti–TNF-α therapies are unavailable. This approach is probably not helpful in patients with significant peripheral synovitis in view of the short half-life of this agent in the periphery. Patients should be advised that treatment benefit is typically delayed for 3 months and that a transient postinfusion reaction is not a source of alarm.

Leflunomide

Leflunomide is a prodrug that is metabolized to its active metabolite, A771726, in the liver and is now well-established as a disease-controlling therapy in RA. Its primary mode of action is to inhibit the enzyme dihydro- orotate dehydrogenase, which is required for the de novo synthesis of pyrimidines. This leads to decreased synthesis of DNA and RNA, particularly in activated T cells, with impairment of T-cell proliferation and B-cell synthesis of autoantibodies.[184] Other actions include decreased activation and expression of NF-κB, decreased generation of TNF-α and IL-1β, and direct inhibition of the COX-2 enzyme.[185]

The results of leflunomide therapy in AS have been reported in two studies. An open-label study of 20 patients over 24 weeks demonstrated an improvement of at least 50% in disease activity (BASDAI) in 5 patients at 3 months although only 10 patients completed the study.[186] Overall, there was no significant benefit at 24 weeks. There was a significant reduction in the number of swollen joints in the subgroup of 10 patients with peripheral arthritis. A second study was a single-center, double-blind, placebo-controlled study of 45 patients over 24 weeks.[187] There was no difference in ASAS20 response rates between the two groups although 11 patients withdrew primarily because of adverse events, and few had peripheral arthritis. This agent may have a role in patients with active peripheral arthritis.

Thalidomide

Thalidomide has been examined for its anti-inflammatory properties in several diseases. It has been shown to possess anti–TNF-α properties by enhancing the degradation of TNF-α mRNA.[188]

An initial study indicated significant improvement in axial and peripheral clinical manifestations of AS in 2 patients with concomitant reductions in acute-phase reactants.[189] Discontinuation of therapy was followed by relapse. Examination of an additional group of 10 patients of whom 7 had AS and 3 had undifferentiated SpA showed modest improvement in disease activity with 4 patients having to withdraw within the first month of treatment because of adverse events.[190] Chinese investigators reported on a 1-year open-label evaluation in 30 male patients with severe refractory AS.[191] Eighty percent were designated as clinical responders, and significant deterioration was noted 3 months after termination of therapy. Common side effects were drowsiness, constipation, and dizziness although peripheral neuropathy, a major side effect of thalidomide, has not yet been reported in AS.

Anakinra

Anakinra, an IL-1 receptor antagonist, has been examined in AS primarily based on its efficacy in RA although IL-1 has a prominent role in osteoclast-mediated bone damage. One open-label study of 20 patients over 24 weeks indicated an ASAS20 response in 26%, which resembles the placebo response in controlled trials of anti–TNF-α therapies, and no effect on the CRP level or the MRI score.[192] In contrast, a second open-label study of 9 patients over 12 weeks showed an ASAS20 response in 6 (67%) patients together with significant improvement in function (BASFI), CRP level, and MRI score.[193] Controlled trials will be required to resolve these discrepancies.

SURGICAL MODALITIES

Despite the remarkable advances in medical therapies for AS, some patients still require surgical intervention after failure of other treatment modalities. One survey of 2452 patients showed that 10% had undergone surgery and of these 50% had undergone two or more operations.[194] Total hip replacements had been performed in 42% followed by spinal surgery in 31%, knee surgery in 15%, and foot surgery in 9%. Hip or knee surgery was more common in patients with a younger age of onset.

The most common indications for surgery include end-stage hip or knee disease, functionally and/or cosmetically unacceptable spinal deformities, a painful spinal deformity, and severe spinal instability, especially at the atlanto-occipital joint. The introduction of minimally invasive techniques and the availability of better implants have greatly improved the results of surgical treatment.[195] Corrective osteotomy in the lumbar and thoracolumbar spine is carried out for severe kyphosis and requires multiple V-shaped osteotomies, transpedicular insertion of screws, and fixation with rods at the most commonly involved segments in the kyphosis through a posterior approach to the spine. A second step includes anterior endoscopically assisted osteotomy through a keyhole incision opposite the apex of the kyphosis. After division of all bony elements anterior to the spinal cord, the trunk is gradually extended to correct the deformity.

Potential complications of surgery include spinal cord injury and/or ischemia leading to paraplegia, injury to spinal nerve roots, and pseudoarthrosis. Consequently, patients requiring surgery should be managed by surgeons at tertiary referral centers with sufficient experience in this highly specialized form of surgery.

CONSENSUS TREATMENT GUIDELINES

Two consensus treatment guidelines have been published: the Spondyloarthritis Research Consortium of Canada guidelines and the ASAS guidelines for the use of anti–TNF-α therapies in AS.[196,197] They present very similar recommendations. Both sets of guidelines were developed after a review of the literature with additional input from experts in the management of AS. The ASAS guidelines also incorporated a Delphi exercise by experts in AS. The guidelines state that such therapy is warranted when the following criteria are met:

1. Active disease for at least 4 weeks as defined by a disease activity score of at least 4 as recorded by the BASDAI instrument (range 0 to 10) together with an expert opinion.
2. Disease that is refractory to at least two NSAIDs that have been used over a single 3-month period plus SSPN and intraarticular steroids, if indicated, in those patients with concomitant peripheral arthritis.

The ASAS guidelines also stipulate criteria for continuation of therapy after patients have had a minimum trial of 6 to 12 weeks:

1. An improvement in disease activity of at least 50% (BASDAI), *and*
2. An absolute improvement of at least 2 on the 0 to 10 BASDAI scale.

CURRENT CONTROVERSIES AND FUTURE DIRECTIONS

A common practice since NSAIDs became available for AS has been to recommend that NSAIDs be taken only as required for relief of symptoms. This recommendation was based on the assumption, largely derived from studies in RA, that NSAIDs were purely symptom-modifying agents. This assumption has recently been challenged in a 2-year randomized study suggesting that patients who took NSAIDs continually as opposed to on demand were less likely to have radiologic progression of disease.[49] This observation was not explained by any discernible effects of therapy on disease activity, which was similar in the two groups throughout the 2-year period or by any apparent differences in disease severity at the start of the study. Although this concept will require further study, it should nevertheless remind physicians to encourage patients to take up to maximum recommended doses to ensure effective symptomatic control.

The advent of MRI and the introduction of highly effective, although very costly, new therapies for AS has raised several new challenges in the treatment of this disease. By analogy with the current treatment paradigm for RA, there is probably an advantage to recognizing and treating patients early in the disease course before the appearance of irreversible structural damage. This may now be possible with the diagnostic sensitivity afforded by MRI. These patients could then be offered anti–TNF-α therapies to ensure effective disease control. Before this strategy can be implemented, further study will be required to address at least two unresolved questions: what is the prognostic significance of lesions identified on MRI and which demographic and disease-related variables predict disease progression despite conventional therapies? Several serologic and urinary biomarkers have impressive predictive validity in RA but have not yet been examined in AS. The emerging area of proteomics together with several ongoing prospective longitudinal cohorts is likely to provide answers to these questions in the near future.

It has been shown that concomitant immunosuppressive therapy with azathioprine in patients with IBD is associated with reduced anti-infliximab antibodies, which are associated with infusion reactions and impaired response to infliximab.[198] Concomitant therapy with MTX is also of benefit in RA. The need for such a strategy in AS remains unclear because both azathioprine and MTX are of unproven efficacy in AS. Further studies should clarify definitively whether MTX is efficacious in AS, justifying consideration of a combination therapeutic strategy including anti–TNF-α.

The importance of cost-benefit considerations in physician decision making regarding therapeutic choices has been increasing. Anti-TNF-α therapy is expensive and is still not available for AS on many formularies. Cost-benefit calculations could be rendered more attractive if reliable predictors of response could be established. Preliminary data point to baseline disease activity, baseline function, CRP levels, and MRI features of inflammation as potential predictors.[199,200] At this time, pharmacogenomic studies have suggested a role for HLA genes in the response of patients with RA to infliximab, although such studies have yet to be performed in AS. Recent studies have shown that anti–TNF-α therapy is associated with significant changes in certain biomarkers, but none have yet been shown to predict response to treatment.[195]

During the past decade breathtaking advances have been seen in the therapy of several inflammatory joint diseases, AS being among these. Patients can now look with some confidence to a future free from pain, disability, and impairment in the enjoyment of life. Physicians can now speak with confidence in saying that severe AS should soon be relegated to the archives of medical history.

REFERENCES

1. Anderson JJ, Baron G, van der Heijde D, et al. Ankylosing spondylitis assessment group preliminary definition of short-term improvement in ankylosing spondylitis. Arthritis Rheum. 2001;44:1876–1886.
2. Barlow J, Turner A, Wright C. A randomized controlled study of the arthritis self-management programme in the UK. Health Educ Res. 2000;15:665–680.
3. Gross M, Brandt KD. Educational support groups of patients with ankylosing spondylitis: a preliminary report. Patient Counseling Health Education. 1981;3(1):6–12.
4. Rehfisch HP, Basler HD. Cognitive behavior therapy in patients with ankylosing spondylitis. Zeitschrift fur Rheumatologie. 1989;48(2):79–85.
5. Basler HD, Rehfisch HP. Cognitive-behavioral therapy in patients with ankylosing spondylitis in a German self-help organization. Journal Psychosomatic Research. 1991;35(2–3):345–354.
6. Basler HD. Group treatment for pain and discomfort. Patient Education Counseling. 1993;20(2–3):167–175.
7. Barlow JH, Barefoot J. Group education for people with arthritis. Patient Education Counseling. 1996;27(3):257–267.
8. Sweeney S, Taylor G, Calin A. The effect of a home based exercise intervention package on outcome in ankylosing spondylitis: a randomized controlled trial. J Rheumatol. 2002;29(4):763–766.
9. Uhrin Z, Kuzis S, Ward MM. Exercise and changes in health status in patients with ankylosing spondylitis. Arch Intern Med. 2000;160:2969–2975.
10. Santos H, Brophy S, Calin A. Exercise in ankylosing spondylitis: how much is optimum? J Rheumatol. 1998;25(11):2156–2160.
11. Hidding A, van der Linden S, de Witte L. Therapeutic effects of individual physical therapy in ankylosing spondylitis related to duration of disease. Clin Rheumatol. 1993;12(3):334–340.
12. Kraag G, Stokes B, Groh J, et al. The effects of comprehensive home physiotherapy and supervision on patients with ankylosing spondylitis—a randomized controlled trial. J Rheumatol. 1990;17(2):228–233.
13. Kraag G, Stokes B, Groh J, et al. The effects of comprehensive home physiotherapy and supervision on patients with ankylosing spondylitis—an 8-month follow up. J Rheumatol. 1994; 21(2): 261–263.
14. Swanell AJ. The case against the value of exercise in the long-term management of ankylosing spondylitis. Clin Rehabilitation. 1988; 2:245–247.
15. Russell P, Unsworth A, Haslock L. The effect of exercise on ankylosing spondylitis—a preliminary study. Br J Rheumatol. 1993; 32(6):498–506.
16. Rasmussen JO, Hansen TM. Physical training for patients with ankylosing spondylitis. Arthritis Care and Research. 1989; 2(1):25–27.
17. Hidding A, van der Linden S, Boers M, et al. Is group physical therapy superior to individualized therapy in ankylosing spondylitis? Arthritis Care Res. 1993;6(3):117–125.
18. Hidding A, van der Linden S, Gielen X, et al. Continuation of group physical therapy is necessary in ankylosing spondylitis: results of a randomized controlled trial. Arthritis Care Res. 1994;7(2):90–96.
19. Analay Y, Ozcan E, Karan A, et al. The effectiveness of intensive group exercise on patients with ankylosing spondylitis. Clinical Rehab. 2003;17(6):631–636.
20. Garrett S, Jenkinson T, Kennedy LG, et al. A new approach to defining disease status in ankylosing spondylitis: the Bath Ankylosing Spondylitis Disease Activity Index. J Rheumatol. 1994;21(12):2286–2291.
21. Calin A, Garrett S, Whitelock H, et al. A new approach to defining functional ability in ankylosing spondylitis: the development of the Bath Ankylosing Spondylitis Functional Index. J Rheumatol. 1994;21(12):2281–2285.
22. Jones SD, Steiner A, Garrett SL, Calin A. The Bath Ankylosing Spondylitis Patient Global Score (BAS-G). Br J Rheumatol. 1996;35(1):66–71.
23. Jenkinson TR, Mallorie PA, Whitelock HC, et al. Defining spinal mobility in ankylosing spondylitis (AS). The Bath AS metrology index. J Rheumatol. 1994;21:1694–1698.
24. Band DA, Jones SD, Kennedy LG, et al. Which patients with ankylosing spondylitis derive most benefit from an inpatient management program? J Rheumatol. 1997;24(12):2381–2384.
25. Viitanen JV, Heikkila S. Functional changes in patients with spondyloarthropathy. A controlled trial of the effects of short-term rehabilitation and 3-year follow up. Rheum International 2001;20:211–214.

26. Roberts WN, Larson MG, Liang MH, et al. Sensitivity of anthropometric techniques for clinical trials in ankylosing spondylitis. Brit J Rheumatol. 1989;28(1):40–45.

27. Heikkila S, Viitanen JV, Kautiainen H, Kauppi M. Sensitivity to change of mobility tests; effect of short term intensive physiotherapy and exercise in spondyloarthropathy. J Rheumatol. 2000;27(5):1251–1256.

28. Viitanen JV, Lehtinen K, Suni J, Kautiainen H. Fifteen months' follow-up of intensive inpatient physiotherapy and exercise in ankylosing spondylitis. Clin Rheumatol. 1995;14(4):413–419.

29. Jayson MI, Baddeley H. Neck movements in ankylosing spondylitis and their responses to physiotherapy. Ann Rheum Dis. 1978;37(1):64–66.

30. Balstrode SJ, Barefoot J, Harrison RA, Clarke AK. The role of passive stretching in the treatment of ankylosing spondyhlitis. Brit J Rheumatol. 1987;26(1):40–42.

31. Helliwell PS, Abbott CA, Chamberlain MA. A randomized trial of three different physiotherapy regimens in ankylosing spondylitis. Physiotherapy. 1996;82:85–90.

32. Van Tubergen A, Landewe R, van der Heijde D, et al. Combined spa-exercise therapy is effective in patients with ankylosing spondylitis: a randomized controlled trial. Arthritis Rheum. 2001;45(5):430–438.

33. Dagfinrud H, Hagen K. Physiotherapy interventions for ankylosing spondylitis (Cochrane Review). Cochrane Database of Systematic Reviews. 2001;4:Cd002822.

34. Dagfinrud H, Kvien TK, Hagen KB. Physiotherapy interventions for ankylosing spondylitis. The Cochrane Database of Systematic Reviews. 2004;4:Cd002822.pub2.

35. Calin A, Elswood J. A prospective nationwide cross-sectional study of NSAID usage in 1331 patients with ankylosing spondylitis. J Rheumatol. 1990;17(6):801–803.

36. Weissmann G, Montesinos MC, Pillinger M, Cronstein BN. Non-prostaglandin effects of aspirin III and salicylate: inhibition of integrin-dependent human neutrophil aggregation and inflammation in COX-2 and NF kappa B (P105)-knockout mice. Adv Expt Med Biol. 2002;507:571–577.

37. Chandrasekharan NV, Dai H, Roos KLT, et al. COX-3, a cyclooxygenase-1 variant inhibited by acetaminophen and other analgesic/antipyretic drugs: cloning, structure and expression. PNAS. 2002;99(21):13926–13931.

38. Catella-Lawson F, Crofford LJ. Cyclooxygenase inhibition and thrombogenicity. Am J Med. 2002;110[suppl 3A]:28S–32S.

39. McAdam BF, Catella-Lawson F, Mardini IA, Kapoor S, Lawson JA, FitzGerald GA. Systemic biosynthesis of prostacyclin by cyclooxygenase (COX-2): the human pharmacology of a selective inhibitor of COX-2. PNAS. 1999;96(1):272–277.

40. Brooks P, Emery P, Evans JF, et al. Interpreting the clinical significance of the differential inhibition of cyclo-oxygenase-1 and cyclo-oxygenase-2. Rheumatology. 1999;38(8):779–788.

41. Boersma JW. Retardation of ossification of the lumbar vertebral column in ankylosing spondylitis by means of phenylbutazone. Scand J Rheumatol. 1976;5(1):60–64.

42. Dougados M, Gueguen A, Nakache JP, et al. Evaluation of a functional index and an articular index in ankylosing spondylitis. J Rheumatol. 1988;15(2):302–307.

43. Dougados M, Caporal R, Doury P, et al. A double blind crossover placebo controlled trial of ximoprofen in AS. J Rheumatol. 1989;16(8):1167–1169.

44. Dougados M, Nguyen M, Caporal R, et al. Ximoprofen in ankylosing spondylitis. A double blind placebo controlled dose ranging study. Scand J Rheumatol. 1994;23(5):243–248.

45. Dougados M, Gueguen A, Nakache JP, et al. Ankylosing spondylitis: what is the optimum duration of a clinical study? A one year versus 6 weeks non-steroidal anti-inflammatory drug trial. Rheumatology. 1999;38(3):235–244.

46. Dougados M, Behier JM, Jolchine I, et al. Efficacy of celecoxib, a cyclo-oxygenase 2-specific inhibitor, in the treatment of ankylosing spondylitis: a six week controlled study with comparison against placebo and against a conventional nonsteroidal anti-inflammatory drug. Arthritis Rheum. 2001;44(1):180–185.

47. Van der Heijde D, Baraf HSB, Ramos-Remus C, et al. Evaluation of the efficacy of etoricoxib in ankylosing spondylitis. Arthritis Rheum 2005;52:1205–1215.

48. Toussirot E, Wendling D. Current guidelines for the drug treatment of ankylosing spondylitis. Drugs. 1998;56(2):225–240.

49. Wanders A, van der Heijde D, Landewe R, et al. Nonsteroidal anti-inflammatory drugs reduce radiographic progression in patients with ankylosing spondylitis: a randomized controlled trial. Arthritis Rheum 2005;52:1756–1765.

50. Coles LS, Fries JF, Kraines RG, Roth SH. From experiment to experience: side effects of nonsteroidal anti-inflammatory drugs. Am J Med. 1983;74:820–828.

51. Paulus HE. FDA arthritis advisory committee: serious gastrointestinal toxicity of nonsteroidal antiinflammatory drugs, etc. Arthritis Rheum. 1988;31:1450–1451.

52. Ward MM, Kuzis S. Medication toxicity among patients with ankylosing spondylitis. Arthritis Rheum. 2002;47(3):234–241.

53. Rostom A, Wells G, Tugwell P, et al. Prevention of NSAID-induced gastroduodenal ulcers (Cochrane Review). In: The Cochrane Library, Issue 3, 2001. Oxford:Update Software.

54. Simon LS, Weaver AL, Graham DY, et al. Anti-inflammatory and upper gastrointestinal effects of celecoxib in rheumatoid arthritis: a randomized controlled trial. JAMA. 1999;282:1921–1928.

55. Solomon DH, Schneeweiss S, Glynn RJ, et al. Relationship between selective cyclooxygenase-2 inhibitors and acute myocardial infarction in older adults. Circulation. 2004;109:2068–2073.

56. Bombardier C, Laine L, Reicin A, et al. Comparison of upper gastrointestinal toxicity of rofecoxib and naproxen in patients with rheumatoid arthritis. N Engl J Med. 2000;343:1520–1528.

57. Amor B, Dougados M, Mijiyawa M, et al. Criteres de classification des spondyloarthropathies. Rev Rhum. 1990;57:85–89.

58. Amor B, Dougados M, Listrat V, et al. Evaluation des critères de spondylarthropathies d'Amor et de l'European Spondylarthropathy Study Group (ESSG). Une etude transversale de 2228 patients. Ann Med Interne (Paris). 1991;142:85–89.

59. Amor B, Santos RS, Nahal R, et al. Predictive factors for the long term outcome of spondyloarthropathies. J Rheum. 1994;21(10):1883–1887.

60. Morgan T, Anderson A. The effect of nonsteroidal anti-inflammatory drugs on blood pressure in patients treated with different antihypertensive drugs. J Clin Hypertension. 2003;5(1):53–57.

61. Hanauer SB, Sandborn W. The Practice Parameters Committee of the American College of Gastroenterology. Am J Gastroenterol. 2001;96(3):635–643.

62. Mahadevan U, Loftus EV JR, Tremain WJ, Sandborn WJ. Safety of selective cyclo-oxygenase-2 inhibitors in inflammatory bowel disease. Am J Gastroenterol. 2002;97(4):910–914.

63. Reinisch W, Miehsler W, Dejaco C, et al. An open-label trial of the selective cyclo-oxygenase-2 inhibitor, Rofecoxib, in inflammatory bowel disease-associated peripheral arthritis and arthralgia. Aliment Pharmacol Therapeutics. 2003;17(11):1371–1380.

64. Biancone L, Tosti C, Geremia A, et al. Rofecoxib and early relapse of inflammatory bowel disease: an open-label trial. Aliment Pharmacol Therapeutics. 2004;19(7):755–764.

65. Pal B. Use of simple analgesics in the treatment of ankylosing spondylitis. Brit J Rheumatol. 1987;26(3):207–209.

66. Ytterberg SR, Mahowald ML, Woods SR. Codeine and oxycodone use in patients with chronic rheumatic disease pain. Arthritis Rheum. 1999;42(4):830–831.

67. Koh WH, Pande I, Samuels A, et al. Low dose amitriptyline in ankylosing spondylitis: a short term, double blind, placebo controlled study. J Rheumatol. 1997;24(11):2158–2161.

68. Amor B, Kahan A, Dougados M, Delrieu F. Sulphasalazine in ankylosing spondylitis. Ann Intern Med. 1984;101:878.

69. Gorman JD, Sack KE, Davis JC. Treatment of ankylosing spondylitis by inhibition of tumor necrosis factor a. N Engl J Med. 2002;346:1349–1356.

70. Davis J.C. Jr., van der Heijde D, Braun J, et al. Recombinant human tumor necrosis factor receptor (Etanercept) for treating ankylosing spondylitis. Arthritis Rheum. 2003;48:3230-3236.

71. Smedegard G, Bjork J. Sulphasalazine: mechanism of action in rheumatoid arthritis. Brit J Rheumatol. 1995;34 Suppl 2:7–15.

72. Gadangi P, Longaker M, Naime D, et al. The anti-inflammatory mechanism of sulfasalazine is related to adenosine release at inflamed sites. J Immunol. 1996;156(5):1937–1941.

73. Cronstein BN, Levin RI, Philips MR, et al. Neutrophil adherence to endothelium is enhanced via adenosine A1 receptors and inhibited by adenosine A2 receptors. J Immunol. 1992;148:2201–2206.

74. Bouma MG, Stad RK, van den Wildenberg FA, Buurman WA. Differential regulatory effects of adenosine on cytokine release by activated human monocytes. J Immunol. 1994;153(9):4159–4168.

75. Doering J, Begue B, Lentze MJ, et al. Induction of T lymphocyte apoptosis by sulphasalazine in patients with Crohn's disease. Gut. 2004;53(11):1632–1638.

76. Mielants H, Veys EM, Joos R. Sulfasalazine (Salazopyrin) in the treatment of enterogenic reactive synovitis and ankylosing spondylitis with peripheral arthritis. Clin Rheumatol. 1986;5:80–83.

77. Mielants H, Veys EM, Joos R, et al. Repeat ileocolonoscopy in reactive arthritis. J Rheumatol. 1987;14:456–458.

78. Dougados M, Boumier P, Amor B. Sulphasalazine in ankylosing spondylitis: a double blind controlled study in 60 patients. Brit Med J. 1986;293:911–914.

79. Feltelius N, Hallgren R. Sulphasalazine in ankylosing spondylitis. Ann Rheum Dis. 1986;45:396–399.

80. Nissila M, Lehtinen K, Leirisalo-Repo M, et al. Sulfasalazine in the treatment of ankylosing spondylitis. Arthritis Rheum. 1988;31:1111–1116.

81. Davis MJ, Dawes PT, Beswick E, et al. Sulphasalazine therapy in ankylosing spondylitis: its effect on disease activity, immunoglobulin A and the complex immunoglobulin A-alpha-1-antitrypsin. Brit J Rheumatol. 1989;28:410–413.

82. Corkill MM, Jobanputra P, Gibson T, Macfarlane DG. A controlled trial of sulphasalazine treatment of chronic ankylosing spondylitis: failure to demonstrate a clinical effect. Brit J Rheumatol. 1990;29:41–45.

83. Taylor HG, Beswick EJ, Dawes PT. Sulphasalazine in ankylosing spondylitis. a radiological, clinical and laboratory assessment. Clin Rheumatol. 1991;10:43–48.

84. Kirwan J, Edwards A, Huitfeldt B, et al. The course of established ankylosing spondylitis and the effects of sulphasalazine over 3 years. Brit J Rheumatol. 1993;32:729–733.

85. Dougados M, van der Linden S, Leirisalo-Repo M, et al. Sulfasalazine in the treatment of spondyloarthropathy. Arthritis Rheum. 1995;38:618–627.

86. Clegg DO, Reda DJ, Weisman MH, et al. Comparison of sulfasalazine and placebo in the treatment of ankylosing spondylitis. Arthritis Rheum. 1996;39:2004–2012.

87. Ferraz MB, Tugwell P, Goldsmith CH, Atra E. Meta-analysis of sulfasalazine in ankylosing spondylitis. J Rheumatol. 1990;17:1482–1486.

88. Thomson GTD, Thomson BRJ, Thomson KS, Ducharme JS. Clinical efficacy of mesalamine in the treatment of the spondyloarthropathies. J Rheumatol. 2000;27:714–718.

89. Dekker-Saeys BJ, Dijkmans BAC, Tytgat GNJ. Treatment of spondyloarthropathy with 5-aminosalicyclic acid (mesalazine): an open trial. J Rheumatol. 1999;27:723–726.

90. Van Denderen JC, van der Horst-Bruinsma I, Bezemer PD, Dijkmans BA. Efficacy and safety of mesalazine (Salofalk) in an open study of 20 patients with ankylosing spondylitis. J Rheumatol. 2003;30(7):1558–1560.

91. Taggart A, Gardiner P, McEvoy F, et al. Which is the active moiety of sulfasalazine in ankylosing spondylitis? Arthritis Rheum. 1996;39:1400–1405.

92. Genestier L, Paillot R, Fournel S, et al. Immunosuppressive properties of methotrexate: apoptosis and clonal deletion of activated peripheral T cells. J Clin Invest. 1998;102(2):322–328.

93. Nesher G, Osborn TG, Moore TL. In vitro effects of methotrexate on polyamine levels in lymphocytes from rheumatoid arthritis patients. Clin Expl Rheumatol. 1996;14(4):395–399.

94. van Ede AE, Laan RF, Rood MJ, et al. Effect of folic or folinic acid supplementation on the toxicity and efficacy of methotrexate in rheumatoid arthritis: a forty-eight week, multicenter, randomized, double-blind, placebo-controlled study. Arthritis Rheum. 2001;44(7):1515–1524.

95. Allegra CJ, Drake JC, Jolivet J, Chabner BA. Inhibition of phosphoribosylaminoimidazolecarboxamide transformylase by methotrexate and dihydrofolic acid polyglutamates. PNAS. 1985;82(15):4881–4885.

96. Laghi Pasini F, Capecchi PL, Di Perri T. Adenosine plasma levels after low dose methotrexate administration. J Rheumatol. 1997;24:2492–2493.

97. Montesinos MC, Desai A, Delano D, et al. Adenosine A2A or A3 receptors are required for inhibition of inflammation by methotrexate and its analog MX-68. Arthritis Rheum. 2003; 48(1):240–247.

98. Becker C, Barbulescu K, Hildner K, et al. Activation and methotrexate-mediated suppression of the TNF alpha promoter in T cells and macrophages. Ann NY Acad Sciences. 1998;859:311–314.

99. Creemers MCW, Franssen MJAM, van de Putte LBA, et al. Methotrexate in severe ankylosing spondylitis: an open study. J Rheumatol. 1995;22:1104–1107.

100. Clavaguera MT, Juanola X, Narvaez FJ, et al. Methotrexate in the treatment of ankylosing spondylitis. Brit J Rheumatol. 1998;37[Suppl 1]:45.

101. Ostendorf B, Specker C, Schneider M. Methotrexate lacks efficacy in the treatment of severe ankylosing spondylitis compared with rheumatoid and psoriatic arthritis. J Clin Rheumatol. 1998; 4:129–136.

102. Biasi D, Carletto A, Caramaschi P, et al. Efficacy of methotrexate in the treatment of ankylosing spondylitis: a 3-year open study. Clin Rheum. 2000;19:114–117.

103. Sampaio-Barros PD, Costallat LT, Bertolo MB, et al. Methotrexate in the treatment of ankylosing spondylitis. Scand J Rheumatol. 2000;29:160–162.

104. Altan L, Bingol U, Karakoc Y, et al. Clinical investigation of methotrexate in the treatment of ankylosing spondylitis. Scand J Rheum. 2001;30:255–259.

105. Roychowdhury B, Bintley-Bagot S, Hunt J, Tunn EJ. Methotrexate in severe ankylosing spondylitis: a randomised placebo controlled, double-blind observer study. Rheumatology. 2001;40[suppl 1]:43.

106. Gonzalez-Lopez L, Garcia-Gonzalez A, Vazquez-del-Mercado M, et al. Efficacy of methotrexate in ankylosing spondylitis: a randomized, double-blind, placebo-controlled trial. J Rheumatol. 2004;31:1568–1574.

107. Chen J, Liu C. Methotrexate for ankylosing spondylitis. The Cochrane Database of Systematic Reviews 2003, Issue 3. Art. No.: CD004524.pub2.

108. Crew MD, Effros RB, Walford RL, et al. Transgenic mice expressing a truncated Peromyscus leucopus TNF-a gene manifest an arthritis resembling ankylosing spondylitis. J Interferon Cytokine Res. 1998;18:219–225.

109. Redlich K, Gortz B, Hayer S, et al. Overexpression of tumor necrosis factor causes bilateral sacroiliitis. Arthritis Rheum. 2004;50:1001–1005.

110. Braun J, Bollow M, Neure L, et al. Use of immunohistologic and in situ hybridization techniques in the examination of sacroiliac joint biopsy specimens from patients with ankylosing spondylitis. Arthritis Rheum. 1995;38:499–505.

111. Laloux L, Voisin M-C, Allain J, et al. Immunohistological study of entheses in spondyloarthropathies: comparison in rheumatoid arthritis and osteoarthritis. Ann Rheum Dis. 2001;60:316–321.

112. Brandt J, Haebel H, Cornely D, et al. Successful treatment of active ankylosing spondylitis with the anti-tumor necrosis factor α monoclonal antibody infliximab. Arthritis Rheum. 2000; 43:1346–1352.

113. Brandt J, Braun J, Sieper J. Infliximab treatment of severe ankylosing spondylitis: one-year followup. Arthritis Rheum. 2001; 44:2936-2937.

114. Van den Bosch F, Kruithof E, Baeten D, et al. Effects of a loading dose regimen of three infusions of chimeric monoclonal antibody to tumour necrosis factor α (infliximab) in spondyloarthropathy: an open pilot study. Ann Rheum Dis. 2000;59:428–433.

115. Kruithof E, Van den Bosch F, Baeten D, et al. Repeated infusions of infliximab, a chimeric anti-TNF α monoclonal antibody, in patients with active spondyloarthropathy: a one-year follow up. Ann Rheum Dis. 2002;61:207–212.

116. Baeten D, Kruithof E, van den Bosch F, et al. Immunomodulatory effects of anti-tumor necrosis factor a therapy on synovium in spondyloarthropathy: histologic findings in eight patients from an open-label pilot study. Arthritis Rheum. 2001;44:186–195.

117. Stone M, Salonen D, Lax M, et al. Clinical and imaging correlates of response to treatment with infliximab in patients with ankylosing spondylitis. J Rheumatol. 2001;28:1605–1614.

118. Maksymowych WP, Jhangri GS, Lambert RG, et al. Infliximab in ankylosing spondylitis: a prospective observational inception cohort analysis of efficacy and safety. J Rheumatol. 2002; 29:959–965.

119. Breban M, Vignon E, Claudepierre P, et al. Efficacy of infliximab in severe refractory ankylosing spondylitis (AS). Results of a 6 month follow-up open-label study. Rheumatology. 2002; 41:1280–1285.

120. Braun J, Brandt J, Listing J, et al. Treatment of active ankylosing spondylitis with infliximab: a randomized controlled multicentre trial. Lancet. 2002;359:1187–1193.

121. Braun J, Baraliakos X, Golder W, et al: Improvement of spinal inflammation in ankylosing spondylitis (AS) by infliximab therapy as assessed by magnetic resonance imaging (MRI) using a novel evaluated spinal scoring system. Arthritis Rheum. 2003; 48:1126–1136.

122. Braun J, Baraliakos X, Brandt J, et al. Persistent clinical response to the anti-TNF-a antibody infliximab in patients with ankylosing spondylitis over 3 years. Rheumatol 2005;44:670–676.

123. Baraliakos X, Listing J, Brandt J, et al. Clinical response to discontinuation of anti-TNF therapy in patients with ankylosing spondylitis after 3 years of continuous treatment with infliximab. Arthritis Res Therapy 2005;7:R439–R444.

124. Van den Bosch F, Kruithof E, Baeten D, et al. Randomised double-blind comparison of chimeric monoclonal antibody to tumor necrosis factor α (infliximab) versus placebo in active spondyloarthropathy. Arthritis Rheum. 2002;46:755–765.

125. Van der Heijde D, Dijkmans B, Geusens P, et al. Efficacy and safety of infliximab in patients with ankylosing spondylitis. Results of a randomized placebo-controlled trial (ASSERT). Arthritis Rheum 2005;52:582–591.

126. Marzo-Ortega H, McGonagle D, O'Connor P, Emery P. Efficacy of etanercept in the treatment of the entheseal pathology in resistant spondyloarthropathy. Arthritis Rheum. 2001;44:2112–2117.

127. Brandt J, Khariouzov A, Listing J, et al. Six-month results of a double-blind, placebo-controlled trial of etanercept treatment in patients with active ankylosing spondylitis. Arthritis Rheum. 2003;48:1667–1675.

128. Baraliakos X, Brandt J, Listing J, et al. Two-years follow up results of a double-blind placebo-controlled trial of etanercept in active ankylosing spondylitis. Arthritis Rheum. 2004; 50[suppl]: S615.

129. Baraliakos, X, Davis J, Tsuji W, Braun J. Magnetic resonance imaging examinations of the spine in patients with ankylosing spondylitis before and after therapy with the tumor necrosis factor alpha receptor fusion protein etanercept. Arthritis Rheum 2005;52:1216–1223.

130. Davis JC, van der Heijde DM, Braun J, et al. Sustained durability and tolerability of etanercept in ankylosing spondylitis for 96 weeks. Ann Rheum Dis 2005;64:1557–1562.

131. Davis JC, van der Heijde DM, Dougados M, Woolley JM. Reductions in health-related quality of life in patients with ankylosing spondylitis and improvements with etanercept therapy. Arthritis Rheum 2005;53:494–501.

132. Calin A, Dijkmans BAC, Emery P, et al. Outcomes of a multicentre randomised clinical trial of etanercept to treat ankylosing spondylitis. Ann Rheum. 2004;63:1587–1593.

133. Haibel H, Brandt H, Rudwaleit M, et al. Results of an open-label 20 week trial of adalimumab in the treatment of active ankylosing spondylitis. Arthritis Rheum. 2004;50[suppl]: S217.

134. Haibel H, Rudwaleit M, Brandt H, et al. Preliminary MRI results in patients with active ankylosing spondylitis treated with adalimumab for 12 weeks. Arthritis Rheum. 2004; 50[suppl]: S618.

135. Maksymowych WP, Rahman P, Keystone E, et al. Efficacy of adalimumab in active ankylosing spondylitis (AS)-Results of the Canadian AS study. Arthritis Rheum 2005;52[suppl]:S217.

136. Davis JC, Kivitz A, Schiff M, et al. Major clinical response and partial remission in ankylosing spondylitis subjects treated with adalimumab: the ATLAS study. Arthritis Rheum 2005:52[suppl]:S208.

137. Baeten D, Kruithof E, Van den Bosch F, et al. Systematic safety follow up in a cohort of 107 patients with spondyloarthropathy treated with infliximab: a new perspective on the role of host defense in the pathogenesis of the disease? Ann Rheum Dis. 2003;62:829–834.

138. Gomez-Reino JJ, Carmona L, Valverde VR, et al. Treatment of rheumatoid arthritis with tumor necrosis factor inhibitors may predispose to significant increase in tuberculosis risk: a multicenter active-surveillance report. Arthritis Rheum. 2003;48: 2122–2127.

139. Brown SL, Greene MH, Gershon SK, et al. Tumor necrosis factor antagonist therapy and lymphoma development: twenty-six cases reported to the Food and Drug Administration. Arthritis Rheum. 2002;46:3151–3158.

140. Hawkins-Holt M, Hochberg MC, Cohen SB, et al. Therapy with biologic agents is not associated with an increased risk of cancer recurrence in patients with rheumatoid arthritis. Arthritis Rheum. 2003;49[suppl]: 806.

141. Marchesoni A, Arreghini M, Panni B, et al. Life-threatening reversible bone marrow toxicity in a rheumatoid arthritis patient switched from leflunomide to infliximab. Rheumatology. 2003;42(1):193–194.

142. Mohan N, Edwards ET, Cupps TR, et al. Demyelination occurring during anti-tumor necrosis factor alpha therapy for inflammatory arthritides. Arthritis Rheum. 2001;44:2862–2869.

143. Kwon HJ, Cote TR, Cuffe MS, et al. Case reports of heart failure after therapy with a tumor necrosis factor antagonist. Ann Intern Med. 2003;138:807–811.

144. Chung ES, Packer M, Lo KH, et al. Anti-TNF therapy against congestive heart failure investigators. Randomized, double-blind, placebo-controlled, pilot trial of infliximab, a chimeric monoclonal antibody to tumor necrosis factor-alpha, in patients with moderate-to-severe heart failure: results of the anti-TNF Therapy against Congestive Heart Failure (ATTACH) trial. Circulation. 2003;107:3133–3140.

145. Wolfe F, Michaud K. Heart failure in rheumatoid arthritis: rates, predictors, and the effect of anti-tumor necrosis factor therapy Amer J Med. 2004;116(5):305–311.

146. De Rycke L, Kruithof E, Van Damme N, et al. Antinuclear antibodies following infliximab treatment in patients with rheumatoid arthritis or spondylarthropathy. Arthritis Rheum. 2003;48:1015–1023.

147. Charles PJ, Smeenk RJT, de Jong J, et al. Assessment of antibodies to double-stranded DNA induced in rheumatoid arthritis patients following treatment with infliximab, a monoclonal antibody to tumor necrosis factor: findings in open-label and randomized placebo-controlled trials. Arthritis Rheum. 2000;43:2383–2390.

148. Jarrett SJ, Cunnane G, Conaghan PG, et al. Anti-tumor necrosis factor-alpha therapy induced vasculitis: case series. J Rheumatol. 2003;30:2287–2291.

149. Cheifetz A, Smedley M, Martin S, et al. The incidence and management of infusion reactions to infliximab: a large center experience. Am J Gastroenterol. 2003;98:1315–1324.

150. Wasserman MJ, Weber DA, Guthrie JA, et al. Infusion-related reactions to infliximab in patients with rheumatoid arthritis in a clinical practice setting: relationship to dose, anti-histamine pretreatment, and infusion number. J Rheumatol. 2004;31:1912–1917.

151. Rudwaleit M, Listing J, Brandt J, et al. Prediction of a major clinical response (BASDAI 50) to tumour necrosis factor a blockers in ankylosing spondylitis. Ann Rheum Dis. 2004;63: 665–670.

152. Adcock IM, Lane SJ. Mechanisms of steroid action and resistance in inflammation: corticosteroid-insensitive asthma, molecular mechanisms. J Endocrinol. 2003;178:347–355.

153. Buttgereit F, Straub RH, Wehling M, Burmester GW. Glucocorticoids in the treatment of rheumatic diseases: an update on their mechanism of action. Arthritis Rheum. 2004;50:3408–3417.

154. Mintz G, Enriquez RD, Mercado U, et al. Intravenous methyl-prednisolone pulse therapy in severe ankylosing spondylitis. Arthritis Rheum. 1981;24:734–736.

155. Richter MB, Woo P, Panayi GS, et al. The effects of intravenous pulse methylprednisolone on immunological and inflammatory processes in ankylosing spondylitis. Clin Exp Rheum. 1983;53:51–59.

156. Ejstrup L, Peters ND. Intravenous methylprednisolone pulse therapy in ankylosing spondylitis. Dan Med Bull. 1985;32: 231–233.

157. Peters ND, Ejstrup L. Intravenous methoylprednisolone pulse therapy in ankylosing spondylitis. Scand J Rheumatol. 1992;21:134–138.

158. Wordsworth BP, Pearcy MJ, Mowat AG. In-patient regime for the treatment of ankylosing spondylitis: an appraisal of improvement in spinal mobility and the effects of corticotrophin. Brit J Rheumatol. 1984;23:39–43.

159. Maugars Y, Mathis C, Vilon P, Prost A. Corticosteroid injection of the sacroiliac joint in patients with seronegative spondylarthropathy. Arthritis Rheum. 1992;35:564–568.

160. Maugars Y, Mathis C, Berthelot JM, et al. Assessment of the efficacy of sacroiliac corticosteroid injections in spondyloarthropathies: a double-blind study. Br J Rheumatol. 1996;35:767–770.

161. Luukkainen R, Nissila M, Asikainen E, et al. Periarticular corticosteroid treatment of the sacroiliac joint in patients with seronegative spondylarthropathy. Clin Exp Rheumatol. 1999;17(1): 88–90.

162. Braun J, Bollow M, Seyrekbasan F, et al. Computed tomography guided corticosteroid injection of the sacroiliac joint in patients with spondyloarthropathy with sacroiliitis: clinical outcome and followup by dynamic magnetic resonance imaging. J Rheumatol. 1996;23(4):659–664.

163. Bollow M, Braun J, Taupitz M, et al. CT-guided intraarticular corticosteroid injection into the sacroiliac joints in patients with spondyloarthropathy: indication and follow-up with contrast-enhanced MRI. J Computer Assist Tom. 1996;20(4):512–521.

164. Hanly JG, Mitchell M, MacMillan L, et al. Efficacy of sacroiliac corticosteroid injections in patients with inflammatory spondyloarthropathy: results of a 6 month controlled study. J Rheumatol. 2000;27(3):719–722.

165. Pereira PL, Gunaydin I, Trubenbach J, et al. Interventional MR imaging for injection of sacroiliac joints in patients with sacroiliitis. Amer J Roentgenology. 2000;175(1):265–266.

166. Gunaydin I, Pereira PL, Daikeler T, et al. Magnetic resonance imaging guided corticosteroid injection of the sacroiliac joints in patients with therapy resistant spondyloarthropathy: a pilot study. J Rheumatol. 2000;27(2):424–428.

167. Pereira PL, Gunaydin I, Duda SH, et al. Corticosteroid injections of the sacroiliac joint during magnetic resonance: preliminary results. J de Radiologie. 2000;81(3):223–226.

168. Cooper C, Carbone L, Michet CJ, et al. Fracture risk in patients with ankylosing spondylitis: a population based study. J Rheumatol. 1994;21(10):1877–1882.

169. Sansoni P, Passeri G, Fagnoni F, et al. Inhibition of antigen-presenting cell function by alendronate in vitro. J Bone Miner Res. 1995;10:1719–1725.

170. Stevenson PH, Stevenson JR. Cytotoxic and migration inhibitory effects of bisphosphonates on macrophages. Calcif Tissue Int. 1986;38:227–233.

171. Pietschmann P, Stohlawetz P, Brosch S, et al. The effect of alendronate on cytokine production, adhesion molecule expression, and transendothelial migration of human peripheral blood mononuclear cells. Calcif Tissue Int. 1998;63:325–330.

172. Van Beek, E, Pieterman E, Cohen L, et al. Farnesyl pyrophosphate synthase is the molecular target of nitrogen-containing bisphosphonates. Biochem Biophys Res Comm. 1999;264: 108–111.

173. Santini D, Vincenzi B, Avvisati G, et al. Pamidronate induces modifications of circulating angiogenic factors in cancer patients. Clin Cancer Res. 2002;8:1080–1084.

174. Maksymowych WP, Jhangri GS, LeClercq S, et al. An open study of pamidronate in the treatment of refractory ankylosing spondylitis. J Rheumatol. 1998;25:714–717.

175. Maksymowych WP, Lambert R, Jhangri GS, et al. Clinical and radiological amelioration of refractory peripheral spondyloarthritis by pulse intravenous pamidronate therapy. J Rheumatol. 2001;28:144–155.

176. Haibel H, Brandt J, Rudwaleit M, et al. Treatment of active ankylosing spondylitis with pamidronate. Rheumatology. 2003;42: 1018–1020.

177. Dumoulin C, Mehsen N, Bentaberry F, et al. Effects of intravenous pamidronate therapy in refractory spondyloarthropathies. Results of an open study. Arthritis Rheum. 2002;46[suppl]: S432.

178. Munoz-Villanueva MC, Perez VC, Castro MC, et al. Potential biological and clinical improvement of refractory ankylosing spondylitis with intravenous pamidronate therapy. Ann Rheum Dis. 2002;61[suppl 1]: 305

179. Houvenagel E, Lormeau C, Solau-Gervais E, et al. Traitement des spondyloarthropathies axiales refractaires par perfusions de pamidronate: resultants preliminaires a 6 mois. Rev Rhum. 2002;69:1026.

180. Gerard D, Flory P, Grisot C, et al. Pamidronate dans le traitement des spondyloarthropathies axiales refractaires: resultants preliminaries a 12 mois. A propos de 24 patients. Rev Rhum. 2003;70:871.

181. Toussirot E, Lohse A, Le Huede G, et al. Treatment of refractory and active spondyloarthropathies with pamidronate. An open study. Ann Rheum Dis. 2004;63[suppl 1]:395.

182. Maksymowych WP, Jhangri GS, Fitzgerald AA, et al. A six-month randomized, controlled, double-blind, dose response comparison of intravenous pamidronate (60 mg versus 10 mg) in the treatment of nonsteroidal antiinflammatory drug-refractory ankylosing spondylitis. Arthritis Rheum. 2002;46(3):766–773

183. Kunzmann V, Bauer E, Wilhelm M. γ/δ T-cell stimulation by pamidronate. N Eng J Med. 1999;340:737–738.

184. Siemasko KF, Chong ASF, Williams JW, et al. Regulation of B cell function by the immunosuppressive agent leflunomide. Transplantation. 1996;61:635–642.

185. Manna SK, Aggarwal BB. Immunosuppressive leflunomide metabolite (A77 1726) blocks TNF-dependent nuclear factor-kappa B activation and gene expression. J Immunol. 1999;162:2095–2102.

186. Haibel H, Rudwaleit M, Braun J, et al. Six month open label trial of leflunomide in ankylosing spondylitis. Ann Rheum Dis. 2005;64:124–126.

187. Van Denderen JC, Van der Paardt M, Nurmohamed MT, et al. Double-blind study of leflunomide in the treatment of active ankylosing spondylitis. Ann Rheum Dis. 2004;63[suppl 1]: SAT0033

188. Moreira AL, Sampaio EP, Zmuidzinas A, et al. Thalidomide exerts its inhibitory action on tumor necrosis factor alpha by enhancing mRNA degradation. J Exp Med. 1993;177:1675–1680.

189. Breban M, Gombert B, Amor B, Dougados M. Efficacy of thalidomide in the treatment of refractory ankylosing spondylitis. Arthritis Rheum. 1999;42:580–581.

190. Breban M, Dougados M. The efficacy of thalidomide in severe refractory seronegative spondyloarthropathy: reply to Lee et al. Arthitis Rheum. 2001;44:2457–2458.

191. Huang F, Gu J, Zhao W, et al. One-year open-label trial of thalidomide in ankylosing spondylitis. Arthritis Rheum. 2002;47:249–254.

192. Haibel H, Rudwaleit M, Listing J, et al. Open-label trial of anakinra in active ankylosing spondylitis over 24 weeks. Ann Rheum Dis 2005;64:296-298.

193. Tan AL, Marzo-Ortega H, O'Connor P, et al. Efficacy of anakinra in active ankylosing spondylitis: a clinical and magnetic resonance imaging study. Ann Rheum Dis. 2004;63:1041–1045.

194. Joshi AB, Markovic L, Hardinge K, Murphy JC. Total hip arthroplasty in ankylosing spondylitis: an analysis of 181 hips. J Arthroplasty. 2002;17(4):427–433.

195. El Saghir H, Boehm H. Surgical options in the treatment of the spinal disorders in ankylosing spondylitis. Clin Exp Rheumatol. 2002;20[suppl 28]:S101–S105.

196. Maksymowych WP, Inman RD, Gladman D, et al. Canadian Rheumatology Association consensus on the use of anti-TNFα-directed therapies in the treatment of spondyloarthritis. J Rheumatol. 2003;30(6);1356–1363.

197. Braun J, Pham T, Sieper J, et al. on behalf of the ASAS Working Group. International ASAS consensus statement for the use of anti-tumour necrosis factor agents in patients with ankylosing spondylitis. Ann Rheum Dis. 2003;62: 817–824.

198. Baert F, Norman M, Vermeire S, et al. Influence of immunogenicity on the long-term efficacy of infliximab in Crohn's disease. N Engl J Med. 2003;348:601–608.

199. Rudwaleit M, Listing J, Brandt J, et al. Prediction of a major clinical response (BASDAI 50) to tumour necrosis factor a blockers in ankylosing spondylitis. Aann Rheum Dis 2004;63:665-670.

200. Davis JC Jr, Van der Heijde DM, Dougados M, et al. Baseline factors that influence ASAS 20 response in patients with ankylosing spondylitis treated with etanercept. Journal of Rheumatol 2005;32:1751–1754.

201. Maksymowych WP, Poole AR, Heibert L, et al. Etanercept suppresses collagenase generated Type II collagen neoepitope and increases cartilage proteoglycan turnover epitope in patients with ankylosing spondylitis. J Rheumatol 2005;32: 1911–1917.

14 Imaging in Ankylosing Spondylitis

Juergen Braun and Xenofon Baraliakos

INTRODUCTION

Imaging has an important role in the diagnosis, classification, and monitoring of ankylosing spondylitis (AS), and several different imaging techniques are available. The standard approach is to use conventional radiography, but magnetic resonance imaging (MRI) and ultrasound also have important roles, which are relevant for clinical practice. The most typical features of AS are inflammation in the sacroiliac joints (SIJs), sacroiliitis (Fig. 14.1), and new bone formation in the spine, leading to syndesmophytes and ankylosis (Fig. 14.2).

Many anatomical structures may be involved in AS. These generally differ according to the stage of the disease.[1] In the first years, the disease is characterized by inflammation affecting the SIJs, which occurs in almost all patients.[2] Less than 5% have no definite sacroiliac changes. In later stages, AS affects the spine in up to 70% of patients. There are different patterns of axial skeleton involvement. The vertebral bodies may be affected by spondylitis and together with the intervertebral discs by spondylodiscitis, entheses and ligaments by spinal enthesitis, and zygapophyseal joints, costovertebral, and costosternal joints by spondylarthritis.[3] Peripheral manifestations of the musculoskeletal system are found mainly in peripheral joints and entheses.

For diagnosis and classification of AS, conventional radiographs of the SIJ and the spine are still the standard for the detection of chronic morphologic changes, whereas MRI has clear advantages in the detection of active inflammatory lesions in the axial skeleton as well as in the periphery. Ultrasound techniques are also being increasingly used to image the periphery.

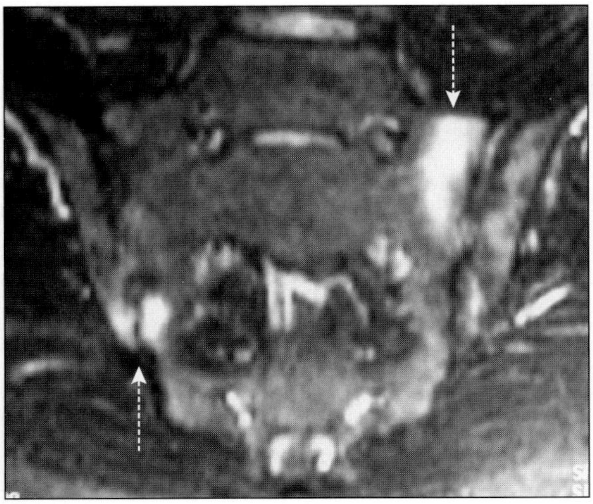

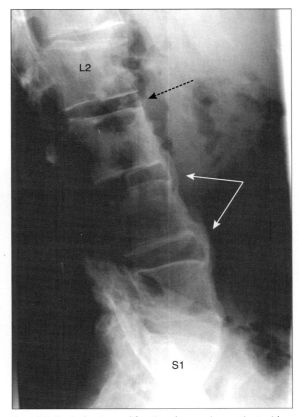

Fig. 14.1 Inflammation in both sacroiliac joints, as detected in the short tau inversion recovery (STIR) MRI sequence in a 35-year-old AS patient with an established disease duration of 11 years.

Fig. 14.2 Typical osteoproliferative changes in a patient with AS. Beginning syndesmophytes (dotted arrow) in L2/3 and bridging syndesmophytes (continuous arrow) in L3-S1.

Imaging is an important part of the classification criteria for AS. The modified New York criteria[4] combine clinical features with definite radiologic criteria. In this system, changes in the SIJs are quantified by a grading between 0 and 4 (Table 14.1). This is relevant for the diagnosis in clinical practice and classification of AS and for the differentiation of AS from undifferentiated spondyloarthropathies (uSpA).[5]

In general, there are two different ways that the musculoskeletal system may be affected in patients with AS: by 1) active inflammatory changes and 2) structural changes, with the latter usually after the former. The structural changes can be further differentiated as a) hyperproliferative changes and b) erosive changes.

Different imaging techniques have different capacities for assessing changes (Table 14.2). Although conventional radiographs and computed tomography (CT) have advantages in the detection of structural changes, MRI and scintigraphy (to a lesser extent) are superior in the detection of active changes. Thus, there are differential indications for the use of the techniques, and therefore they are often used complementarily.

There are two different aims for the quantification of changes by imaging: 1) to define the disease status of the patient and 2) to assess change. The latter is relevant in both daily clinical practice and clinical studies.

IMAGING OF THE SACROILIAC JOINT IN ANKYLOSING SPONDYLITIS

Imaging of the SIJ is important in AS because almost all patients with AS have involvement of the SIJs. In addition, imaging of the SIJ is a major point in the modified New York criteria for classification and diagnosis of AS[4] (see Table 14.1).

TABLE 14.1 GRADING OF CHRONIC RADIOGRAPHIC CHANGES OF THE SIJ IN AS

Grade	Evaluation
0	Normal
1	Suspicious
2	Sclerosis, some erosions
3	Severe erosions, widening of joint space, minor ankylosis
4	Complete ankylosis

This aspect includes the differentiation of rheumatic from septic sacroiliitis in patients with back pain.[5] The quantification of inflammation may be important in patients with SpAs and AS to assess the activity and the extent of the disease, including both current status and also changes.

Conventional Radiography of the Sacroiliac Joints in Ankylosing Spondylitis

Conventional radiographs of the axial skeleton comprise anteroposterior (AP) radiographs of the pelvis (including the hip joints) and AP and lateral views of the three spinal segments. The SIJs may be combined with a view of the lower lumbar spine and the thoracolumbar junction. Special views of the SIJ are oblique, Ferguson, and Barsony.

In advanced stages of disease, x-ray films are the standard for assessing SIJ changes. Sclerosis, erosions, pseudodilatation, and ankylosis (Fig. 14.3A and B) are the major features. The value of the findings depends on the age of the patient because erosions and ankylosis are increasingly found in people of older age and are thus regarded as a consequence of osteoarthritis.

TABLE 14.2 IMAGING TECHNIQUES AND SENSITIVITY OF ASSESSMENT OF ACTIVE AND CHRONIC CHANGES IN AS

	Active Changes	Chronic Changes	Inflammatory Changes	Bony Changes
Conventional radiographs	–	+	(+)	+
CT	–	++	(+)	++
Scintigraphy	+	–	+	–
MRI	++	+	++	+
MRI—T1-weighted sequence	(+)	+	(+)	+
MRI—post-T1-weighted and STIR sequence		++	–	++	–

CT, computed tomography; MRI, magnetic resonance imaging; STIR, short tau inversion recovery.

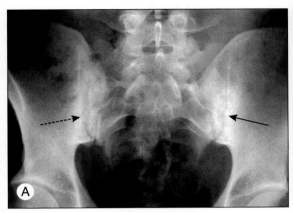
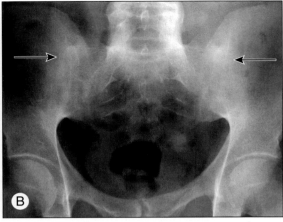

Fig. 14.3 Typical AS related changes of the sacroiliac joint in AS. A: Pseudodilatation (dotted arrow) and sclerotic lesion (continuous arrow). **B:** Fusion of the SI joints.

Conventional radiography has limited value for diagnosis in early disease stages because of its poor sensitivity and specificity.[6] In later disease stages, the identification of definite SIJ changes is very useful because more than 95% of patients with AS have such changes.

Nevertheless, conventional radiographs have limited capacity to give insight into the complicated anatomy of the SIJ because of the irregular **S**-shaped orientation and the resulting overlap of sacral and iliac joint structures.[7] To overcome this structural problem, techniques with the patient in the prone position using the posteroanterior projection with the tube angled at 25 to 30 degrees are preferred in Anglo-American countries.[8] In Europe, AP radiographs of the lumbar spine, which are also capable of detecting SI changes, are widely used. Additional prone radiographs of the SIJ do not provide substantial additional information.[9] However, this situation may differ in younger patients with inflammatory back pain (IBP) and probable SpA,[10] but has not been studied. Special imaging views, such as the Barsony technique (a special tilted view for better insight into the SIJ) proposed in 1928 are still often used for imaging of the SIJs, especially if MRI is not available. This view provides a better insight into the SIJ space than AP radiographs do. No controlled studies to compare the different techniques and projections have been performed, mainly because of the patient's exposure to radiation. Thus, there is as yet no international consensus on which technique should be used for imaging of the SIJ by use of conventional radiography.

Scintigraphy of the Sacroiliac Joints in Ankylosing Spondylitis

In scintigraphy the radionuclide technetium-99 is used to enrich areas of increased metabolism or inflammation. Therefore, scintigraphy of the SIJ has often been used to screen for SIJ and/or spinal inflammation. Nowadays scintigraphic images are used mainly for comparison with former examinations,[11–15] because the sensitivity and specificity of other imaging techniques such as MRI have been shown to be superior.[16] Scintigraphic results in the SIJ are mainly reliable if there is unilateral involvement (Fig. 14.4). However, as a tool to detect sacroiliitis this technique has clear limitations, and it is not suitable for diagnosing AS. In special cases, scintigraphy can be useful as a screening method for detecting bony or entheseal inflammation in different regions at separate times.

Computed Tomography of the Sacroiliac Joints in Ankylosing Spondylitis

The main advantage of CT is the ability to image the anatomic structure more dimensionally by cutting the SIJ in slices. This is advantageous because of the complicated anatomy of the SIJ. Thus, CT is especially useful for the detection of structural changes. CT is superior to conventional radiography for the diagnosis of bony changes in the SIJ caused by sacroiliitis.[17–19] However, it is crucial to know that subchondral sclerosis of the iliac part of the SIJ is a phenomenon of aging similar to joint space narrowing and erosions, which occur often with increasing age of patients.[20] Thus, findings of sclerosis, joint space narrowing, erosions, and ankylosis may be misleading in elderly patients,[21] Overall, CT is a reliable method for the detection of early bone changes such as erosions and small areas of ankylosis. When one is searching for inflammation in the SIJ, MRI is superior. CT-guided techniques to obtain biopsy specimens and inject axial structures such as the SIJ[22] have been used by experienced operators with some success.[23] However, the radiation exposure associated with CT technology needs to be considered.

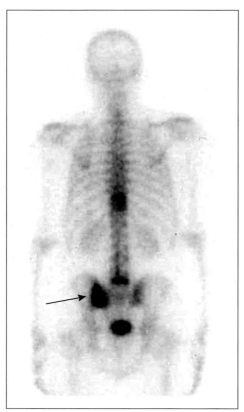

Fig. 14. 4 Unilateral involvement of the SIJ in a patient with AS as a typical sign of active disease.

Magnetic Resonance Imaging of the Sacroiliac Joints in Ankylosing Spondylitis

MRI is an advantageous method to visualize the complicated irregular anatomy of the SIJ, including abnormalities of the periarticular tissues such as joint capsule, subchondral bone, and surrounding ligaments, which are difficult to detect by other methods. A systematic comparison of MRI scans with histologic results showed good correlation of the findings.[24]

In contrast to all other imaging techniques, there is no radiation exposure associated with MRI. This makes use of this technique favorable, especially in young women, children, or patients who need frequent examinations. However, routine access to MRI, optimal technical equipment, and a skilled staff are still not widely available, and the costs are still rather high.[25] Patients with claustrophobia, pacemakers, and metal implants cannot be examined by MRI. Furthermore, the rather long duration of the procedure (about 20 to 30 min) makes the technique not applicable for some patients with AS because of intolerable pain and stiffness when they are in the supine position.[20]

In general, oblique transaxial sections are used[24] (Fig. 14.5A to D). Paraxial slices may provide additional information on the SIJ in some patients.[26]

For the assessment of *active* lesions, the appropriate MRI techniques are the T2-weighted gradient-echo sequence after fat suppression (T2-FS) (Fig. 14.5A), the short tau inversion recovery (STIR) technique (Fig. 14.5B), and the T1-weighted turbo spin-echo sequence after application of contrast agent (gadolinium diethylenetriamine-pentaacetic acid [T1/Gd-DTPA]) (Fig.14.5C).[27,28] The T1/Gd-DTPA turbo spin-echo sequence depicts inflammation in the SIJ by the detection of enhancement of contrast agents, especially in the regions where inflammation is due to hypervascularization (Fig. 14.5C). The T2-FS and the STIR techniques assess inflammatory lesions by depiction of bone edema, without the use of contrast agents. Although the T2-FS sequence has been used more often, the new STIR technique is now usually preferred because of its superior fat/water contrast obtained by total suppression of the fat signal.[20] However, in contrast to MRI of the spine, the question whether application of contrast agents provides additional information has not been resolved. Preliminary results suggest that STIR imaging is 90% compatible with techniques using post-gadolinium T1-weighted MRI.[20] The use of dynamic MRI of the SIJ on the basis of an early scoring proposal[27] should not be considered anymore in routine care because its performance has caused problems resulting from too many positive but nonspecific results.

Because grading of SIJ changes is essential for the classification criteria for AS, MRI examinations may also be of interest to assess chronic SIJ changes[22,29,30] (Figs. 14.5D and 14.6). However, this grading has not been standardized to date. Currently, the most commonly used MRI sequences for quantification and assessment of structural SIJ lesions are the T1-weighted turbo spin-echo sequence (usually performed before application of contrast material) (Fig. 14.5D) and gradient-echo techniques.[20] Suggestions for scoring systems have been published in abstract form,[31–33] and a systematic comparison is in press.[34] The whole topic is currently being evaluated by the Assessments in Ankylosing Spondylitis (ASAS)/Outcome Measures in Rheumatoid Arthritis Clinical Trials (OMERACT) MRI in the ASAS Working Group, with the aim of developing and validating scoring systems for the use of MRI of the SIJ in AS. This is an important aim, because several recent studies have shown that biologic agents, such as infliximab and etanercept,[35,36] have definite clinical efficacy on disease activity and improve inflammation of the SIJs and the spine.[35,37–39]

Magnetic Resonance Imaging of the Pubic Symphysis in Ankylosing Spondylitis

Involvement of the pubic symphysis in AS occurs in up to 25% of patients. In most patients, this is only detected in late stages of the disease when advanced

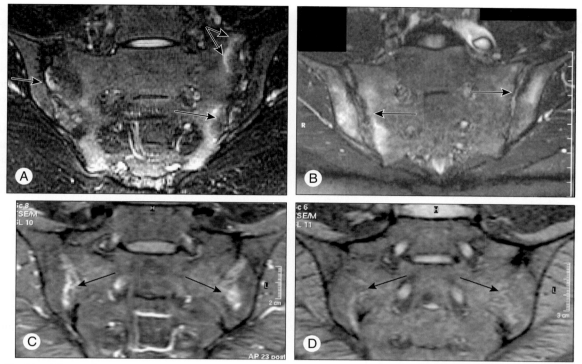

Fig. 14.5 MRI examinations of the sacroiliac in patients with AS. A: T2-weighted MRI of the SIJ after fat suppression. **B:** Short tau inversion recovery (STIR) MRI. **C:** T1-weighted MRI of the SIJ after application of contrast agent with typical hyperdensity due to contrast agent enhancement in inflammatory regions. **D:** T1-weighted MRI of the SIJ of the same patient as in Fig. 14.5c, before application of contrast agent. Enhancement of contrast agent due to inflammation (hypervascularization) shows the typical hypodensity, as compared to post-enhancement images.

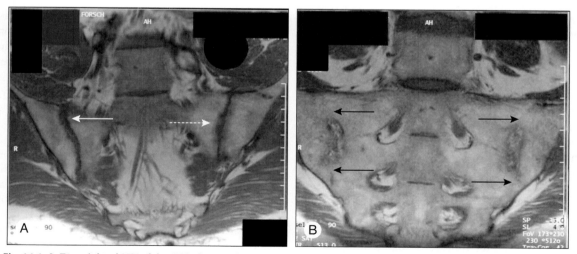

Fig. 14.6 A: T1-weighted MRI of the SIJ before application of contrast agent. Typical signs of the disease are the irregular course of the joint (right SIJ, continuous line) or the pseudodilatation (left SIJ, dotted line). **B:** Ankylosis of the SIJ, as detected by T1-weighted MRI. The joint space is no longer detectable (arrows).

abnormalities in the SIJ have already been detected.[40] Involvement of the pubic symphysis detected by conventional radiography ranges from minimal changes to erosions, parasymphyseal osteosclerosis, apparent destruction, and ankylosis.[40] A symphysitis in earlier stages of disease may be detected by scintigraphy or by MRI using T1/Gd-DTPA, T2-FS, or STIR techniques with which it appears as subcortical, anteriorly located bone marrow edema, indicating either enthesitis or pelvic instability with a correspondingly decreased signal on T1-weighted images.

Comparative Studies of Available Imaging Techniques for Sacroiliac Joints in Ankylosing Spondylitis

There are several studies in which the available techniques for imaging the SIJ have been directly compared. Scintigraphy has been compared with MRI and MRI with CT and conventional radiography.[16,41,42] All studies indicate that MRI is the most sensitive and specific method for evaluating inflammation in the SIJ. The sensitivity of the techniques for the detection of active sacroiliitis has been reported to range from 95% to 100% for MRI, 48% to 71% for scintigraphy, and 19% to 38% for CT and conventional radiography. Thus, Gd-DTPA–enhanced MRI is about 75% more sensitive for detecting active sacroiliitis than conventional radiographs are. On the other hand, CT was found to be superior for the detection of sclerosis,[42] indicating that this imaging method might be most appropriate for the assessment of structural changes in the SIJ.

However, for the diagnosis of AS, conventional x-ray films are the method of choice.[4,5] MRI techniques should be used in patients with possible early spondyloarthritis (SA) and IBP to clarify the diagnosis on a more objective basis and possibly exclude infections if appropriate. To determine the degree of structural changes, for example, for insurance purposes, T1-weighted turbospin-echo- or gradient-echo MRI sequences or CT may be used. Finally, scintigraphy may be used for the evaluation of patients with widespread pain, for example, on the basis of polyenthesitis, because it allows for the localization of active processes at different sites at the same time.[20]

Differential Diagnoses of Sacroiliitis

Sacroiliitis is not a totally specific feature of SA and may also occur in other rheumatic diseases, such as the synovitis acne pustulosis hyperostosis osteitis syndrome (SAPHO), which is closely related to SpA, but, although rarely, also in clearly different conditions such as in rheumatoid arthritis, systemic lupus erythematosus, Sjögren's syndrome, and sarcoidosis; in infectious diseases, such as tuberculosis and brucellosis; or in malignancy. With septic sacroiliitis conventional radiographs are usually rather normal in the first 2 weeks of disease,[20] whereas MRI can show the pathologic findings substantially earlier.[43,44] Thus, MRI is now the standard for making a diagnosis of septic sacroiliitis. A differential diagnostic criterion is that proximal parasacroiliac structures, such as the iliopsoas muscle, may be infiltrated. Similarly, sequestration of bone can be seen in septic sacroiliitis but not in SA.[20] Furthermore, sacroiliitis as an initial feature of AS usually starts in the iliac part of the SIJ.[45] This is in contrast to other inflammatory conditions such as septic sacroiliitis, which might start in the sacral part of the SIJ.

Some patients have evidence of moderate sacroiliitis shown by MRI but not by x-ray films and have no additional clinical features of SA. Such patients, mostly elderly women, can be classified using the term *undifferentiated sacroiliitis*.[5] There is no evidence of a later progression to SA.

Local Sacroiliac Joint Therapy: Guidance by Imaging Procedures

In some patients with SA, the local symptom of IBP on the basis of a clinical manifestation of sacroiliitis is more important than the systemic features of the disease. The primary target of therapy in those patients may be the clinically most relevant complaint of the patient and the reduction of pain at that site. Because intraarticular corticosteroid injections, guided by CT and fluoroscopy[22,46–49] and recently also by MRI,[49,50] have benefitted patients with severe active sacroiliitis, their use is an option for this particular clinical situation. Significant improvement of clinical symptoms has been reported in the majority of the patients in all studies. Thus, imaging-guided intraarticular injections may benefit patients with SA including those with AS who have local symptoms due to active sacroiliitis. Accordingly, this procedure is a relevant treatment option, especially in patients who do not have a sufficient response to NSAIDs or who have side effects from this therapy.

IMAGING OF THE SPINE IN ANKYLOSING SPONDYLITIS

The classification of AS is usually based on the modified 1984 New York criteria,[4] which rely mainly on the detection and the degree of SI changes obtained by conventional x-ray films. However, conventional radiographs are known to have a rather low sensitivity to detect sacroiliitis and spondylitis in the early stages of disease.[51] In one study, the mean time between the first symptoms and the diagnosis of AS ranged between 5 and 9 years.[52] The other problem with the New York criteria is that about 3% to 5% of patients with AS do not have unequivocal x-ray changes[53] but rather spinal changes in the form of the classical syndesmophytes.

Another problem with the criteria in patient care is that 10% to 20% of patients with AS have nothing but chronic SIJ changes and thus no spinal radiographic changes and no symptoms.

Conventional radiographs are still the standard for the assessment and quantification of structural spinal lesions, similar to the SIJ. However, T1-weighted MRI has also been successfully used to assess structural spinal lesions.[54] Overall, spinal MRI performs best for the identification and quantification of active spinal lesions and it has proved to be superior to other imaging techniques.[37,39,55–58]

Conventional Radiography of the Spine

Conventional x-ray films of the spine serving as a cumulative image of osteodestructive and osteoproliferative processes in the vertebral bodies may be useful to reflect the course of the disease. AS-related spinal changes can be differentiated in active (spondylitis and spondylodiscitis), structural osteodestructive (erosions) (Fig. 14.7A), and structural hyperproliferative (enthesophytes, vertebral squaring, disc calcifications, spondylophytes, syndesmophytes, bony bridging, and vertebral ankylosis) changes (Fig. 14.7B). Syndesmophytes are characterized by a typical axial growth that may lead to

bridging phenomena in the outer but sometimes also in the central part of the annulus fibrosus (annulus fibrosus type). Furthermore, syndesmophytes may appear in the prediscal region between the intervertebral disc and the anterior intervertebral ligament (prediscal type) (Fig. 14.7B).[59–61]

The differentiation of hyperproliferative/hyperostotic and ankylosing processes, which are typical for AS, from the so-called diffuse idiopathic skeletal hyperostosis (DISH) syndrome[62] is sometimes difficult. In the DISH syndrome, the pattern of ankylosis is different, and spondylophytes grow more laterally or in the horizontal direction, most often on the right side of the thoracic spine. In contrast, syndesmophytes in AS show cranial and caudal growth, and they tend to build bony bridges (Fig. 14.7B).

Furthermore, the zygapophyseal (ZA) joints deserve attention, because they are often affected in AS and rather early in the disease (Fig. 14.8). Involvement of the ZA joints is often underdiagnosed, simply because they are difficult to assess by most imaging procedures. Ankylosis of the ZA joints was described to be discordantly associated with the presence of bridging syndesmophytes in AS.[63] This description suggests that the ZA joints are involved primarily and early in patients

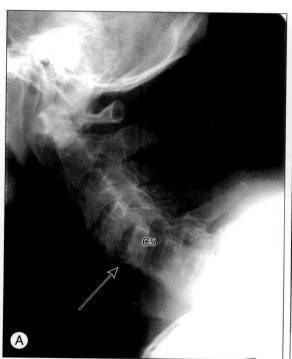

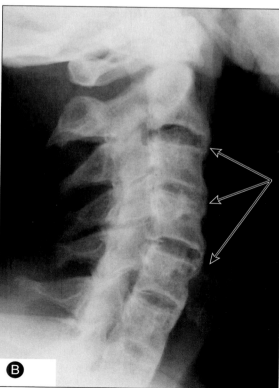

Fig. 14.7 Structural spinal changes in AS as assessed by conventional x-rays. A: Erosive spinal changes in the upper border of C5. **B:** Bridging syndesmophytes and ankylosis in the cervical spine.

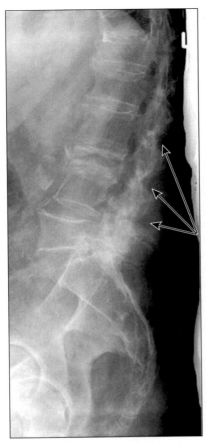

Fig. 14.8 Ankylosis of the zygapophyseal joints in a 57-year-old male patient with AS.

with AS. The consequence is that syndesmophytes and bony bridging then represent advanced stages of the disease.

SCORING OF STRUCTURAL SPINAL CHANGES

Currently, there are two methods for scoring of structural spinal changes when conventional x-ray films are used for patients with AS: the modified Stokes Ankylosing Spondylitis Scoring System (mSASSS),[64] which is a modification of the original SASSS[65,66] and the Bath Ankylosing Spondylitis Radiology Index (BASRI).[67] Both scoring systems are widely used for quantification of structural spinal changes in patients with AS in both daily practice and clinical trials. However, the mSASSS has been the most reliable scoring method for this purpose.[68] It also has excellent sensitivity to change,[69] and it is the preferred instrument for clinical trials.[68] The best sensitivity to change is reached when the reader is aware of the sequence; however, paired reading also provides sufficient sensitivity to change. About 100 patients per treatment arm need to be

included in a 2-year trial for sufficient power if the paired reading order is used.[68]

For scoring with the mSASSS, lateral radiographs of the cervical and the lumbar spine are needed. The mSASSS is used to evaluate the anterior part of the lumbar and the cervical spine by assessing structural changes using a score between 0 and 3 (Table 14.3 and Fig. 14.9). The cervical spine is scored from the lower border of C2 to the upper border of T1 and the lumbar spine is scored from the lower border of T12 to the upper border of S1. Thus, the mSASSS includes the evaluation of 24 vertebrae overall, and the number of scoring points range from 0 to 72.

The BASRI is a composite score (BASRI-total) comprised of the BASRI-spine and the BASRI-hip. The former includes the evaluation of the SIJ (scored according to the New York criteria) and a scoring of the lumbar and the cervical spine, ranging between 0 and 4 per vertebral segment (Table 14.4). It is used to evaluate the cervical spine from the upper border of C1 to the lower border of C7 and the lumbar spine from T12 to the upper border of S1. The cervical spine is evaluated on the lateral view and the lumbar spine is evaluated on both AP and lateral views. The final BASRI score is a composite score of the scorings of the cervical and the lumbar spine, adding the mean score of the right and left SIJ. Because according to the New York criteria patients need to have radiographic evidence of sacroiliitis for the diagnosis of AS, the range of the total BASRI (spinal score plus SIJ score) is 2 to 12. The BASRI has a ceiling effect and is less sensitive to change. The BASRI-hip is scored in accordance to the BASRI-spine by using the same grading and by the mean of the right and the left hip for the final score. Finally, the BASRI-total is the total score of the addition of the BASRI-spine and the BASRI-hip.

MAGNETIC RESONANCE IMAGING OF THE SPINE IN ANKYLOSING SPONDYLITIS

MRI is currently considered the most sensitive method for the imaging of spinal inflammation.[1,10] Positron

TABLE 14.3 THE MODIFIED SASSS	
Grade	Evaluation
0	Normal
1	Erosion, sclerosis, or squaring
2	Syndesmophyte
3	Bridging syndesmophyte

Grading of the modified SASSS (mSASSS). Each vertebral edge in the cervical and lumbar spine is graded with 0–3, the score ranges from 0–72. See text for further explanation of the scoring system.

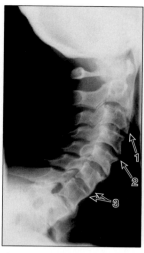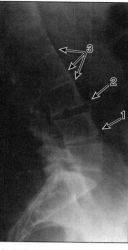

0 =	Normal
1 =	Erosion, sclerosis or squaring
2 =	Syndesmophyte
3 =	Bridging syndesmophyte

Fig. 14.9 The modified Stokes Ankylosing Spondylitis Spinal Score (mSASSS) for assessment of structural spinal changes in patients with AS.

emission tomography techniques have not been evaluated for this purpose to a sufficient degree. MRI is now being increasingly tested to classify and diagnose patients with SA and predominant axial involvement (Fig. 14.10A–B). In patients with AS, spinal MRI has been used to assess spinal inflammation as an indicator of disease activity and a possible predictor of response to therapy. The evaluation of MRI as a tool to define allocation to different therapeutic strategies, such as treatment with biologic agents, is currently ongoing.[37,39,55,58]

Spondylitis

Inflammation of the vertebral body and adjacent structures (called *spondylitis anterior, Romanus lesion, shiny corner sign,* or *vertebral osteitis*) has been considered as a rather early sign of spinal involvement in patients with AS. First described by Romanus and Yden in 1952,[70] it represents a rather typical radiographic sign of spinal involvement in AS, which is most often seen in the thoracolumbar region at T10 to T12 (Fig. 14.11).[10] When MRI is used, spondylitis anterior is typically seen as a decreased signal on T1-weighted MRI scans before contrast agent enhancement and, in correspondence, it turns into an increased signal in T1-weighted MRI scans due to enhancement after application of the contrast agent. The findings are similar to those for T2-weighted or STIR MRI (Fig. 14.11). The typical appearance of spondylitis is not always limited to the vertebral edges but may also spread to the entire vertebral body as a sign of generalized inflammation.[71–73]

The signal intensity within the disc may remain normal during vertebral osteitis. In the postinflammatory healing phase T1- and T2-weighted MRI scans may show hyperintensity of the MRI signal, discordant to a low T1 signal after Gd-DTPA, owing to accumulation of yellow fat marrow.[71] Discovertebral junctions may display a low signal intensity on T1- and T2-weighted images when a marginal sclerosis occurs after a spondylitis.[71]

Spondylitis anterior is an active osteitis and enthesitis at the junction of the annulus fibrosus and the longitudinal ligaments with the anterior ligament, the vertebral body, and the intervertebral disc. In later stages, active inflammation may result in erosive changes and later in sclerotic changes and in reactive new bone formation including syndesmophytes at the corner of the affected vertebral bodies. Less commonly, these changes are also seen at the posterior vertebral edges.[10,71]

TABLE 14.4 THE BASRI-SPINE	
Grade	**Evaluation**
0	Normal
1	Suspicious (no definite change)
2	Mild (any number of erosions, squaring or sclerosis, with or without syndesmophytes, on two vertebrae)
3	Moderate (syndesmophytes on three vertebrae, with or without fusion involving two vertebrae)
4	Severe (fusion in three vertebrae)

Grading of the BASRI-spine. Each vertebral body (anterior and posterior edge in the cervical (C1-C7) and lumbar (Th12-S1) spine is graded with 0-4. After inclusion of the sacroiliac joints and according to the NY criteria, patients with ankylosing spondylitis are supposed to range from 2-12. See text for further explanation of the scoring system.

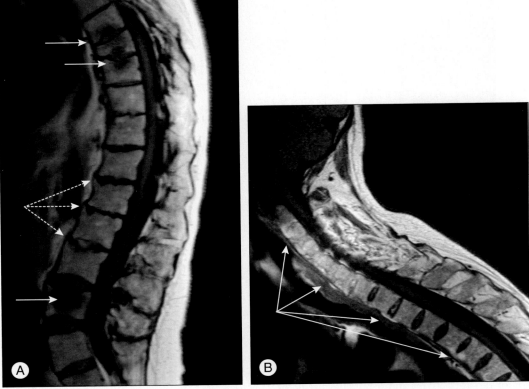

Fig. 14.10 Structural spinal changes in AS, as detected by T1-weighted MRI. A: Severe erosions (continuous arrows) and hyperproliferative changes (syndesmophytes) (dotted arrows). **B:** Hyperproliferation in the cervical spine in a patient with AS. The arrows indicate regions with bridging syndesmophytes and ankylosing.

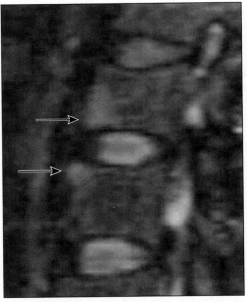

Fig. 14.11 Romanus lesions in the anterior and the posterior edge of the vertebral body, as depicted by short tau inversion recovery (STIR) MRI in the lumbar spine of an AS patient.

Spondylitis anterior has rarely been seen in patients with SA without an established diagnosis of AS.[72]

Spondylodiscitis and Discitis

Inflammation of the intervertebral space (discitis) and the disc together with the vertebral body (called *spondylodiscitis* or *Andersson lesion*) is also a rather typical sign of spinal inflammation in patients with AS. In contrast to conventional radiographs, on which only the consequences of spondylodiscitis are visible in later disease stages, with MRI such changes can be detected in early phases.[74,75] Accordingly, negative radiographic findings are sometimes accompanied by positive MRI findings indicative of spondylodiscitis[74,75] (Fig. 14.12A). Asymptomatic spondylodiscitis may occur in multiple spinal segments in approximately 8% of patients in early disease.[76] The incidence of spondylodiscitis, which may occur without major clinical symptoms, has been estimated to be 15% in patients with AS.[51,76] The first radiologic description of spondylodiscitis was published by Andersson in 1937,[77] and in 1978 Dihlmann

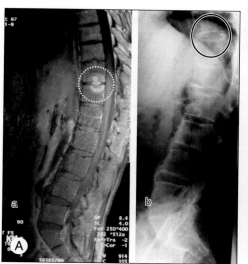
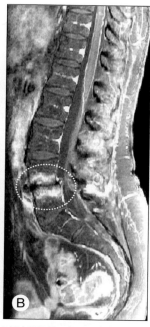

Fig. 14.12 A: Anderson lesion, as detected by contrast agent (Gd-DTPA) enhanced MRI with the typical circumscribed hemispherical erosive lesion (dotted circle) which is often surrounded by an area of low signal intensity in one of two neighbored vertebral bodies. In contrast to the MRI, the corresponding x-ray image does not show any pathological sign (continuous circle). **B:** Modic-I lesion as a sign of erosive osteochondrosis. The dotted circle indicates the inflamed area in the lumbar spine. This pathognomonic sign is not AS related and should be taken into account as a differential diagnostic sign of AS.

and Delling[78] proposed a distinction between inflammatory and noninflammatory spondylodiscitis. With MRI, spondylodiscitis (Fig. 14.12A) is characterized by a circumscribed hemispherical erosive lesion that is often surrounded by an area of low signal intensity in one of two neighboring vertebral bodies. In the course of the disease, spondylodiscitis may develop into transdiscal ossification processes without marginal syndesmophytes. In contrast, the "noninflammatory" spondylodiscal lesion is a transdiscal fracture due to an osteoporotic process,[79] which may occur spontaneously or after certain rapid movements. It should be noted that the early lesions described, whether inflammatory or noninflammatory, are very similar to Modic I lesions, which have been known to lead to erosive osteochondrosis[80] (Fig. 14.12B), whereas late spondylodiscitis is similar to Modic II lesions on MRI scans. Therefore, spondylodiscal lesions cannot be used for diagnosis per se without clinical evidence of AS-related symptoms.[51]

Costovertebral Joints

Inflammatory lesions in the costovertebral joints are also characterized by low-density signals on T1-weighted MRI sequences and high-density signals in MRI sequences that are sensitive for detection of inflammation. Involvement of the costovertebral joints in AS leads to reduced chest expansion, a frequent finding and even a diagnostic tool in patients with AS.[4] This symptom may be explained by both active and structural spinal changes.

C1/C2 Atlantoaxial Subluxation

Atlantoaxial subluxations (AASs) may occur as the presenting symptom of AS,[81] leading to atlantoaxial instability and dislocation associated with a neurologic deficit, often making surgical management mandatory.[82] The incidence of AASs is not low, and they may occur in young male patients with a relatively short mean disease duration.[82] Anterior AASs may progress in a number of patients with AS after 2 years from its detection, and surgical management is thought appropriate in a considerable number of patients, with or without neurologic signs.

Scoring of Spinal Magnetic Resonance Imaging Sequences in Ankylosing Spondylitis

MRI is now being increasingly used for the evaluation of the influence of anti-inflammatory drugs (such as anti–tumor necrosis factor-α agents) on spinal inflammation in randomized clinical trials.[55,58] To quantify active spondylitic changes in patients with AS, MRI scoring methods have been developed: the best system is the

197

AS spinal MRI scoring system (ASspiMRI)[20,54,55,58,59,83–85] (Tables 14.5 and 14.6). This scoring system is based on grading on a 0 to 6 scale for both disease activity (ASspiMRI-a, Table 14.5) and chronicity (ASspiMRI-c, Table 14.6). Inflammatory activity as assessed by the ASspiMRI-a 1) quantifies either enhancement after T1/Gd-DTPA or 2) the bone marrow edema detected by the STIR or the T2-FS technique. Disease chronicity is assessed by the ASspiMRI-c by grading structural lesions in T1-weighted MRI sequences (before application of contrast agents). For the quantification of active and structural spinal lesions, the ASspiMRI evaluates vertebral units (VU), which are defined as the region between two virtual lines drawn through the middle of each vertebra.

Almost the complete spine is included in the ASspiMRI assessment, from C2/3 to L5/S1, comprising 23 vertebral units. Thus, the range of the scoring system is from 0 to 138 for both the activity and the chronicity index. A possible modification of the ASspiMRI-a is a concentration on the scores 0 to 3, leaving out 4 to 6.[86]

TABLE 14.5 THE ASsPIMRI-a	
Grade	**Evaluation**
0	Normal, no lesions
1	Mild enhancement and bone marrow edema, covering 25% of a VU
2	Moderate bone marrow edema, covering 50% of a VU
3	Severe bone marrow edema, covering >50% of a VU
4	Bone marrow edema and erosion covering 25% of a VU
5	Bone marrow edema and erosion covering 50% of a VU
6	Bone marrow edema and erosion covering >50% of a VU

Grading of the Ankylosing Spondylitis spinal MRI score for active changes (ASspiMRI-a). Each vertebral unit in the cervical (C1-Th1), thoracic (Th1-L1) and lumbar (L1-S1) spine is graded with 0-6, the score ranges from 0-138. See text for further explanation of the scoring system.

TABLE 14.6 THE ASspiMRI-c	
Grade	**Evaluation**
0	Normal, no lesions
1	Minor sclerosis/suspicion of relevant changes
2	Sclerosis/vertebral squaring/ton-shaped vertebrae/possible syndesmophyte
3	One or two syndesmophytes/minor erosion
4	More than two syndesmophytes/spondylodiscitis/severe erosions
5	Vertebral bridging
6	Vertebral fusion

Grading of the Ankylosing Spondylitis spinal MRI score for chronic changes (ASspiMRI-c). Each vertebral unit in the cervical (C1-Th1), thoracic (Th1-L1) and lumbar (L1-S1) spine is graded with 0-6, the score ranges from 0-138. See text for further explanation of the scoring system.

Spinal Fractures in Ankylosing Spondylitis

Owing to osteoporosis and rigid stiffness of the spine there is an increased risk of spinal fractures in AS,[87,88] especially in patients with long disease duration and a high degree of spinal involvement.[91,92] Overall, there are three different patterns of spinal fractures in AS patients[93]: simple compression fractures, stress fractures, and acute shear fractures. Simple compression fractures occur mainly as a result of low bone density and quality. They can usually be found in early disease but occur much more often in later stages when they contribute to the characteristic hyperkyphosis of the patients. Stress fractures associated with pseudarthroses are due to an underlying spondylodiscitis. The transversely oriented acute shear fractures are often associated with rupture of ossified paraspinal ligaments. If the posterior spinal column is involved the fracture may lead to vertebral displacement and neurologic sequelae[94,95] (Fig. 14.13). Spinal fractures usually occur in the cervical spine[96,97] and in the cervicothoracic and the thoracolumbar regions, mostly due to hyperextension injuries.[76,91] Because of osteopenia and severe structural changes, nondisplaced spinal fractures may not be easily diagnosed by conventional x-rays (Fig. 14.14). The shear forces resulting from spinal movements may lead to dislocation of the injured spinal segment,[94] and a CT scan is necessary to diagnose a possible dislocation in patients with persistent or progressive symptoms after injury, especially if the symptoms are related to movement. Neurologic symptoms are further evaluated by MRI.[87,96] Acute fractures show an increased signal intensity on T2-weighted MRI or STIR MRI sequences and variable enhancement on T1-weighted MRI sequences after contrast agent application, indicating the location of the fracture line though the vertebral body.[97] On T1-weighted MRI sequences without application of contrast material fracture lines display a signal of decreased intensity.[91] Rarely, fracture lines may show a decreased signal intensity on both T1- and T2-weighted MRI sequences.[97] Finally, a disruption of the anterior longitudinal ligament is detected as a discontinuation and step-off of the low signal intensity structure along the anterior side of the vertebral body.[97]

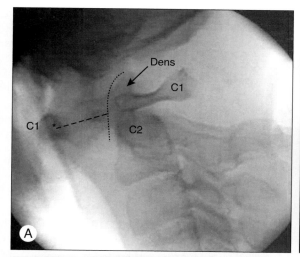

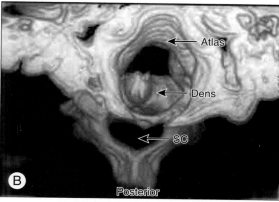

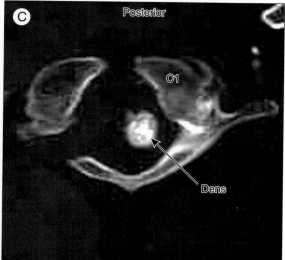

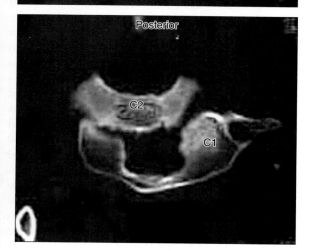

Fig. 14.13 A: Conventional x-ray of the upper lateral cervical spine of an AS patient showing pathologic changes in the C1/C2 segment with a galloping phenomenon. The atlantodental distance (dashed line) which is measured from the posterior surface of the anterior ring of the atlas (*) to the anterior surface of the dens axis (dotted line) is extremely extended to > 2 cm (normal distance • 0.4 cm). **B** and **C:** 3D computed tomography (CT) and conventional CT images of C1 and C2 showing shearing of atlas and axis in the transversal view. C1 = atlas, C2 = axis, SC = spinal canal (Images provided by Dr. H. Böhm, Bad Berka, Germany).

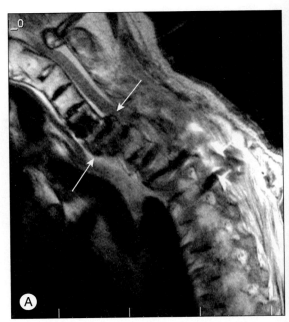
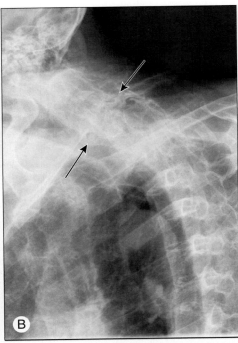

Fig. 14.14 A: Fracture in the posterior spinal column of the cervical spine in an AS patient, leading to vertebral displacement, as detected by T1-weighted MRI. **B:** As depicted by conventional x-rays in the same patient, such fractures are very difficult to be diagnosed, due to the severe overlapping structural changes in this region. (Images provided by H. Böhm, Bad Berka, Germany).

Calcification of the Spinal Disc

Calcification of the intervertebral disc is a common finding in older patients with long-standing AS. However, a diagnosis of disc calcification does not affect the management of the disease.

The correlation between conventional radiographs and T1-weighted MRI sequences for a diagnosis of disk calcification was 78%.[83] Variable degrees of disc calcification may appear. The localization is mainly in the thoracolumbar region, especially at the T12 to L1 level.[91] Four different patterns of increased signal intensity within the discs termed type A (marginal), type B (annular), type C (central), and type D (solid) can be differentiated.[98] The increased signal intensity on T1-weighted MRI sequences is likely to be related to the surface area of the calcium crystal. End-plate marrow changes may also be detected in addition to disk calcifications, but these are not correlated with signal changes within the discs; in some patients they are related to bony bridging.[98] Intervertebral discs may also show a decreased signal intensity on T2-weighted images; this is possibly related to decreased water content.[98]

Ossification of Paraspinal Ligaments in Ankylosing Spondylitis

Patients with AS tend to develop ossification of the posterior longitudinal ligament, mainly in structural disease stages. Typically, this sign is seen as a linear band of decreased signal intensity on all MRI sequences in the posterior side of the vertebra.[99] Paraspinal ligament ossification is usually mild to moderate and does not cause clinical symptoms in most patients.

Cauda Equina Syndrome

The cauda equina syndrome (CES) is a specific but rare feature, seen mainly in patients with advanced AS.[100] The pathophysiologic sources are arachnoid cysts that may cause nerve compression symptoms such as irradiating pain and limb numbness. Furthermore, patients with AS and CES often have dural ectasia in the lumbar spine. The ultimate cause of CES in AS is not completely known, but arachnoiditis due to inflammation of the posterior facet joints leading to adhesions within the thecal sac is one possible explanation of the pathogenesis.[101] CES is characterized by slow and progressive sensorimotor loss, possibly leading to sphincter disturbances and incontinence. The prevalence of neurologic symptoms in patients with AS has been reported to be approximately 2.1%,[102] and CES seems to be among the most common causes of neurologic disturbances in AS.[103]

Imaging of the CES can be performed by conventional radiographs (Fig. 14.15), myelography, and CT by showing enlargement of the caudal sac and dorsal arachnoid diverticula with erosions of the lamina and spinous

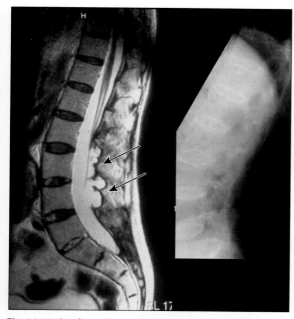

Fig. 14.15 Cauda equina syndrome in a patient with AS. The characteristic expansion of the lumbar spinal canal with scalloping of the laminae and spinous processes related to the presence of dorsal dural diverticulae, as also the dilatation of lumbosacral nerve roots can be seen on MRI. In contrast, imaging with conventional x-rays is limited, showing only evidence of a possible cause cauda equina syndrome.

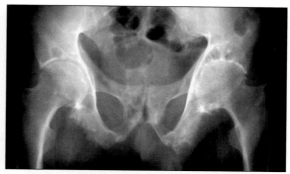

Fig. 14.16 Typical extravertebral manifestations of AS, with enthesitis of the attaching pelvic ligaments, coxitis and symphysitis.

processes and widening of the neural canal at one or more levels.[104] Both CT and MRI can be used to show the characteristic expansion of the lumbar spinal canal with scalloping of the laminae and spinous processes related to the presence of dorsal dural diverticula (Fig. 14.14).[105,106] However, MRI is superior for permitting confident exclusion of other intradural pathologic changes without recourse to invasive investigations.[106] Displacement of the lower spinal cord and clumping of nerve roots as well as dilatation of lumbosacral nerve roots may be seen on MRI scans (Fig. 14.15, *dotted circle*).[105–107]

Extravertebral Manifestations of Ankylosing Spondylitis

Peripheral extravertebral manifestations, such as enthesitis (Fig. 14.16) and bursitis, are a clinical hallmark of the spondyloarthritides. A common extravertebral manifestation of AS that is often detected on conventional x-rays is an enthesitis of attaching pelvic ligaments, also referred to as *fibroosteitis*. This is characterized by proliferative changes of bone and cartilage. If active inflammation is present, MRI shows a hypodense signal on T1-weighted sequences and a hyperdense signal on T2-weighted sequences or STIR sequences.

These signs of enthesitis may also be seen with involvement of the trochanter major or calcaneus (Fig. 14.17A) in SA. Often, there is also involvement of the retrocalcaneal bursa (Fig. 14.17B) and the Achilles tendon,[108] which can be depicted as areas of hyperintensity on T2-weighted and STIR sequences and show strong signal increase after contrast agent enhancement due to hypervascularization of the retrocalcaneal bursa.[51] These are similarly well detected by ultrasound. Ultrasound of the joints and tendons may play an increasing role as a diagnostic tool in clinical practice, especially in cases of doubtful clinical findings. Here, not only conventional but also power Doppler-techniques are especially recommended (Fig. 14.19).[108–110]

In juvenile forms of AS, patients may show asymmetrical synovitis, especially of the lower extremities.[111] Inflammation of the tarsus[112] can occur as the first symptoms of AS, before any other manifestation of the axial skeleton. Similar to sacroiliitis, inflammatory lesions of the tarsus may develop into ankylosis of the ankle and the intertarsal joints.[51]

Finally, perichondritis and synchondrosis of the pubic symphysis and the sternum (Fig. 14.20), mainly in the manubrium sterni, may occur as signs of extravertebral manifestations in AS. Those are not always accompanied by clinical symptoms and are therefore diagnosed in later stages of the disease as a synostosis on conventional radiographs. However, partial synostoses in these areas may also occur in arthrotic conditions.

SUMMARY

In summary, x-ray films are still the standard method for diagnosis of structural changes in SIJs. For assessment of active sacroiliitis, MRI sequences are preferred.

Conventional radiographs of the spine are the basis for diagnosis of AS-related structural spinal changes, such as syndesmophytes, erosions, or ankylosis. MRI examinations of the spine are useful for assessment of

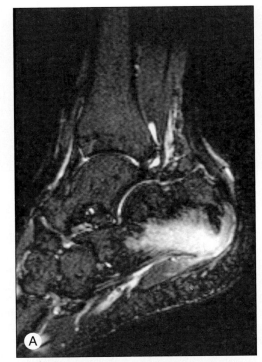

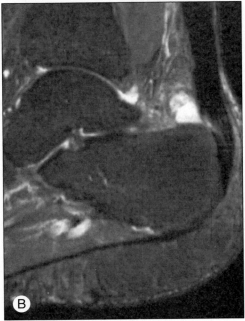

Fig. 14.17 Affection of the calcaneus in the short tau inversion recovery (STIR) MRI sequence (Fig. 17a) and involvement of the retrocalcanear bursa in the gadolinium-enhanced MRI sequence (Fig. 17b) as a sign of extraspinal manifestation in 2 patients with AS.

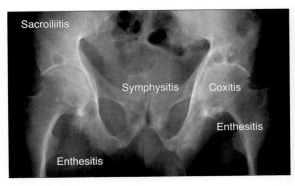

Fig. 14.18

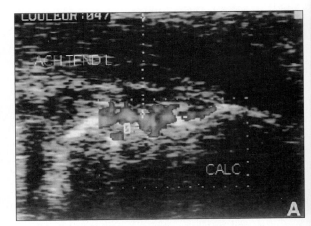

Fig. 14.19 Ultrasonography of the left calcaneal (CALC) enthesitis in a spondyloarthropathy patient. The Power Doppler sonography shows hypoechoic thickening of the Achilles tendon (ACH TEND) at the entheses, with increased blood flow.

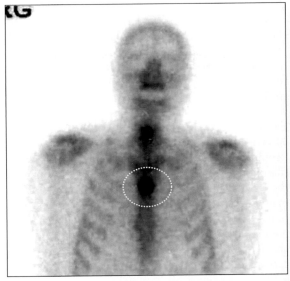

Fig. 14.20 Perichondritis of the sternum, as detected by scintigraphy, as a typical extraspinal manifestation of inflammatory lesions in patients with AS.

inflammatory changes or for diagnosis of early stages of the disease.

MRI sequences for assessment of active disease are the STIR, T2-fat saturated, and gadolinium-enhanced. For assessment of structural changes, the T1-weighted MRI sequence is used.

Both SIJ and spinal changes can be quantified by validated scoring systems. However, these systems are mostly used in clinical trials for quantification of the efficacy of new treatment options, such as anti–tumor necrosis factor-α compounds.

The main extraspinal manifestation of AS is peripheral enthesitis. This can be reliably diagnosed by ultrasound. Atlantoaxial dislocations of the spine occur in very late stages of the disease and may lead to severe neurologic complications.

REFERENCES

1. Bollow M, Enzeiler C, Taupitz M, et al. Use of contrast enhanced magnetic resonance imaging to detect spinal inflammation in patients with spondyloarthritides. Clin Exp Rheumatol. 2002;20(6 suppl 28):S167–S174.

2. Braun J, Sieper J. The sacroiliac joint in the spondyloarthropathies. Curr Opin Rheumatol. 1996;8:275–287.

3. Hermann KG, Bollow M. Magnetic resonance imaging of the axial skeleton in rheumatoid disease. Best Pract Res Clin Rheumatol. 2004;18:881–907.

4. van der Linden S, Valkenburg HA, Cats A. Evaluation of diagnostic criteria for ankylosing spondylitis. A proposal for modification of the New York criteria. Arthritis Rheum. 1984;27:361–368.

5. Brandt J, Bollow M, Haberle J, et al. Studying patients with inflammatory back pain and arthritis of the lower limbs clinically and by magnetic resonance imaging: many, but not all patients with sacroiliitis have spondyloarthropathy. Rheumatology (Oxford). 1999;38:831–836.

6. Hollingsworth PN, Cheah PS, Dawkins RL, Owen ET, Calin A, Wood PH. Observer variation in grading sacroiliac radiographs in HLA-B27 positive individuals. J Rheumatol. 1983;10: 247–254.

7. Bellamy N, Park W, Rooney PJ. What do we know about the sacroiliac joint? Semin Arthritis Rheum. 1983;12:282–313.

8. Forrester DM. Imaging of the sacroiliac joints. Radiol Clin North Am. 1990;28:1055–1072.

9. Robbins SE, Morse MH. Is the acquisition of a separate view of the sacroiliac joints in the prone position justified in patients with back pain? Clin Radiol. 1996;51:637–638.

10. Braun J, Bollow M, Sieper J. Radiologic diagnosis and pathology of the spondyloarthropathies. Rheum Dis Clin North Am. 1998; 24:697–735.

11. Russell AS, Lentle BC, Percy JS. Investigation of sacroiliac disease: comparative evaluation of radiological and radionuclide techniques. J Rheumatol. 1975;2:45–51.

12. Dequeker J, Goddeeris T, Walravens M, De Roo M. Evaluation of sacroiliitis: comparison of radiological and radionuclide techniques. Radiology. 1978;128:687–689.

13. Ho G Jr, Sadovnikoff N, Malhotra CM, Claunch BC. Quantitative sacroiliac joint scintigraphy. A critical assessment. Arthritis Rheum. 1979;22:837–844.

14. Ryan PJ, Fogelman I. The bone scan: where are we now? Semin Nucl Med. 1995;25:76–91.

15. de Vlam K, Van de Wiele C, Mielants H, Dierckx RA, Vays EM. Is 99mTc human immunoglobulin G scintigraphy (HIG-scan) useful for the detection of spinal inflammation in ankylosing spondylitis? Clin Exp Rheumatol. 2000;18:379–382.

16. Battafarano DF, West SG, Rak KM, Fortenbery EJ, Chantelois AD. Comparison of bone scan, computed tomography, and magnetic resonance imaging in the diagnosis of active sacroiliitis. Semin Arthritis Rheum. 1993;23:161–176.

17. Lawson TL, Foley WD, Berland LL, Lawson TL, Varma RR. The sacroiliac joints: anatomic, plain roentgenographic, and computed tomographic analysis. J Comput Assist Tomogr. 1982; 6:307–314.

18. Ryan LM, Carrera GF, Lightfoot RW Jr, Hoffman RG, Kozin F. The radiographic diagnosis of sacroiliitis. A comparison of different views with computed tomograms of the sacroiliac joint. Arthritis Rheum. 1983;26:760–763.

19. Fam AG, Rubenstein JD, Chin-Sang H, Leung FY. Computed tomography in the diagnosis of early ankylosing spondylitis. Arthritis Rheum. 1985;28:930–937.

20. Braun J, van der Heijde D. Imaging and scoring in ankylosing spondylitis. Best Pract Res Clin Rheumatol. 2002;16: 573–604.

21. Vogler JB III, Brown WH, Helms CA, Genant HK. The normal sacroiliac joint: a CT study of asymptomatic patients. Radiology. 1984;151:433–437.

22. Braun J, Bollow M, Seyrekbasan F, et al. Computed tomography guided corticosteroid injection of the sacroiliac joint in patients with spondyloarthropathy with sacroiliitis: clinical outcome and followup by dynamic magnetic resonance imaging. J Rheumatol. 1996;23:659–664.

23. Bollow M, Braun J, Taupitz M, et al. CT-guided intraarticular corticosteroid injection into the sacroiliac joints in patients with spondyloarthropathy: indication and follow-up with contrast-enhanced MRI. J Comput Assist Tomogr. 1996;20: 512–521.

24. Puhakka KB, Melsen F, Jurik AG, Boel LW, Vesterby A, Egund N. MR imaging of the normal sacroiliac joint with correlation to histology. Skeletal Radiol. 2004;33:15–28.

25. Fenton P. Magnetic resonance imaging of the sacroiliac joints: worth the cost? J Rheumatol. 1996;23:2020–2021.

26. Remy M, Bouillry ZP, Bertin P, et al. Evaluation of magnetic resonance imaging for the detection of sacroiliitis in patients with early seronegative spondylarthropathy. Rev Rhum Engl Ed. 1996;63:577–583.

27. Braun J, Bollow M, Eggens U, Konig H, Distler A, Sieper J. Use of dynamic magnetic resonance imaging with fast imaging in the detection of early and advanced sacroiliitis in spondylarthropathy patients. Arthritis Rheum. 1994;37:1039–1045.

28. Bollow M, Braun J, Neure L, et al. Early sacroiliitis in patients with spondyloarthropathy: evaluation with dynamic gadolinium-enhanced MR imaging. Radiology. 1995;194:529–536.

29. Marzo-Ortega H, Braun J, Maksymowych WP, et al. Interreader agreement in the assessment of magnetic resonance imaging of the sacroiliac joints in spondyloarthropathy—the 1st MISS study [abstract]. Arthritis Rheum. 2002;46:S428.

30. Braun J, Sieper J, Bollow M. Imaging of sacroiliitis. Clin Rheumatol. 2000;19:51–57.

31. Puhakka KB, Jurik AG, Egund N, et al. Imaging of sacroiliitis in early seronegative spondylarthropathy. Assessment of abnormalities by MR in comparison with radiography and CT. Acta Radiol. 2003;44:218–229.

32. Hermann KG, Braun J, Fischer T, Reisshauer H, Bollow M. Magnetic resonance tomography of sacroiliitis: anatomy, histological pathology, MR-morphology, and grading. Radiologe. 2004;44:217–228.

33. Maksymowych WP, et al. Spondyloarthritis Research Consortium of Canada Magnetic Resonance Imaging Index for assessment spinal inflammation in ankylosing spondylitis. Arthritis Rheum. 2005;15:502–509.

34. Landewé R, Hermann KG, van der Heijde DM, et al. Scoring sacroiliac joints by magnetic resonance imaging—A multiple-reader reliability experiment. J Rheumatol. 2005; 32(10):2050–2055.

35. Braun J, Brandt H, Listing J, et al. Treatment of active ankylosing spondylitis with infliximab: a randomised controlled multicentre trial. Lancet. 2002;359:1187–1193.

36. Brandt J, Khariouzov A, Listing J, et al. Six-month results of a double-blind, placebo-controlled trial of etanercept treatment in patients with active ankylosing spondylitis. Arthritis Rheum. 2003;48:1667–1675.

37. Marzo-Ortega H, McGonagle D, O'Connor P, Emery P. Efficacy of etanercept in the treatment of the entheseal pathology in resistant spondylarthropathy: a clinical and magnetic resonance imaging study. Arthritis Rheum. 2001;44:2112–2117.

38. Rudwaleit M, Baraliakos X, Listing J, et al. Magnetic resonance imaging (MRI) of the spine and the sacroiliac joints (SIJ) in ankylosing spondylitis (AS) before and during therapy with the anti-TNF agent etanercept. Ann Rheum Dis. 2005;64(9):1305–1310.

39. Stone M, Salonen D, Lax M, Payne U, Lapp V, Inman R. Clinical and imaging correlates of response to treatment with infliximab in patients with ankylosing spondylitis. J Rheumatol. 2001;28: 1605–1614.

40. Jajic Z, Jajic I, Grazio S. Radiological changes of the symphysis in ankylosing spondylitis. Acta Radiol. 2000;41:307–309.

41. Blum U, Buitrago-Tellez C, Mundinger A, et al. Magnetic resonance imaging (MRI) for detection of active sacroiliitis—a prospective study comparing conventional radiography, scintigraphy, and contrast enhanced MRI. J Rheumatol. 1996;23: 2107–2115.

42. Yu W, Feng F, Dion E, Yang H, Jiang M, Genant HK. Comparison of radiography, computed tomography and magnetic resonance imaging in the detection of sacroiliitis accompanying ankylosing spondylitis. Skeletal Radiol. 1998;27: 311–320.

43. Sackett D. Rules of evidence and clinical recommendations on use of antithrombotic agents. Chest. 1986;89 (2 suppl):2–3.

44. Sturzenbecher A, Braun J, Paris S, Biedermann T, Hamm B, Bollow M. MR imaging of septic sacroiliitis. Skeletal Radiol. 2000;29:439–446.

45. Muche B, Bollow M, Francois RJ, Sieper J, Hamm B, Braun J. Anatomic structures involved in early- and late-stage sacroiliitis in spondylarthritis: a detailed analysis by contrast-enhanced magnetic resonance imaging. Arthritis Rheum. 2003;48:1374–1384.

46. Braun J, Bollow M, Neure L, et al. Use of immunohistologic and in situ hybridization techniques in the examination of sacroiliac joint biopsy specimens from patients with ankylosing spondylitis. Arthritis Rheum. 1995;38:499–505.

47. Bollow M, Fischer T, Reisshauer H, et al. Quantitative analyses of sacroiliac biopsies in spondyloarthropathies: T cells and macrophages predominate in early and active sacroiliitis—cellularity correlates with the degree of enhancement detected by magnetic resonance imaging. Ann Rheum Dis. 2000;59:135–140.

48. Maugars Y, Berthelot JM, Forestier R, et al. Assessment of the efficacy of sacroiliac corticosteroid injections in spondylarthropathies: a double-blind study. Br J Rheumatol. 1996;35: 767–770.

49. Gunaydin I, Pereira PL, Daikeler T, et al. Magnetic resonance imaging guided corticosteroid injection of the sacroiliac joints in patients with therapy resistant spondyloarthropathy: a pilot study. J Rheumatol. 2000;27:424–428.

50. Pereira PL, Gunaydin I, Trubenback J, et al. Interventional MR imaging for injection of sacroiliac joints in patients with ankylosing spondylitis. AJR Am J Roentgenol. 2000;175:265–266.

51. Bollow M. Magnetic resonance imaging in ankylosing spondylitis (Marie-Struempell-Bechterew disease). Rofo. 2002; 174:1489–1499.

52. Feldtkeller E. Age at disease onset and delayed diagnosis of spondyloarthropathies. Z Rheumatol. 1999;58:21–30.

53. Khan MA, van der Linden SM, Kushner I, Valkenburg VA, Cats A. Spondylitic disease without radiologic evidence of sacroiliitis in relatives of HLA-B27 positive ankylosing spondylitis patients. Arthritis Rheum. 1985;28:40–43.

54. Braun J, Baraliakos X, Golder W, et al. Analysing chronic spinal changes in ankylosing spondylitis: a systematic comparison of conventional x rays with magnetic resonance imaging using established and new scoring systems. Ann Rheum Dis. 2004;63: 1046–1055.

55. Braun J, Baraliakos X, Golder W, et al. Magnetic resonance imaging examinations of the spine in patients with ankylosing spondylitis, before and after successful therapy with infliximab: evaluation of a new scoring system. Arthritis Rheum. 2003;48: 1126–1136.

56. Baraliakos X, Landewe R, Hermann KG, et al. Inflammation in ankylosing spondylitis—a systematic description of the extension and frequency of acute spinal changes using magnetic resonance imaging (MRI). Ann Rheum Dis. 2005;64:730–734.

57. Baraliakos X, Hermann KG, Landewe R, et al. Assessment of acute spinal inflammation in patients with ankylosing spondylitis by magnetic resonance imaging (MRI)—a comparison between contrast enhanced T1 and short-tau inversion recovery (STIR) sequences. Ann Rheum Dis. 2005;64:1141–1144.

58. Baraliakos X, Davis J, Tsuji W, Braun J. Magnetic resonance imaging examinations of the spine in patients with ankylosing spondylitis before and after therapy with the tumor necrosis factor α receptor fusion protein etanercept. Arthritis Rheum. 2005;52:1216–1233.

59. Dihlmann W. Current radiodiagnostic concept of ankylosing spondylitis. Skeletal Radiol. 1979;4:179–188.

60. Calin A. Radiology and spondylarthritis. Baillieres Clin Rheumatol. 1996;10:455–476.

61. Gaucher AA, Pere PG, Gillet PM. From ankylosing spondylitis to Forestier's disease: ossifying enthesopathy, a unifying concept. J Rheumatol. 1990;17:854–856.

62. Cammisa M, De Serio A, Guglielmi G. Diffuse idiopathic skeletal hyperostosis. Eur J Radiol. 1998;27(suppl 1):S7–S11.

63. de Vlam K, Mielants H, Veys EM. Involvement of the zygapophyseal joint in ankylosing spondylitis: relation to the bridging syndesmophyte. J Rheumatol. 1999;26:1738–1745.

64. Creemers MC, Franssen MJ, van't Hof MA, Gribnau FW, van de Putte LB, van Riel PL. Assessment of outcome in ankylosing spondylitis: an extended radiographic scoring system. Ann Rheum Dis. 2005;64:127–129.

65. Averns HL, Oxtoby J, Taylor HG, Jones PW, Dziedzic K, Dawes PT. Radiological outcome in ankylosing spondylitis: use of the Stoke Ankylosing Spondylitis Spine Score (SASSS). Br J Rheumatol. 1996;35:373–376.

66. Taylor HG, Beswick EJ, Dawes PT. Sulphasalazine in ankylosing spondylitis. A radiological, clinical and laboratory assessment. Clin Rheumatol. 1991;10:43–48.

67. MacKay K, Mack C, Brophy S, Calin A. The Bath Ankylosing Spondylitis Radiology Index (BASRI): a new, validated approach to disease assessment. Arthritis Rheum. 1998;41:2263–2270.

68. Wanders AJ, Landewe RB, Spoorenberg A, et al. What is the most appropriate radiologic scoring method for ankylosing spondylitis? A comparison of the available methods based on the Outcome Measures in Rheumatology Clinical Trials filter. Arthritis Rheum. 2004;50:2622–2632.

69. Spoorenberg A, de Vlam K, van der Linden S, et al. Radiological scoring methods in ankylosing spondylitis. Reliability and change over 1 and 2 years. J Rheumatol. 2004;31:125–132.

70. Romanus R, Yden S. Destructive and ossifying spondylitic changes in rheumatoid ankylosing spondylitis. Acta Orthop Scand. 1952;22:89.

71. Jevtic V, Kos-Golja M, Rozman B, McCall I. Marginal erosive discovertebral "Romanus" lesions in ankylosing spondylitis demonstrated by contrast enhanced Gd-DTPA magnetic resonance imaging. Skeletal Radiol. 2000;29:27–33.

72. Kurugoglu S, Kanberoglu K, Kanberoglu A, Mihmanli I, Cokyuksel O. MRI appearances of inflammatory vertebral osteitis in early ankylosing spondylitis. Pediatr Radiol. 2002;32:191–194.

73. Remedios D, Natali C, Saifuddin A. Case report: MRI of vertebral osteitis in early ankylosing spondylitis. Clin Radiol. 1998;53:534–536.

74. Rasker JJ, Prevo RL, Lanting PJ. Spondylodiscitis in ankylosing spondylitis, inflammation or trauma? A description of six cases. Scand J Rheumatol. 1996;25:52–57.

75. Wienands K, Lukas P, Albrecht HJ. Clinical value of MR tomography of spondylodiscitis in ankylosing spondylitis. Z Rheumatol. 1990;49:356–360.

76. Kabasakal Y, Garrett SL, Calin A. The epidemiology of spondylodiscitis in ankylosing spondylitis—a controlled study. Br J Rheumatol. 1996;35:660–663.

77. Andersson O. Röntgenbilden vid spondylarthritis ankylopoetica. Nord Med Tidskr. 1937;14:2000.

78. Dihlmann W, Delling G. Disco-vertebral destructive lesions (so called Andersson lesions) associated with ankylosing spondylitis. Skeletal Radiol. 1978;3:10–15.

79. Cooper C, Carbone L, Michet CJ, Atkinson EJ, O'Fallon WM, Melton LJ III. Fracture risk in patients with ankylosing spondylitis: a population based study. J Rheumatol. 1994;21: 1877–1882.

80. Modic MT, Steinberg PM, Ross JS, Masaryk TJ, Carter JR. Degenerative disk disease: assessment of changes in vertebral body marrow with MR imaging. Radiology. 1988;166(1 Pt 1): 193–199.

81. Hamilton MG, MacRae ME. Atlantoaxial dislocation as the presenting symptom of ankylosing spondylitis. Spine. 1993;18: 2344–2346.

82. Ramos-Remus C, Gomez-Vargas A, Hernandez-Chavez A, Gomez-Nava JI, Gonzalez-Lopez L, Russell AS. Two year followup of anterior and vertical atlantoaxial subluxation in ankylosing spondylitis. J Rheumatol. 1997;24:507–510.

83. Baraliakos X, Davis J, Tsuji W, Braun J. Magnetic resonance imaging examinations of the spine in patients with ankylosing spondylitis before and after therapy with the tumor necrosis factor alpha receptor fusion protein etanercept. Arthritis Rheum. 2005;52:1216–1223.

84. Rudwaleit M, Baraliakos X, Listing J, et al. Magnetic resonance imaging of the spine and the sacroiliac joints in ankylosing spondylitis before and during therapy with etanercept. Ann Rheum Dis. 2005;64:1305–1310.

85. Hermann KG, Landewé R, Braun J, van der Heijde D, et al. Magnetic resonance imaging of inflammatory lesions in the spine in ankylosing spondylitis clinical trials: Is paramagnetic contrast medium necessary? J Rheumatol. In press.

86. Haibel H, Rudwaleit M, Brandt HC, et al. Preliminary MRI results in patients with active ankylosing spondylitis treated with adalimumab for 12 weeks. Arthritis Rheum. 2004;50(9 suppl):S618.

87. Goldberg AL, Keaton NL, Rothfus WE, Daffner RH. Ankylosing spondylitis complicated by trauma: MR findings correlated with plain radiographs and CT. Skeletal Radiol. 1993;22: 333–336.

88. Fitt G, Hennessy O, Thomas D. Case report 709: Transverse fracture with epidural and small paravertebral hematomata, in a patient with ankylosing spondylitis. Skeletal Radiol. 1992;21: 61–63.

89. Fox MW, Onofrio BM, Kilgore JE. Neurological complications of ankylosing spondylitis. J Neurosurg. 1993;78:871–878.

90. Mitra D, Elvins DM, Speden DJ, Collins AJ. The prevalence of vertebral fractures in mild ankylosing spondylitis and their relationship to bone mineral density. Rheumatology (Oxford). 2000;39:85–89.

91. Vinson EN, Major NM. MR imaging of ankylosing spondylitis. Semin Musculoskelet Radiol. 2003;7:103–113.

92. Hanson JA, Mirza S. Predisposition for spinal fracture in ankylosing spondylitis. AJR Am J Roentgenol. 2000;174:150.

93. Grisolia A, Bell RL, Peltier LF. Fractures and dislocations of the spine complicating ankylosing spondylitis: a report of six cases. Clin Orthop Relat Res. 2004 May;(422):129–134.

94. Bernd L, Blasius K, Lukoschek M. Spinal fractures in ankylosing spondylitis. Z Orthop Ihre Grenzgeb. 1992;130:59–63.

95. Broom MJ, Raycroft JF. Complications of fractures of the cervical spine in ankylosing spondylitis. Spine. 1988;13:763–766.

96. Karasick D, Schweitzer ME, Abidi NA, Cotler JM. Fractures of the vertebrae with spinal cord injuries in patients with ankylosing spondylitis: imaging findings. AJR Am J Roentgenol. 1995;165: 1205–1208.

97. Shih TT, Chen PQ, Li YW, Hsu CY. Spinal fractures and pseudoarthrosis complicating ankylosing spondylitis: MRI manifestation and clinical significance. J Comput Assist Tomogr. 2001;25:164–170.

98. Tyrrell PN, Davies AM, Evans N, Jubb RW. Signal changes in the intervertebral discs on MRI of the thoracolumbar spine in ankylosing spondylitis. Clin Radiol. 1995;50:377–383.

99. Olivieri I, Fiandra E, Muscat C, Barozzi L, Tomassini D, Gerli R. Cervical myelopathy caused by ossification of the posterior longitudinal ligament in ankylosing spondylitis. Arthritis Rheum. 1996;39:2074–2077.

100. Sant SM, O'Connell D. Cauda equina syndrome in ankylosing spondylitis: a case report and review of the literature. Clin Rheumatol. 1995;14:224–226.

101. Abello R, Rovira M, Sanz MP. MRI and CT of ankylosing spondylitis with vertebral scalloping. Neuroradiology. 1988;30:272–275.

102. Edgar MA. Letter: Nervous system involvement in ankylosing spondylitis. BMJ. 1974;1:394.

103. Ahn NU, Ahn UM, Nallamshetty L, et al. Cauda equina syndrome in ankylosing spondylitis (the CES-AS syndrome): meta-analysis of outcomes after medical and surgical treatments. J Spinal Disord. 2001;14:427–433.

104. Mitchell MJ, Sartoris DJ, Moody D, Resnick D. Cauda equina syndrome complicating ankylosing spondylitis. Radiology. 1990;175:521–525.

105. Sparling MJ, Bartleson JD, McLeod RA, Cohen MD, Ginsburg WW. Magnetic resonance imaging of arachnoid diverticula associated with cauda equina syndrome in ankylosing spondylitis. J Rheumatol. 1989;16:1335–1337.

106. Kerslake RW, Mitchell LA, Worthington BS. Case report: CT and MRI of the cauda equina syndrome in ankylosing spondylitis. Clin Radiol. 1992;45:134–136.

107. Tullous MW, Skerhut HE, Story JL, et al. Cauda equina syndrome of long-standing ankylosing spondylitis. Case report and review of the literature. J Neurosurg. 1990;73:441–447.

108. Olivieri I, Barozzi L, Padula A, et al. Retrocalcaneal bursitis in spondyloarthropathy: assessment by ultrasonography and magnetic resonance imaging. J Rheumatol. 1998;25:1352–1357.

109. Olivieri I, Barozzi L, Padula A. Enthesopathy: clinical manifestations, imaging and treatment. Baillieres Clin Rheumatol. 1998;12:665–681.

110. D'Agostino MA, Said-Nahal R, Hacquard-Bouder C, Brasseur JL, Dougados M, Breban M. Assessment of peripheral enthesitis in the spondylarthropathies by ultrasonography combined with power Doppler: a cross-sectional study. Arthritis Rheum. 2003;48:523–533.

111. Barozzi L, Olivieri I, De Matteis M, Padula A, Pavlica P. Seronegative spondylarthropathies: imaging of spondylitis, enthesitis and dactylitis. Eur J Radiol. 1998;27(suppl 1):S12–S17.

112. Remedios D, Martin K, Kaplan G, Mitchell R, Woo P, Rooney M. Juvenile chronic arthritis: diagnosis and management of tibio-talar and sub-talar disease. Br J Rheumatol. 1997;36: 1214–1217.

15

Assessment of Disease Activity, Function, and Quality of Life

Désirée van der Heijde and Robert Landewé

INTRODUCTION

Patients with ankylosing spondylitis (AS) may have symptoms of axial, peripheral joint, and entheseal involvement, as well as extraarticular features such as uveitis, psoriasis, and gut inflammation. These symptoms can either be present simultaneously or in a consecutive order during the course of the disease. All of these different localizations and manifestations need to be taken into account in the assessment of the disease. The heterogeneous presentation of AS makes it impossible to use a single measure appropriately to capture the consequences of the disease: the outcome. In general, we distinguish two types of outcome variables: variables measuring actual disease activity (often referred to as *process variables*), and variables measuring structural changes (often referred to as *outcome variables*). Disease activity may be reversible; structural changes are (largely) irreversible. Both have an impact on the functioning and quality of life of patients. It is essential to assess both the reversible and irreversible consequences of the disease.

Researchers are well aware of the fact that they need validated, reliable, and relevant instruments that are sensitive to change. But for clinicians also it is becoming increasingly important to use this type of instrument in clinical practice. Especially since highly effective treatments have become available recently, it is key for clinicians to know when to start these drugs and how to assess their efficacy. The usefulness of instruments in clinical practice depends on feasibility, even more so than in clinical trials. Another difference between clinical practice and clinical trials is that the instruments should be applicable to an individual patient: Measuring a reliable change in an individual puts demands on instruments with regard to reliability other than just measuring change in a group of patients.

The need to use outcome measures in both research and clinical practice, as well as the fact that the various expressions of the disease should be covered, led the Assessment in Ankylosing Spondylitis (ASAS) International Working Group to develop core sets of outcome assessments, both for use in clinical practice and for research purposes.[1] These sets are partially overlapping but differ on other points. In this chapter we describe the most commonly used outcome assessments for the evaluation of AS, based mainly on the recommendations by the ASAS Working Group.

COMMON ASPECTS OF INSTRUMENTS

Most of the instruments that are used in the assessment of AS are patient derived and completed by the patient.

Answer Modalities

In principal, there are several scales on which they answer questions to present to patients. The simplest is the yes/no or true/false statement (Fig. 15.1). Another commonly used answer modality is the verbal rating scale. Patients pick the word that most closely resembles the status of, e.g., their pain (such as no pain, little pain, moderate pain, severe pain, or unbearable pain). This scale is often preferred by patients, but causes problems for researchers. For example, the answers are difficult to translate into different languages while keeping exactly the same meaning. Another problem is that a change from one state to another state (e.g., no pain to little pain) is not necessarily of the same magnitude as a change at another part of the scale (e.g., from severe pain to unbearable pain), and a change from no pain to moderate pain is not necessarily exactly twice the change from little to severe pain. This methodologic fallacy is often disregarded: in calculations based on verbal rating scales it is usually assumed that the distances between the various categories reflect similar status differences. Moreover, translations into different languages may cause problems, with unintended differences in the performance of the scale in the various languages as a consequence.

A widely used scale is the visual analog scale (VAS). This is a (usually horizontal) line of 10 cm with two anchors. The left anchor represents the best situation (a score of 0) and the right anchor represents the worst situation (a score of 10). Patients are asked to put a vertical mark at the position on the line that best represents the severity of their symptoms or the quality of their status. The distance between the left anchor and the vertical mark is measured and recorded to one decimal point.

An alternative to a VAS is a numerical rating scale (NRS), which consists of a row of numbers from 0 to 10. Patients are asked to put a cross through the number that best reflects their symptoms. The anchors (0 and 10) have the same meaning as on the VAS. A NRS has several advantages over a VAS: it is better understood and accepted by patients, the results are immediately clear without measuring and therefore there are no additional sources of measurement error, and an NRS can be assessed by telephone. Many of the questionnaires used in AS are developed with a VAS. However, it has been proven that this can easily and validly be replaced by an NRS without loosing information.[2] Especially in clinical practice, an NRS is much more feasible than a VAS.

Individual Patient versus Group Level Analysis

In evaluating research, the focus of the primary analysis is often on the group level. Most often, the question is whether one group of patients has a better outcome than another group of patients. This type of analysis may give us important information with regard to the efficacy of an intervention or the contribution of a prognostic factor, and it is important to test the hypothesis of treatment efficacy in randomized clinical trials. However, it only provides limited information to the clinician who has to make decisions regarding an individual patient. Taking the group analysis of a clinical trial as an example, it remains largely unclear if there is a small but homogeneous effect in all patients or a major effect in a small proportion of patients and no effect in the remainder. And if the latter were the case, it is often not possible to investigate further what characterizes the patients with a good response.

Analysis to define whether an individual patient could expect improvement is therefore critical for a good understanding of the treatment effect and the appropriate application of the treatment in clinical practice. In trying to define improvement for an individual patient the clinician must take into consideration the variation due to biologic fluctuation of the disease, errors in assessment, and the influence of other factors such as comorbidity. Consequently, a certain cutoff needs to be defined as the minimum improvement that is considered *real* improvement. For analyses on the average improvement in a clinical trial context, this is of less importance, because the errors are balanced in both groups (assuming that groups were formed by randomization). Often such cutoffs are based on an estimation of measurement error from repeated measures, obtained under conditions in which no change is assumed.[3] Another aid in selecting an appropriate instrument to define improvement in an individual patient is to combine several assessments into one index or use a combined response measure. An example of an index is the Disease Activity Score in rheumatoid arthritis: the values of four different assessments are combined according to a certain formula to obtain one number.[4] A good index is composed of several measures that correlate to some extent with each other, but not too strongly. Indices have the advantage of lower measurement error so that a smaller cutoff can be used than with the use of a single measure. Moreover, indices can also be used to assess an absolute level of disease activity compared with a combined response measure, which can only be used to assess change over time. An example of such a response measure is the ASAS20 response.[5] To fulfill an ASAS20 response, a consistent improvement in at least three domains should be present. The advantage of such a response measure is that if the change in the various assessments points in the same direction (and is of a similar magnitude), it is more likely that the result is based on a real change than on fluctuation by chance only. Consequently, a smaller cutoff can be used (e.g., an improvement of 3.5 on a 10-point scale for a single instrument and a 2-point improvement if changes in three different measures are consistent).

Change versus Status Scores

In addition, to know whether an individual patient has improved, it is also important to know whether the patient has achieved an acceptably low level of discomfort or impairment. Improvement refers to the concept "Do you feel better?"; *acceptable low level* refers to the concept "Do you feel good?" Both are essential and give additional information. The first category is often captured by response or improvement criteria and the second by (partial) remission or low disease activity criteria. These two types of criteria have been developed

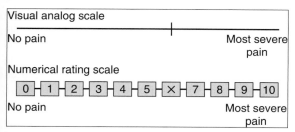

Fig. 15.1 Example of a VAS and NRS for the assessment of pain.

and validated for the assessment of AS (see later for a detailed description).

CORE SETS OF INSTRUMENTS

The ASAS Working Group defined core sets for both research and clinical practice.[1] A core set is the minimum information that should be collected in each study for every patient. Depending on the research question or clinical presentation of the patient, additional data might be collected. For use in research separate core sets were defined for different types of treatment. The following three settings were differentiated: research for the evaluation of disease-controlling antirheumatic therapy (DC-ART), research for the evaluation of symptom-modifying antirheumatic drugs and/or physical therapy, and clinical record keeping. First, the domains that cover the various expressions of AS were defined.[6] Thereafter, for each domain the most appropriate instruments were selected.[7] The domains similar for all three core sets are physical function, pain, spinal mobility, spinal stiffness, fatigue, and patient global assessment. The core sets for clinical record keeping and DC-ART were extended with the domains acute-phase reactants, peripheral joints, and entheses. The DC-ART core set also includes radiographic assessment (Fig. 15.2). For each domain within the core sets, one or several instruments were selected. The definition of core sets including specified instruments helps to create uniformity and comparability in AS clinical trials.

Specific Instruments

The instruments are grouped to reflect first the overall assessment of the disease followed by the assessments of the various presentations of the disease (Table 15.1).

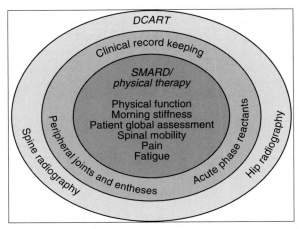

Fig. 15.2 Domains included in the core sets for the assessment of symptom-modifying drugs (SMARD) and/or physical therapy (inner circle), clinical record keeping (inner two circles), and disease-controlling antirheumatic therapy (DC-ART) (all three circles).

TABLE 15.1 SPECIFIC INSTRUMENTS FOR EACH DOMAIN IN CORE SETS FOR DCART, SMARD, PHYSICAL THERAPY, AND CLINICAL RECORD KEEPING (FROM VAN DER HEIJDE ET AL., 1999)

Domain	Instrument
Physical function*	BASFI or Dougados Functional Index
Pain*	VAS/NRS, last week, in spine, at night, due to AS and VAS/NRS, last week, in spine, due to AS
Spinal mobility*	Chest expansion and modified Schober and occiput-to-wall distance and lateral spinal flexion or BASMI
Patient global assessment*	VAS/NRS, last week
Morning stiffness*	Duration of morning stiffness, in spine, last week
Fatigue*	VAS/NRS, last week
Peripheral joints and entheses†	Number of swollen joints (44-joint count) Validated enthesis indexes
Acute phase reactants†	ESR
Spine radiographs‡	Aneroposterior + lateral lumbar and lateral cervical spine and x-ray pelvis (to visualize sacroiliac joint and hips)
Hip radiographs‡	As above

AS, ankylosing spondylitis; BASFI, Bath Ankylosing Spondylitis Functional Index; BASMI, Bath Ankylosing Spondylitis Metrology Index; CRP, C-reactive protein; DCART, disease-controlling antirheumatic therapy; ESR, erythrocyte sedimentation rate; NRS, numerical rating scale; SMARD, symptom-modifying antirheumatic drug; VAS, visual analog scale.
*Included in core sets for DCART, SMARD/physical therapy, and clinical record keeping.
†Included in core sets for DCART and clinical record keeping.
‡Included in core sets for DCART.

Overall level of disease activity and functioning

The domains patient global assessment of disease activity, pain, morning stiffness, fatigue, and physical functioning give an overall view of the activity of the disease. Physical functioning has a special position in this scheme, because it is influenced both by disease activity and by disease severity. Many instruments are answered on a VAS, but as explained earlier, the VAS can easily be changed into the NRS if preferred. All VASs are horizontal and 10 cm long and all NRSs are 11-point scales. The anchors on the left always represent the best clinical situation and those on the right represent the worst clinical situation. The time horizon for the question is defined as "on average last week."

The instruments recommended for the various domains are assessed as follows:

Patient global assessment

The question is answered on a VAS: "How active was your spondylitis on average last week?"

Pain

There are two questions related to pain, one related to the overall level of spinal pain, and one limited to the spinal pain at night. The first question is "How much pain of your spine due to AS did you have?" and the second is "How much pain of your spine due to AS did you have at night?"

Stiffness

Stiffness is assessed by the question: "How long did the morning stiffness of your spine last on average from the time you woke up last week?" This answer is recorded in minutes or on a VAS where the maximum score represents 2 hours. This last VAS is one of the questions of the Bath Ankylosing Spondylitis Disease Activity Index (BASDAI).[8] In the BASDAI the severity of morning stiffness is also included. The overall impact of morning stiffness in the BASDAI is defined as the average of the scale on duration and severity. Often, this combined score is used to define the domain morning stiffness.

Fatigue

There is one general question on the level of fatigue worded as "How would you describe the overall level of fatigue/tiredness you have experienced?" This is again one of the questions of the BASDAI. It has been proved that the information obtained by this simple overall question gives sufficient knowledge on the overall level of fatigue. Only if knowing more about the various aspects of fatigue is important, is it appropriate to use one of the extensive fatigue scales.[9]

Function

To capture functional capacity, two functional indexes are the most widely used: the Bath Ankylosing Spondylitis Functional Index (BASFI) and the Dougados functional index.[10,11] The BASFI consists of 10 questions, answered on a VAS. The final score is the average of the questions, ranging from 0 (no limitation) to 10 (maximal limitation in function). The Dougados functional index has 20 questions answered on a 3- or 5-point verbal rating scale and summed to get the total score. The answers are coded 0, 1, and 2 or 0, 0.5, 1, 1.5, and 2, respectively, to ensure the same range of the final score (0 to 40). Both functional indexes have been shown to be valid and sensitive to differentiate between groups of patients with a different level and/or improvement in physical function. There seems to be little difference in sensitivity to change between the two instruments. Another functional index is the Health Assessment Questionnaire Spine (HAQ-S), which is a version of the HAQ adapted for AS.[12] Although there are some theoretical advantages to use this questionnaire, it is not widely applied in AS.

Axial involvement

Sacroiliitis and spinal features are involved in the concept of axial involvement. However, the anterior chest wall and root joints (shoulders and hips) are also often considered to belong to this concept. The domain spinal mobility comprises four instruments and is assessed as follows.

Chest expansion

With the patient's hands resting on or behind the head, the difference between maximal inspiration and expiration at the fourth intercostal level anteriorly (e.g., 4.4 cm) is assessed. The better of two tries is recorded.

Modified Schober test

A mark is made on the skin on the imaginary line between the two superior, posterior iliac spines, and a second mark is made 10 cm higher than the first mark. The patient bends forward maximally and the distance between the two marks on the skin is measured. The increase above 10 cm should be noted (e.g., 3.4 cm). The better of two tries is recorded.

Occiput-to-wall test

The patient stands with the heels and back against the wall, with hips and knees as straight as possible. The chin should be held at the usual carrying level. The patient should undertake maximal effort to touch the head against the wall. The distance between the wall and the occiput is measured in centimeters (e.g., 9.2 cm). The better of two tries is recorded. Another comparable test is the tragus-to-wall test. The theoretical advantage of this test is that it is less influenced by rotation of the head. This is also the test that is included in the Bath Ankylosing Metrology Index (BASMI).[13] However, in a formal comparison of the two tests, there was no difference in performance of the occiput-to-wall test compared with the tragus-to-wall test.[14] The advantage of the occiput-to-wall test is that a normal test is clearly defined by a result of 0, whereas a tragus-to-wall test result of 12 cm could be normal or abnormal, depending on the magnitude of the head.

Lateral spinal flexion

This is measured by the fingertip-to-floor distance with the patient in full lateral flexion without flexing forward or bending the knees. The patient stands as close to the wall as possible with shoulders level. The distance between patient's middle fingertip and the floor is measured with a tape measure. The patient is asked to bend sideways without bending the knees or lifting the heels and attempting to keep the shoulders in the same plane. A second reading is taken, and the difference between the two is recorded. The better of two tries is recorded for left and right. The mean of left and right gives the final result for lateral spinal flexion (in centimeters to the nearest 0.1 cm).

Peripheral involvement

The 44 swollen joint count should be assessed. Joints included are acromioclavicular joints, humeroscapular joints, sternoclavicular joints, elbows, wrists, metacarpophalangeal joints, proximal interphalangeal joints, knees, ankles, and metatarsophalangeal joints. In clinical practice it is important also to check for involvement of the manubriosternal and sternocostal joints, hips, and distal interphalangeal joints in patients with concomitant psoriasis.

Enthesitis

For clinical studies a few validated enthesitis scores exist. In recent treatment studies an index developed by the Berlin group and another one developed in San Francisco have been used.[15,16] The group in Maastricht derived another index (the Maastricht Ankylosing Spondylitis Enthesitis Score [MASES]) from a large patient cohort based on the prevalence of involvement of the various sites,[17] which was then validated. In clinical practice painful sites should be examined. Frequently involved sites are the plantar fascia (heel pain) and the Achilles tendon. Other commonly involved sites are the pelvis, symphysis, thorax, spine, and large joints. In fact, all entheses can be involved.

Laboratory assessments

Except for acute-phase reactants, laboratory tests are of little value in assessing AS. Both the erythrocyte sedimentation rate after 1 hour according to Westergren (ESR) and C-reactive protein level (CRP) work equally well in following the patient. The absence of an increased ESR or CRP is common in patients with AS and does not rule out inflammation. For reasons of feasibility (mainly costs), the ASAS core sets have a preference for the ESR.

Imaging

For the domain imaging, radiographs of the lateral cervical and lumbar spine should be scored by the modified Stoke Ankylosing Spondylitis Spine Score (mSASSS).[18] The pelvis is important in making the diagnosis and in assessing hip involvement but is less important in following patients over time. More detailed information on imaging is provided in Chapter 14.

Measures not included in the ASAS core set

For the ASAS core set, only single-item variables have been selected. However, in recent years several combined instruments (indices) have become available, especially

from the Bath group in the United Kingdom. These are pooled instruments developed to assess the various aspects of the disease process. The BASDAI is a measure for assessing signs and symptoms of disease activity including fatigue, axial pain, peripheral pain and swelling, entheseal pain, and morning stiffness (duration and severity) (Table 15.2). These items are scored on a VAS, and the average of the five items gives the final score. The ASAS International Working Group advocates use of the BASDAI in clinical practice to evaluate the indication and monitoring of tumor necrosis factor (TNF)–blocking agents.

The metrology index (BASMI) combines information on various aspects of mobility of the spine and hips: tragus to wall distance, modified Schober test, cervical rotation, lateral spinal flexion, and intermalleolar distance. All of these assessments are measured in their usual metric units. Thereafter, each needs to be converted into either a 3-point (0 to 2) or an 11-point (0 to 10) scale using a conversion table. In using the 3-point scale the five measures have to be added to get the final BASMI score. For the 11-point scale the average of the five measures has to be taken. In recent research, the performance of the lateral spinal flexion measurement and the BASMI turned out to be very similar. ASAS recommendations leave it open to the investigator to use either the lateral spinal flexion test alone or the entire BASMI.

Assessment of quality of life

Physical function is a subset of health-related quality of life, and disability is a concept that includes social functioning and adaptation. It is increasingly recognized that disability reflects a multidimensional construct. This view is reflected in the International Classification of

TABLE 15.2 SIX QUESTIONS INCLUDED IN THE BASDAI ANSWERED ON A 10-CM VAS OR A 0 TO 10 NRS*
1. How would you describe the overall level of fatigue/tiredness you have experienced?
2. How would you describe the overall level of AS neck, back, or hip pain you have had?
3. How would you describe the overall level of pain/swelling in joints other than neck, back, or hips you have had?
4. How would you describe the overall level of discomfort you have had from any areas tender to touch or pressure?
5. How would you describe the overall level of discomfort you have had from the time you wake up?
6. How long does your morning stiffness last from the time you wake up?

*To obtain the score calculate the mean of questions 5 and 6. Total the results of questions 1 to 4 and the average of 5 and 6. Divide this by 5 for the BASDAI score (range 0 to 10).

Functioning by the World Health Organization (WHO).[19] However, health-related quality of life and disability are less disease-specific than physical function. In general, there are two groups of instruments: generic instruments, applicable to persons with various conditions, and disease-specific instruments for use in patients with a specific disease. The advantage of generic instruments is that data from persons with different conditions can be compared with each other. A disadvantage is that many questions might not be applicable to the patient category under investigation. Conversely, disease-specific questionnaires are highly accepted and recognized by patients, but the results cannot be directly compared with those for other diseases or for the normal population. Several generic instruments are also applied to patients with AS. These include the World Health Organization Disability Assessment Schedule II (WHODAS) II and the 36-item Medical Outcomes Study Short-Form Health Survey (SF-36).[20,21] The Arthritis Impact Measurement Scales 2 (AIMS-2) is an instrument directed to musculoskeletal disorders and is validated for AS.[22] An instrument specifically developed for use in AS in collaboration with patients with AS is the Ankylosing Spondylitis Quality of Life Questionnaire (ASQoL).[23] This instrument is highly appreciated by patients, sensitive to change over time, and feasible (it takes only 5 minutes to complete). There is insufficient information on the comparison of the performance of the above-mentioned instruments to prefer one for use in trials. The use of both a generic and a disease-specific instrument could yield additive information.

Response criteria

For the evaluation of a response within a trial on an individual patient level, response criteria have been developed. The ASAS20 response criteria were based on the best discrimination between nonsteroidal anti-inflammatory drugs (NSAIDs) and placebo in a combination of a large number of clinical trials and further validated in relation to expert opinion (Box 15.1).[5] The value of the ASAS20 criteria in daily practice is unknown. The following four instruments are included: BASFI or Dougados Functional Index (domain function), morning stiffness (domain inflammation), patient global assessment of disease activity on a VAS (domain patient global assessment), and overall pain on a VAS (domain pain). In summary, three of four domains should be improved by 20% and a minimum of 1 unit on a 0 to 10 scale, and there should be no worsening of 20% and a minimum of 1 unit in the remaining domain. Applying these response criteria resulted in a response rate of 49% in patients in the NSAID-treated arms of clinical trials, compared with 24% in the placebo-treated arms.

With the availability of TNF blocking treatment, an ASAS20 response was achieved in large proportions of patients and also higher levels of response were seen. Therefore, additional response criteria were developed and validated. Two sets of criteria were proposed (Box 15.1).[24] First were the ASAS40 criteria that require a 40% improvement with a minimum of 2 units in at least three of the same four domains as assessed for the

---

BOX 15.1 DEFINITION OF ASAS20, ASAS40, ASAS5/6, AND ASAS PARTIAL REMISSION CRITERIA*

ASAS20 response criteria

Improvement of at least 20% and 1 unit in at least three of the following four domains

Patient global assessment of disease activity

Inflammation assessed as morning stiffness

Function

Pain

Without worsening of 20% and 1 unit in the possible remaining domain

ASAS40 response criteria

Improvement of at least 40% and 2 units in at least three of the following four domains

Patient global assessment of disease activity

Inflammation assessed as morning stiffness

Function

Pain

Without worsening at all in the possible remaining domain

ASAS5/6 response criteria

Improvement of at least 20% in at least five of the following 6 domains

Patient global assessment of disease activity

Inflammation assessed as morning stiffness

Function

Pain

CRP

Spinal mobility

ASAS partial remission criteria

A value below 2 units in all of the four following domains

Patient global assessment of disease activity

Inflammation assessed as morning stiffness

Function

Pain

*All patient reported assessments are assessed on a 0 to 10 scale.

ASAS20 criteria, with no worsening at all in the fourth domain. Second were the ASAS5/6 criteria that require an improvement of at least 20% in at least five of six domains. In addition to the already mentioned four domains, the domains spinal mobility and acute-phase reactants are included. There is no definition of a minimum absolute value of improvement, and the criteria are fulfilled whatever the improvement or worsening is in the sixth domain. Both the ASAS40 and the ASAS5/6 criteria performed better in discriminating patients treated with TNF-blocking agents from patients treated with placebo than many other combinations tried, including, e.g., a 50% improvement in BASDAI or ASAS50. Compared with ASAS20, ASAS40 is merely a quantitative difference: a large improvement in the same domains. The advantage is its simplicity of application and interpretation. In contrast, the ASAS5/6 criteria are qualitatively different: an improvement in at least one additional domain needs to be fulfilled. Because these two domains are objective measures, which are difficult to influence by weak therapies over relatively short periods of time, these data suggest a qualitatively different effect. On the other hand, the meaning of a 20% improvement in ESR/CRP or in spinal mobility is not well known. Further research is needed to define clearly the performance of these two new types of response criteria.

Response criteria are developed and validated for use in clinical trials to discriminate groups of patients. How they perform in following patients in clinical practice is not known; therefore, their use is not recommended to assess effectiveness of treatment in clinical practice. For the purpose of the evaluation of TNF-blocking agents, the ASAS International Working Group has advised the use of improvement of at least 50% in the BASDAI with a minimum of 2 units, in addition to the core set for clinical record keeping.[25]

Status criteria

Apart from the response criteria, the ASAS has proposed a state of *partial remission* as an indication of very low disease activity (see Box 15.1).[5] Partial remission is defined as a value of less than 2 (on a 0 to 10 scale) in all four domains (function, inflammation, patient global assessment, and pain). Stopping therapy is not a prerequisite for fulfilling these criteria, but it will be helpful information to add if patients fulfill the partial remission criteria while using treatment or not.

CONCLUSION

In this chapter, important aspects of assessing disease in general and measuring different aspects of disease in AS in particular, both in the context of research as in the context of clinical practice, have been outlined.

REFERENCES

1. van der Heijde D, van der Linden S, Dougados M, Dougados M, Bellamy N, Russell AS. Ankylosing spondylitis: plenary discussion and results of voting on selection of domains and some specific instruments. J Rheumatol. 1999;26:1003–1005.
2. van Tubergen A, Debats I, Ryser L, et al. Use of a numerical rating scale as an answer modality in ankylosing spondylitis-specific questionnaires. Arthritis Rheum. 2002;47:242–248.
3. Auléley GR, Benbouazza K, Spoorenberg A, et al. Evaluation of the smallest detectable difference in outcome or process variables in ankylosing spondylitis. Arthritis Rheum. 2002;47:582–587.
4. van der Heijde DM, van 't Hof M, van Riel PL, van de Putte LB. Development of a disease activity score based on judgment in clinical practice by rheumatologists. J Rheumatol. 1993;20:579–581.
5. Anderson JJ, Baron G, van der Heijde D, Felson DT, Dougados M. Ankylosing spondylitis assessment group preliminary definition of short-term improvement in ankylosing spondylitis. Arthritis Rheum. 2001;44:1876–1886.
6. van der Heijde D, Bellamy N, Calin A, Dougados M, Khan MA, van der Linden S. Preliminary core sets for endpoints in ankylosing spondylitis. J Rheumatol. 1997;24:2225–2229.
7. van der Heijde D, Calin A, Dougados M, Khan MA, van der Linden S, Bellamy N. Selection of instruments in the core set for DC-ART, SMARD, physical therapy, and clinical record keeping in ankylosing spondylitis. Progress report of the ASAS Working Group. Assessments in Ankylosing Spondylitis. J Rheumatol. 1999;26:951–954.
8. Garrett S, Jenkinson T, Kennedy LG, Whitelock H, Gaisford P, Calin A. A new approach to defining disease status in ankylosing spondylitis: the Bath Ankylosing Spondylitis Disease Activity Index. J Rheumatol. 1994;21:2286–2291.
9. van Tubergen A, Coenen J, Landewé R, et al. Assessment of fatigue in patients with ankylosing spondylitis: a psychometric analysis. Arthritis Rheum. 2002;47:8–16.
10. Calin A, Garrett S, Whitelock H, et al. A new approach to defining functional ability in ankylosing spondylitis: the development of the Bath Ankylosing Spondylitis Functional Index. J Rheumatol. 1994;21:2281–2285.
11. Dougados M, Gueguen A, Nakache JP, Nguyen M, Mery C, Amor B. Evaluation of a functional index and an articular index in ankylosing spondylitis. J Rheumatol. 1988;15:302–307.
12. Daltroy LH, Larson MG, Roberts NW, Liang MH. A modification of the Health Assessment Questionnaire for the spondyloarthropathies. J Rheumatol. 1990;17:946–950.
13. Jenkinson TR, Mallorie PA, Whitelock HC, Kennedy LG, Garrett SL, Calin A. Defining spinal mobility in ankylosing spondylitis (AS). The Bath AS Metrology Index. J Rheumatol. 1994;21:1694–1698.
14. Heuft-Dorenbosch L, Vosse D, Landewé R, et al. Measurement of spinal mobility in ankylosing spondylitis: comparison of occiput-to-wall and tragus-to-wall distance. J Rheumatol. 2004;31:1779–1784.
15. Gorman JD, Sack KE, Davis JC, Jr. Treatment of ankylosing spondylitis by inhibition of tumor necrosis factor alpha. N Engl J Med. 2002;346:1349–1356.
16. Braun J, Brandt J, Listing J, et al. Treatment of active ankylosing spondylitis with infliximab: a randomised controlled multicentre trial. Lancet. 2002;359:1187–1193.
17. Heuft-Dorenbosch L, Spoorenberg A, van Tubergen A, et al. Assessment of enthesitis in ankylosing spondylitis. Ann Rheum Dis. 2003;62:127–132.

18. Wanders AJ, Landewé RB, Spoorenberg A, et al. What is the most appropriate radiologic scoring method for ankylosing spondylitis? A comparison of the available methods based on the Outcome Measures in Rheumatology Clinical Trials filter. Arthritis Rheum. 2004;50:2622–2632.

19. Stucki G. Understanding disability. Ann Rheum Dis. 2003;62: 289–290.

20. van Tubergen A, Landewé R, Heuft-Dorenbosch L, et al. Assessment of disability with the World Health Organisation Disability Assessment Schedule II in patients with ankylosing spondylitis. Ann Rheum Dis. 2003;62:140–145.

21. Ware JE Jr, Sherbourne CD. The MOS 36-item Short-Form Health Survey (SF-36). I. Conceptual framework and item selection. Med Care. 1992;30:473–483.

22. Guillemin F, Challier B, Urlacher F, Vancon G, Pourel J. Quality of life in ankylosing spondylitis: validation of the ankylosing spondylitis Arthritis Impact Measurement Scales 2, a modified Arthritis Impact Measurement Scales Questionnaire. Arthritis Care Res. 1999;12:157–162.

23. Doward LC, Spoorenberg A, Cook SA, et al. Development of the ASQoL: a quality of life instrument specific to ankylosing spondylitis. Ann Rheum Dis. 2003;62:20–26.

24. Brandt J, Listing J, Sieper J, Rudwaleit M, van der Heijde D, Braun J. Development and preselection of criteria for short term improvement after anti-TNFα treatment in ankylosing spondylitis. Ann Rheum Dis. 2004;63:1438–1444.

25. Braun J, Davis J, Dougados M, Sieper J, van der Linden Sj, van der Heijide D. First update of the international ASAS consensus statement for the use of anti-TNF agents in patients with ankylosing spondylitis. Ann Rheum Dis. 2005;doi:10.1136/ard.2005.040758

16 Social and Economic Consequences

Michael M. Ward

INTRODUCTION

As is the case for most chronic illnesses, ankylosing spondylitis (AS) can have profound social and economic consequences for those affected. Symptoms of pain, stiffness, fatigue, functional limitations, and the psychological adjustment to illness can affect how people with AS function at school, home, and work and how they interact with spouses, family members, friends, coworkers, and employers. In this chapter I examine the impact of AS on a person's roles in society, focusing on schooling, interpersonal relationships, participation in recreation and community activities, and employment, using the World Health Organization International Classification of Functioning model.[1] In addition, the economic costs of AS are examined.

In evaluating studies of the socioeconomic consequences of AS, it is important to note the sample of patients. To obtain a true assessment of social and economic consequences, population-based samples should be studied. Population-based studies identify all patients in a given locality, ensuring that the sample represents, in correct proportions, patients across the entire range of severity of AS. Because population-based studies are difficult to perform, community-based studies, which draw participants from multiple different sources in the community, are often used as approximations. Clinic-based samples are convenient but less representative, because the sample is shaped by the factors that promote certain patients to attend the clinic that is studied and that limit other patients from attending. Samples of patients from rheumatology clinics or academic medical centers are probably not representative, because they tend to include higher proportions of patients with AS that is more severe or more difficult to treat. Population-based or community-based samples have rarely been used for studies of the socioeconomic consequences of AS but rather clinic-based samples or surveys of members of patient advocacy groups have been used. The selected nature of these samples should be considered when one evaluates the findings.

SCHOOLING

AS typically begins in late adolescence or young adulthood, by which time most people have completed or are nearing completion of their formal education. Therefore, it might be expected that AS would not influence educational attainment or school performance in most patients. No researchers have examined if AS affects whether individuals continue in school or causes them to shorten their educational careers. Similarly, researchers have not examined the extent to which AS may be responsible for missed days, prolonged absences, limited participation in activities, or poor academic performance in high school or college.

AS begins in childhood or early adolescence in up to 10% of patients.[2] Most studies of juvenile-onset AS focus on medical aspects of the disease, rather than on its socioeconomic consequences.[3–6] Studies of educational outcomes in children with chronic arthritis have included small numbers of patients with juvenile-onset AS, but results for these patients were not reported separately. In general, educational attainment was similar to that of population control subjects, although educational goals may have been affected in 25% of patients.[7,8] Of children, 50% to 60% reported that their arthritis had affected their school performance, but it is not clear whether this association was present among those with juvenile-onset AS or only among those with polyarticular juvenile chronic arthritis.[8,9] Poor school performance was associated with the severity of functional limitations in these children.[9]

Pediatric quality-of-life measures include assessment of functioning in school.[10–13] As these measures become more widely used, more information on the impact of AS on school performance will be available. Additional studies are needed on the effect of AS on educational plans and performance in young adults.

MARRIAGE AND FAMILY LIFE

Marriage

Two of the major social roles of adulthood are those of spouse and parent. Pain, functional limitations, and depression may cause some people with AS to limit social interactions and concerns about body image may influence perceptions of sexual attractiveness. However, there are no data suggesting that AS affects the likelihood of marriage or stable life partnership. The presence of a chronic illness can cause stress in interpersonal relationships. Up to 14% of patients with AS report problems in their relationship with their spouse, and for 7% of patients these problems were rated as very important[14–16] (Table 16.1). These problems were reported three times more often by patients with a high school education or less than by those with at least some college education but were not associated with age, sex, or the duration of AS.[14] However, many other life concerns were more common and had greater importance[14,16] (Table 16.1). It is not known whether the likelihood of divorce differs between people with AS and those without AS.

Social support, most often provided by spouses, can have an important influence on the course of a chronic illness. Better social support predicts improvement in physical functioning over time in persons with AS.[17]

Sexual Relations

The sexual functioning of patients with AS has not been studied extensively. Surveys of men with AS, which included between 17 and 79 men, indicated sexual problems in 32% to 71%, including decreased sexual interest in 39% and pain during intercourse in 25%.[15,18–20] In a larger survey of 303 people with AS (74% men) living in the United Kingdom, only 8.8% endorsed sexual functioning as an area of concern.[16] Patients with more active AS symptoms or more advanced AS would be predicted to report more problems, but in these surveys the presence of sexual problems was not correlated with the severity of AS. One controlled study showed no difference in sexual motivation or satisfaction between 50 men aged 18 to 55 with AS and unaffected men in the same age group, whereas a second study of 65 men with AS showed poorer self-reported ratings of erectile function, orgasmic function, and sexual satisfaction among men with AS compared with unaffected control subjects.[21,22] Erectile dysfunction has been reported by 12% to 13% of men with AS.[19,22] Rare organic causes of ED in AS are cauda equina syndrome and paraplegia after spinal fracture.

Women with AS report more problems with sexual functioning, sexual motivation, and discomfort during sexual activity than do men with AS, and more problems compared with unaffected women.[15,20,21] In a survey of 21 women with AS, one third reported mild pain during intercourse, whereas 19% reported severe pain.[15] Associations with the severity of AS were not examined in these studies. Among patients with hip arthritis, sexual functioning often improves after total hip arthroplasty, although modifications in position may be needed.[23,24]

Activity	Ward[14]		Haywood et al.[16]	
	Proportion Reporting (%)	Rank	Proportion Reporting (%)	Rank
Sports/leisure	31	11	23	4
Household tasks	25	14	15	6
Job performance	24	15	40	1
Participation in community groups	15	18	NA	NA
Relationship with spouse	14	19	13	15
Relationship with family members	12	20	8	22
Social activities/relationship with friends	8	22	13	14
Hobbies	NA	NA	10	19
Sex life	NA	NA	9	21

TABLE 16.1 PREVALENCE OF CONCERNS IN SPECIFIC AREAS OF HEALTH-RELATED QUALITY OF LIFE IN TWO LARGE SURVEYS OF PATIENTS WITH AS*

*In the study by Ward,[14] the rank is the order of prevalences among 23 general areas of health-related quality of life. In the study by Haywood et al.,[16] the rank is the order of prevalences among 67 specific activities nominated by respondents. NA, not available.

Reproductive Decisions and Parenting

Fertility is normal in people with AS, but men treated with sulfasalazine may develop oligospermia and decreased fertility.[25] Although many people with AS are concerned about the possibility of having children who develop AS, the limited data available suggest that this concern does not influence the decision to have children or decisions about family size.[25] Mothers with AS often have problems caring for newborns and young children, particularly lifting, carrying, and bathing them.[20,26] These difficulties may be compounded by postpartum flares of AS.[27,28] A need for assistance with child-care tasks was reported by 30% of mothers with AS.[26] Because caring for newborns can be physically demanding, attention should be paid to the spacing of pregnancies.

Family Life

In two large surveys of 175 and 303 people with AS, relationships with family members were noted as areas of concern for 12% and 8%, respectively, and the ability to look after or play with children or grandchildren was a concern for 12%[14,16] (Table 16.1). Illness in a child can also contribute to problems in family life. In a study of 12 children with juvenile spondyloarthropathy, the degree of chronic family stress and support was rated as moderate and was similar to that for families with children who have with juvenile chronic arthritis.[29] These findings suggest that family life may be affected for a small proportion of people with AS. Demands on caregivers have not been explored, but complete dependency or nursing home placement because of physical limitations or a need for care is rare.

SOCIAL INTERACTIONS AND LEISURE

Social Interactions

Limitations in social life can occur in interactions with friends or coworkers, with participation in social, professional, or volunteer organizations, or with participation in neighborhood or civic life. In two surveys of people with AS, 6% to 13% of respondents reported a problem or concern with relationships with friends or coworkers[14,16] (Table 16.1). Participation in community groups was noted as a problem by 15%.[14] Although problems in social interactions may have been reported by only a small proportion, people with AS have worse social functioning than the general public, as measured by the Medical Outcomes Study Short-Form 36 (SF-36).[30] In cross-sectional studies, poorer social functioning has been associated with lower levels of education, more functional limitations, more active AS, and more fatigue but was similar between men and women and was not associated with age.[14,30–33] The potential impact of social interactions on quality of life in AS has been highlighted by the inclusion of three items on social interactions (activities with family and friends, missing out on activities, and letting people down) in the AS Quality of Life Questionnaire.[34]

Leisure

Leisure activities may be affected earlier and more universally in AS than work activities. In surveys of patients, concerns about participation in sports and leisure activities were noted by 23% to 31%, although fewer expressed concerns about hobbies and pastimes[14,16] (Table 16.1). Because leisure activities are discretionary, individuals may sacrifice participation in sports and hobbies to focus more attention on maintaining energy and controlling symptoms to allow themselves to work. For younger individuals with active AS, this may apply particularly to physically demanding sports. Patients are often advised not to participate in contact sports or activities that have a potential for spinal injury, such as horseback riding or skydiving. It is not known how commonly individuals with AS modify their participation in sports, change activities, or give up favored activities to accommodate their illness.

EMPLOYMENT

Choice of Career and Vocational Rehabilitation

Many people have made vocational plans or have begun their careers by the time symptoms of AS develop. For people whose AS begins in adolescence or young adulthood, it is not known how often the diagnosis influences their initial choice of career. However, changes in type of work over the course of AS are not uncommon. In surveys of clinic-based cohorts, 8% to 28% of employed people report having changed jobs sometime during the first 20 to 25 years of AS, most often to less strenuous work.[15,35–38] A large survey of patients in the Netherlands found that half changed job activities after diagnosis, and for 30% of individuals, job choice was influenced by AS.[39] In a 4-year prospective study of work ability in patients with AS, women and those with physically demanding jobs were more likely to change their type of work than were men and those with less strenuous jobs.[38] Patients with higher levels of self-reported pain were also more likely to change their type of work.

Job counseling, vocational rehabilitation, and workplace accommodations can help maintain employment when it is threatened by illness. Whether vocational rehabilitation is effective may depend on appropriate timing of the intervention and appropriate selection of candidates. In a French study of patients with AS followed during the 1970s and 1980s, vocational counseling and job training were used by 36% of patients and were associated with a 62% decrease in risk of work disability after 20 years of AS.[40] In contrast, in a California study of patients followed in the 1980s and 1990s, only 8% of patients received vocational rehabilitation, and its use was associated with a greater than threefold increased risk of permanent work disability.[38] In the latter setting, rehabilitation may have been used too late in the course of disablement to effect much change, serving only as a marker of those destined for work disability. In a recent Dutch study it was estimated that 25% of withdrawals from the labor force could be prevented by job training after the diagnosis of AS and 73% of withdrawals could be prevented by technical or ergonomic adjustments in job tasks.[39]

Employment discrimination due to AS has not been systematically examined but may occur for some potentially hazardous occupations. Legal protections have been established in many countries to prevent employment discrimination based on physical limitations, such as those that might be associated with AS. Difficulty obtaining medical or life insurance, or securing full coverage, may occur after AS is diagnosed.[41]

Job Performance

Illness may affect job performance by causing affected individuals to take days off work, reduce their hours of work, or require help from coworkers to complete certain tasks. These limitations in job performance represent interactions between the nature of the illness and the health status of the worker, his or her social situation, and the type of work. Risks differ between manual workers and those with professional or clerical jobs, between those who need to provide for themselves and those who can depend on others for economic support, and between those whose employers have supportive policies regarding sick leave and those with restrictive workplace policies, as well as between those with active AS or functional limitations and those without active AS or functional limitations. The proportion of people with AS who have problems in job performance will depend on the characteristics of the work and the social setting as well as the characteristics of AS in the groups that are studied.

Sick leaves are common among people with AS. In studies from the 1980s that examined groups with high proportions of manual workers, sick leaves had been taken by 60% to 70% of patients at some time during their work history.[15,42] These leaves often lasted longer than 2 months. In a French study, sick leaves lasting longer than 4 weeks were taken by 32% of workers with a mean duration of AS of 14 years, half of whom had physically demanding jobs.[40] In two more recent studies, which included higher proportions of white-collar workers, sick leaves had been taken by 50% of patients followed over 2 years and by 14% of patients followed

over 6 months.[38,43] The number of sick days per year ranged from 6 to 18.5, but the number of sick days attributed specifically to AS has been estimated to be 10 days per year.[43,44] These estimates are derived from reports of patients treated by rheumatologists and therefore probably represent a subset of patients with more severe AS.[45] Sick leaves and a higher number of days lost from work are more common among people with more active AS, higher levels of self-reported pain, more functional limitations, peripheral arthritis, and concomitant inflammatory bowel disease (IBD) and those employed in manual labor.[38,40,43]

Of patients with AS who are employed, 11% to 30% work part-time or have reduced work hours.[37-39,46,47] Part-time employment is more common among women with AS and is associated with more active symptoms, greater functional limitations, lower levels of formal education, and employment in manual jobs.[37,38,46]

Of workers with AS, 24% report needing help from coworkers.[38,39] This occurs more often for those with physically demanding jobs or during periods of more active symptoms.[38] Having supportive coworkers may help prevent permanent work disability.[39]

Work Disability

The likelihood of permanent work disability is also determined by the severity of a person's AS, his or her social situation, the characteristics of the work, and societal responses to disability. Estimates of the frequency of work disability are based mainly on cross-sectional studies of patients of diverse ages and durations of AS* (Table 16.2). Because permanent work disability is a cumulative process and increases with age, these cross-sectional estimates are less helpful in judging the impact of AS on work ability. Individuals in these studies had not been observed for the same length of time, and some may not have had AS long enough to manifest work disability. A more accurate picture comes from studies showing the proportion of individuals with work disability after a specific number of years of AS, as in a life table analysis, because these proportions are standardized for the length of observation.[35,36,38,51] Ideally, these studies should include only people who were employed at the onset of AS. This criterion removes from consideration individuals who are not susceptible to work loss due to AS.

Studies also differ in how work disability is represented. Although some researchers report the proportion of work-disabled people, most report the proportion employed. The proportion employed may be a misleading reflection of work disability if homemakers, those out of work because of economic downturns, or

---

*References 15, 35–38, 40, 42, 43, 45–54

TABLE 16.2 EMPLOYMENT AND WORK DISABILITY IN PERSONS WITH AS

Study (Ref.)	Country	N	Mean Age (years)	Mean Duration of AS (years)	% Male	% Professional	% Manual Labor	% Employed	Employed at 20 years	Employed at 30 years	% Work Disabled
Lehtinen, 1981[35]	Finland	76	—	30.5	89	—	84	—	82	53	16
Carette et al., 1983[48]	Canada	51	62	38	100	—	—	54	—	—	—
Urbanek et al., 1984[42]	Czechoslovakia	170	—	—	83	—	56	61	—	—	—
McGuigan et al., 1984[36]	New Zealand	60	44	24	78	15	—	85	79	73	15
Gran and Husby, 1984[45]	Norway—hospital based	74	37	13.6	74	—	—	63	—	—	—
Gran and Husby, 1984[45]	Norway—population based	27	42	17.7	81	—	—	89	—	—	—
Gran and Husby, 1984[45]	Norway	126	38	13.9	65	—	—	68	—	—	—
Wordsworth and Mowat, 1986[15]	United Kingdom	100	42	20	79	26	26	84	—	—	9
Kaarela et al., 1987[50]	Finland	20	38	—	—	—	—	85	—	—	15

Guillemin et al., 1990[40]	France	182	—	14	88	—	—	64	—	—	36
Ringsdal et al., 1991[51]	Denmark	193	45	21	63	46	—	72	85	81	28
Edmunds et al., 1991[52]	United Kingdom	120	48	24	78	—	—	68	—	—	—
Gran and Skomsvoll, 1997[46]	Norway	100	42	16	67	—	—	63	—	—	—
Roussou et al., 1997[53]	United Kingdom	1044	43	21	100	37	10	85	—	—	—
Zink et al., 2000[54]	Germany	8776	44	15	69	—	—	71	—	—	—
Ward and Kuzis, 2001[38]	United States	234	48	21	70	45	—	87	87	84	13
Boonen et al., 2001[37]	Netherlands	529	44	11.7	76	—	34	71	—	—	23
Barlow et al., 2001[47]	United Kingdom	133	49	28	73	—	—	80	—	—	20
Boonen et al., 2002[43]	Europe	209	43	11	70	—	39	54	—	—	29

those retired because of old age are included in the group studied. These other categories of employment status deplete the proportion employed, but do not add to the proportion work disabled. In addition, most researchers consider only whether or not the person is work disabled and do not make a specific attribution to AS, although this would probably be the cause for most individuals. Early retirement prompted by AS is also not captured well.

Almost all studies of employment in AS are from Europe, with many from the 1980s or early 1990s* (Table 16.2). Sixteen studies included patients from rheumatology clinics or members of patient support groups. Although the results are heterogeneous, between 80% and 90% of people are employed at a median duration of AS of 20 years. Findings are similar for those studies that report the proportion employed at 20 years.[35,36,38,51] There was no obvious trend of higher employment percentages in more recent studies, although differences in the nature of the patients studied make such comparisons difficult. The results of studies with longer times of observation are also heterogeneous, but more recent studies indicate that more than 80% of patients remain employed at 30 years of AS.[38,51] The importance of the sample of patients is highlighted by a study from Norway comparing employment between a group of patients at a referral hospital and a group from an epidemiologic study.[45] The employment rate was 63% in the hospital-based group and 89% in the population-based group, despite a longer mean duration of AS in the population-based group.

Despite low absolute levels of work disability, people with AS are estimated to have three times the risk of permanent work disability than an age- and sex-matched group of the general population.[37] This risk is somewhat higher for men than women and decreases with age. This high relative risk of permanent work disability is a consequence of the young age of many people with AS and the very low rates of work disability in the general population at these ages.

Risk Factors for Work Disability

Although the cumulative risk of work disability increases with the duration of AS, it is not clear whether work disability develops at a constant rate or whether certain times in the course of AS pose more risk than others. Two studies indicated that the risk is fairly uniform throughout the course of AS, but an early study suggested that the risk was greatest in the first 15 years.[36,38,51] In contrast, an association between work disability and complete spinal fusion suggests

that the risk may be higher among patients with more long-standing AS.[46] Onset of AS at an older age increases the risk of work disability, perhaps because these patients are less able to accommodate to their new circumstances.[37,38]

The risk factors identified most consistently are socioeconomic status and occupation. People with university-level educations are 1.4 to 4 times more likely to remain employed than people with lower levels of education.[38,42,46,47,54] This association is probably related to occupational status and the greater likelihood of manual labor or heavy physical activity among those with less formal education. Higher occupational status has also been associated with lower risks of work disability, and heavy physical activity at work or prolonged standing at work increases the risk of work disability.[35,37,38,40,53,55]

More active AS, more depressive symptoms, and greater functional limitations have been associated with work disability in cross-sectional studies, but assessment of these symptoms postdated the loss of work in these studies.[47,53] Hip arthritis and particularly total hip arthroplasty have been linked to work disability in some studies, as has the presence of comorbid medical conditions.[36,46,47]

In two studies a broad range of potential risk factors for work disability in large cohorts of patients have been examined with multivariate analyses to identify independent predictors of work disability. In a retrospective cohort study of 234 patients followed for a median of 21 years, 31 patients developed permanent work disability.[38] Among these patients, independent risk factors for work disability were older age at onset of AS and having a more physically demanding job, whereas higher levels of formal education were protective. In a second retrospective cohort study of 529 patients followed for a mean of 12 years, 123 patients developed permanent work disability due to AS.[37] Independent risk factors for work disability in this study were older age at onset of AS, working in a manual job, and unfavorable coping with pain and functional limitations. These findings indicate that avoidance of physically demanding work is likely to be an effective strategy to maintain employment for people with AS.

COSTS AND HEALTH CARE UTILIZATION

Components of Costs and Cost Measurement

The total costs of an illness are composed of direct costs, indirect costs, and intangible costs.[56] Direct costs represent the resources used in the provision of medical care and the costs of obtaining care. These include the costs of visits to physicians and other health care

---

*References 15, 35–38, 40, 42, 43, 45–54

providers, hospitalizations, medications and other treatments, assistive devices, and diagnostic tests, as well as the costs of transportation and child care to allow medical appointments to be kept. In the most common approach to estimating costs of illness, patients report the number and types of health care services or treatments used. Each service or treatment is assigned a standard dollar cost, and the number of services or treatments used are multiplied by unit costs. These are then summed to obtain an estimate of direct costs. Health care use thus forms the basis of direct cost estimates.

Indirect costs represent the costs of lost productivity. For people in the workforce, indirect costs represent the costs associated with time off work due to illness, either in the form of sick days, temporary sick leaves, or permanent work disability. These costs may be estimated using the people's preabsence wages or, to obtain more generalized estimates, by the age- and sex-specific wages of full-time workers in the local area. Using the human capital approach, indirect costs accrue for the duration of work loss. Indirect costs for people not in the workforce (homemakers and retirees) can be estimated for the time lost from household work due to illness, valued either at the level of wages of full-time workers of the same age and sex (opportunity costs) or the wages of domestic workers (replacement costs). Intangible costs represent the costs of reductions in quality of life associated with having an illness. Because these costs are difficult to value economically, intangible costs are rarely estimated.

Because the costs of medical care are, in many instances, shared by patients, insurers, and the government, the costs of illness borne by the patient (out-of-pocket expenses) or by the insurer differ from the costs to society as a whole. Most researchers use the societal perspective and calculate costs regardless of the payer. Costs may also be calculated as those attributable to AS or as costs regardless of whether they were due to AS or to a comorbid medical condition. This distinction may be important if the group studied includes many older patients with comorbid conditions or many patients with coexisting IBD.

Cost Identification

Two comprehensive cost identification studies in AS have been reported. Both studies, one American and one European, were prospective studies conducted in the mid- to late-1990s and were based on patient-reported health resource use and lost productivity.[43,57,58] In both studies costs attributed to AS were examined using the societal perspective. In the European study average costs over 2 years were examined, whereas in the American study costs over 1 year were examined. Yearly costs were stable over time in a subset of patients in the American study who were followed for 5 years. The American study included 241 patients, with a mean age of 47 years and mean duration of AS of 19.8 years. The European study included 209 patients, with a mean age of 43 years and mean duration of AS of 11.1 years. Seven percent of patients in the European study had IBD (with its costs attributed to AS), whereas such patients were excluded from the American study. In a third study of the costs of AS from France the perspective of the payer rather than society was used and several categories of direct costs were omitted, resulting in cost estimates that are less relevant than those of the more recent studies.[59]

In the American study, mean annual total costs associated with AS were $6720 per patient (in 1999 U.S. dollars), and the median annual total costs were $1495 per patient (Table 16.3).[58] Indirect costs accounted for 74% of the total costs. Of the indirect costs, 86% were due to permanent work disability experienced by 30 patients.

Mean annual total costs in the European study were €9452 per patient (in 1998 €; $8079); median total costs were not reported.[57] Indirect costs accounted for 72% of the total costs. Most of the indirect costs in this study were also due to permanent work disability.[43] Costs from the perspective of the payer (insurer) or the patient (out-of-pocket expenses) were substantially lower than when costs were computed from the societal perspective.[57,60]

In the American study, annual direct costs averaged $1775 per patient (median $1113).[58] Medication costs,

	TABLE 16.3 COSTS OF AS FROM THE SOCIETAL PERSPECTIVE*					
	Ward[58]			Boonen et al.[43,55]		
	Mean ($)	Median ($)	% Mean Total Costs	Mean (€)	Median (€)	% Mean Total Costs
Total costs	6720	1495	—	9452	NR	—
Direct costs	1775	1113	26	2640	1242	28
Indirect costs	4945	0	74	6812	NR	72

*Costs are reported in 1999 U.S. dollars, and 1998 Euros. NR, not reported.

mostly for nonsteroidal anti-inflammatory drugs, comprised the largest portion of direct costs (42%; Fig. 16.1). Hospitalizations and ambulatory care visits contributed 16% and 15% of direct costs, respectively, whereas diagnostic tests and paid household help each contributed 11% of direct costs. Costs for assistive devices, alternative treatments, and transportation to visits made minor contributions.

Annual direct costs in the European study averaged €2640 per patient (median €1242).[57] The largest contributors to direct costs were hospitalizations, ambulatory care visits, and household help, each of which comprised more than 20% of total costs (Fig. 16.1). In contrast to the American study, medication costs comprised only 13% of total costs. Differences between the American and European study could arise from differences in characteristics of the patients studied or the costs assigned to services or treatments used but also serve to highlight different strategies for managing AS. Inpatient care and physical therapy were much more commonly used by the European patients than by the American patients, whereas the frequency of outpatient visits to physicians was comparable[57,58] (Table 16.4). Of the 28 European patients who received inpatient care, 12 patients were admitted for treatment of active AS, 6 for orthopedic

procedures, and 9 for IBD. Four of the 7 patients in the American study who were hospitalized were admitted for treatment of complications of nonsteroidal anti-inflammatory drug use, and none was admitted for active AS. A similar emphasis on inpatient care and physical therapy was present among patients with early AS in a Dutch study conducted in the late 1980s.[61]

Direct medical costs, regardless of whether the costs were related to AS treatment or to other medical conditions, in the American study averaged $2674 per patient.[58] AS was the predominant cause of health care utilization and treatment costs for most patients in this cohort. In half of patients, AS-related direct costs accounted for 90% of their all-cause direct costs, and for two-thirds of patients, AS-related direct costs accounted for 75% of their all-cause direct costs.

Both cost identification studies were performed before the use of anti–tumor necrosis factor (TNF) medications in AS. Use of these medications will increase direct costs for medications and ambulatory care visits and possibly costs of hospitalizations to treat medication-related toxicities. Cost-benefit analyses will need to be done to assess whether these medications can decrease or prevent work loss, particularly permanent work disability, to offset these increased direct costs. In Europe, use of these medications may decrease hospitalizations for the treatment of active AS, a benefit not applicable in the United States. Therefore, cost-benefit analyses of anti-TNF medications might differ between Europe or other areas where inpatient care is used for active AS, and the United States and areas where inpatient care is uncommonly used.

The increasing emphasis on early diagnosis could increase direct costs if magnetic resonance imaging of the sacroiliac joints is used more routinely for this purpose in the future. However, because repeated imaging is not usually done, the costs of these procedures are not sustained and would likely contribute little to cumulative costs. Recurrent and high costs, such as those associated with anti-TNF medications, would have a much greater impact. Use of these medications early in the course of AS would need to be targeted to those patients most at risk for poor outcomes, particularly those with severe functional limitations and work disability, to be economically justifiable. Prognostic markers that are highly specific for these outcomes, yet are present early in the course of illness, are needed to guide this treatment strategy.

Predictors of Costs of Illness

Because indirect costs comprise the majority of total costs of AS, the predictors of total costs are similar to the predictors of work disability, which is the major determinant of indirect costs. The degree of functional limitation is the major predictor of total costs.[43,58] Each

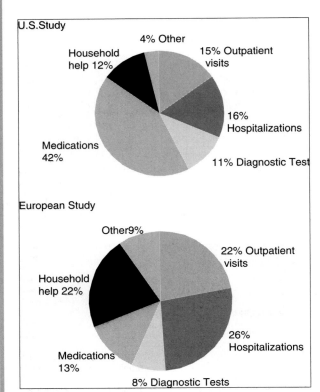

Fig. 16.1 Proportion of direct costs of AS contributed by categories of health care use, treatments, or services.

TABLE 16-4 HEALTH CARE UTILIZATION PER YEAR BY PATIENTS WITH AS				
	Ward[58]		Boonen et al.[43,55]	
	Proportion of Patients With Any Use	Mean Number of Visits/Days*	Proportion of Patients With Any Use	Mean Number of Visits/Days*
Rheumatologist visits	68	2.1	NR	NR
Other physician visits	48	2.1	NR	NR
Specialist visits	NR	NR	77	2.7
General practitioner visits	NR	NR	64	1.9
Other health care provider visits	12	0.6	21	0.4
Physical therapy or occupational therapy visits	16	1.3	60	19.1
Inpatient hospital days	3	0.03	6-8[†]	2.3

*Mean for all patients, regardless of use of service. NR = not reported.
[†]Proportion hospitalized varied between 6% and 8% over the 2 years of the study.

1-point increase in the Health Assessment Questionnaire Disability Index increased the likelihood that annual total costs were greater than $10,000 by threefold.[58] The severity of stiffness was also associated with higher total costs.

Functional limitation is also an important predictor of direct costs, along with greater AS activity, longer duration of AS, and lower levels of formal education.[57,58] Women also tend to have higher direct costs than men, even after adjustments for the severity of AS. Given the strong association of functional limitations with both direct and indirect costs, treatments that reduced functional disability would be the most effective means to decrease the costs of AS.

REFERENCES

1. World Health Organization. International Classification of Functioning, Disability, and Health (ICF). Geneva, Switzerland: World Health Organization, 2001.
2. Burgos-Vargas R, Pacheco-Tena C, Vasquez-Mellado J. Juvenile-onset spondyloarthropathies. Rheum Dis Clin North Am. 1997;23:569–598.
3. Garcia-Morteo O, Maldonada-Cocco JA, Suarez-Almazor ME, Garay E. Ankylosing spondylitis of juvenile onset: comparison with adult onset disease. Scand J Rheumatol. 1983;12:246–248.
4. Calin A, Elswood J. The natural history of juvenile-onset ankylosing spondylitis: a 24 year retrospective case-control study. Br J Rheumatol. 1988;27:91–93.
5. Burgos-Vargas R, Vazquez-Mellado J, Cassis N, et al. Genuine ankylosing spondylitis in children: a case-control study of patients with early definite disease according to adult onset criteria. J Rheumatol. 1996;23:2140–2147.
6. Minden K, Kiessling U, Listing J, Zink A. German Study Group of Pediatric Rheumatologists. Prognosis of patients with juvenile chronic arthritis and juvenile spondyloarthropathy. J Rheumatol 2000;27:2256–2263.
7. Minden K, Niewerth M, Listing J, et al. Long-term outcome in patients with juvenile idiopathic arthritis. Arthritis Rheum 2002;46:2392–2401.
8. Gare BA, Fasth A. The natural history of juvenile chronic arthritis: a population-based cohort study. II. Outcome. J Rheumatol. 1995;22:308–319.
9. Flatø B, Aasland A, Vinje O, Førre Ø. Outcome and predictive factors in juvenile rheumatoid arthritis and juvenile spondyloarthropathy. J Rheumatol. 1998;25:366–375.
10. Duffy CM, Arsenault L, Duffy KNW, Paquin JD, Strawczynski H. The Juvenile Arthritis Quality of Life Questionnaire—Development of a new responsive index for juvenile rheumatoid arthritis and juvenile spondyloarthritides. J Rheumatol. 1997;24:738–746.
11. Landgraf JM, Abetz L, Ware JE. The CHQ User's Manual. Boston, Mass: The Health Institute, New England Medical Center, 1996.
12. Raat H, Bonsel GJ, Essink-Bot M-L, Landgraf JM, Gemke RJBJ. Reliability and validity of comprehensive health status measures in children: the Child Health Questionnaire in relation to the Health Utilities Index. J Clin Epidemiol 2002;55:67–76.
13. Varni JW, Seid M, Knight TS, Burwinkle T, Brown J, Szer IS. The PedsOL in pediatric rheumatology. Reliability, validity, and responsiveness of the Pediatric Quality of Life Inventory Generic Core scales and Rheumatology module. Arthritis Rheum 2002;46:714–725.
14. Ward MM. Health-related quality of life in ankylosing spondylitis: a survey of 175 patients. Arthritis Care Res. 1999;12:247–255.
15. Wordsworth BP, Mowat AG. A review of 100 patients with ankylosing spondylitis with particular reference to socioeconomic effects. Br J Rheumatol. 1986;25:175–180.
16. Haywood KL, Garratt AM, Dziedzic K, Dawes PT. Patient centered assessment of ankylosing spondylitis-specific health related quality of life: evaluation of the Patient Generated Index. J Rheumatol. 2003;30:764–773.
17. Ward MM. Predictors of the progression of functional disability in patients with ankylosing spondylitis. J Rheumatol 2002;29:1420–1425.
18. Brown GMM, Dare CM, Smith PR, Meyers OL. Important problems identified by patients with chronic arthritis. S Afr Med J. 1987;72:126–128.
19. Gordon D, Beastall GH, Thomson JA, Sturrock RD. Androgenic status and sexual function in males with rheumatoid arthritis and ankylosing spondylitis. Q J Med. 1986;60:671–679.

20. Chamberlain MA. Socioeconomic effects of ankylosing spondylitis in females: a comparison of 25 female with 25 male subjects. Int Rehabil Med. 1983;5:149–153.

21. Elst P, Sybesma T, van der Stadt RJ, Prins APA, Hissink Muller W, den Butter A. Sexual problems in rheumatoid arthritis and ankylosing spondylitis. Arthritis Rheum. 1984;27:217–220.

22. Pirildar T, Muezzinoglu T, Pirildar S. Sexual function in ankylosing spondylitis: a study of 65 men. J Urol 2004;171:1598–600.

23. Stern SH, Fuchs MD, Ganz SB, Classi P, Sculco TP, Salvati EA. Sexual function after total hip arthroplasty. Clin Orthop. 1991;269:228–235.

24. Wiklund I, Romanus B. A comparison of quality of life before and after arthroplasty in patients who had arthrosis of the hip joint. J Bone Joint Surg Am. 1991;73:765–769.

25. Østensen M, Husby G. Ankylosing spondylitis and pregnancy. Rheum Dis Clin North Am. 1989;15:241–254.

26. Østensen M, Østensen H. Ankylosing spondylitis—the female aspect. J Rheumatol. 1998;25:120–124.

27. Østensen M, Husby G. A prospective clinical study of the effect of pregnancy on rheumatoid arthritis and ankylosing spondylitis. Arthritis Rheum. 1983;26:1155–1159.

28. Østensen M, Fuhrer L, Mathieu R, Seitz M, Villiger PM. A prospective study of pregnant patients with rheumatoid arthritis and ankylosing spondylitis using validated clinical instruments. Ann Rheum Dis. 2004;63:1212–1217.

29. Vandvik IH, Høyeraal HM, Fagertun H. Chronic family difficulties and stressful life events in recent onset juvenile arthritis. J Rheumatol. 1989;16:1088–1092.

30. Dagfinrud H, Mengshoel AM, Hagen KB, Loge JH, Kvien TK. Health status of patients with ankylosing spondylitis: a comparison with the general population. Ann Rheum Dis. 2004;63:1605–1610.

31. van Tubergen A, Landewe R, Heuft-Dorenbosch L, et al. Assessment of disability with the World Health Organisation Disability Assessment Schedule II in patients with ankylosing spondylitis. Ann Rheum Dis. 2003;62:140–145.

32. Bostan EE, Borman P, Bodue H, Barca N. Functional disability and quality of life in patients with ankylosing spondylitis. Rheumatol Int. 2003;23:121–126.

33. van Tubergen A, Coenen J, Landewe R, et al. Assessment of fatigue in patients with ankylosing spondylitis: a psychometric analysis. Arthritis Care Res. 2002;47:8–16.

34. Haywood KL, Garratt AM, Jordan K, Dziedzic K, Dawes PT. Disease-specific, patient-assessed measures of health outcome in ankylosing spondylitis: reliability, validity and responsiveness. Rheumatology (Oxford). 2002;41:1295–1302.

35. Lehtinen K. Working ability of 76 patients with ankylosing spondylitis. Scand J Rheumatol. 1981;10:263–265.

36. McGuigan LE, Hart HH, Gow PJ, Kidd BL, Grigor RR, Moore TE. Employment in ankylosing spondylitis. Ann Rheum Dis. 1984;43:604–606.

37. Boonen A, Chorus A, Miedema H, et al. Withdrawal from labour force due to work disability in patients with ankylosing spondylitis. Ann Rheum Dis. 2001;60:1033–1039.

38. Ward MM, Kuzis S. Risk factors for work disability in patients with ankylosing spondylitis. J Rheumatol. 2001;28:315–321.

39. Chorus AMJ, Boonen A, Miedema HS, van der Linden S. Employment perspectives of patients with ankylosing spondylitis. Ann Rheum Dis. 2002;61:693–699.

40. Guillemin F, Braincon S, Pourel J, Gaucher A. Long-term disability and prolonged sick leaves as outcome measurements in ankylosing spondylitis. Possible predictive factors. Arthritis Rheum. 1990;33:1001–1006.

41. Boonen A, van Tubergen A, van der Linden S. Insurance problems among patients with ankylosing spondylitis. Ann Rheum Dis. 2003;62:1242–1243.

42. Urbanek T, Sitajova H, Hudakova G. Problems of rheumatoid arthritis and ankylosing spondylitis patients in their labor and life environments. Czech Med. 1984;7:78–89.

43. Boonen A, van der Heijde D, Landewe R, et al. Work status and productivity costs due to ankylosing spondylitis: comparison of three European countries. Ann Rheum Dis. 2002;61:429–437.

44. Boonen A, Chorus A, Miedema H, van der Heijde D, van der Tempel H, van der Linden S. Employment, work disability, and work days lost in patients with ankylosing spondylitis: a cross sectional study of Dutch patients. Ann Rheum Dis. 2001;60:353–358.

45. Gran JT, Husby G. Ankylosing spondylitis: a comparative study of patients in an epidemiological survey, and those admitted to a department of rheumatology. J Rheumatol. 1984;11:788–793.

46. Gran JT, Skomsvoll JF. The outcome of ankylosing spondylitis: a study of 100 patients. Br J Rheuamtol. 1997;36:766–771.

47. Barlow JH, Wright CC, Williams B, Keat A. Work disability among people with ankylosing spondylitis. Arthritis Care Res. 2001;45:424–429.

48. Carette S, Graham D, Little H, Rubenstein J, Rosen P. The natural disease course of ankylosing spondylitis. Arthritis Rheum. 1983;26:186–190.

49. Gran JT, Østensen M, Husby G. A clinical comparison between males and females with ankylosing spondylitis. J Rheumatol. 1985;12:126–129.

50. Kaarela K, Lehtinen K, Luukkainen R. Work capacity of patients with inflammatory joint diseases. Scand J Rheumatol. 1987;16:403–406.

51. Ringsdal VS, Helin P. Ankylosing spondylitis—education, employment and invalidity. Dan Med Bull. 1991;38:282–284.

52. Edmunds L, Elswood J, Kennedy LG, Calin A. Primary ankylosing spondylitis, psoriatic and enteropathic spondyloarthropathy: a controlled analysis. J Rheumatol. 1991;18:696–698.

53. Roussou E, Kennedy LG, Garrett S, Calin A. Socioeconomic status in ankylosing spondylitis: relationship between occupation and disease activity. J Rheumatol. 1997;24:908–911.

54. Zink A, Braun J, Listing J, Wollenhaupt J. Disability and handicap in rheumatoid arthritis and ankylosing spondylitis—results from the German Rheumatological Database. J Rheumatol. 2000;27:613–622.

55. Boonen A, Chorus A, Landewe R, et al. Manual jobs increase the risk of patients with ankylosing spondylitis withdrawing from the labour force, also when adjusted for job related withdrawal in the general population. Ann Rheum Dis. 2002;61:658.

56. Gold MR, Siegel JE, Russell LB, et al. Cost-Effectiveness in Health and Medicine. New York, NY: Oxford University Press, 1996.

57. Boonen A, van der Heijde D, Landewe R, et al. Direct costs of ankylosing spondylitis and its determinants: an analysis among three European countries. Ann Rheum Dis. 2003;62:732–740.

58. Ward MM. Functional disability predicts total costs in patients with ankylosing spondylitis. Arthritis Rheum. 2002;46:223–231.

59. Sailly JC, Lebrun T. Les conséquences économiques et sociales de la pelvispondylite rhumatismale. Rev Epidemiol Sante Publique. 1982;30:305–324.

60. Boonen A, van der Heijde D, Landewe R, et al. Costs of ankylosing spondylitis in three European countries: the patient's perspective. Ann Rheum Dis. 2003;62:741–747.

61. Bakker C, Hidding A, van der Linden S, van Doorslaer E. Cost effectiveness of group physical therapy compared to individualized therapy for ankylosing spondylitis. A randomized controlled trial. J Rheumatol. 1994;21:264–268.

Index

A

acetaminophen for AS, 165
acute anterior uveitis (AAU), 146
acute ReA. *See* Reactive arthritis (ReA)
adalimumab for AS, 175
5-aminosalicylic acid for AS, 168–169
amitriptyline for AS, 165
Amor criteria, 118, 138–139
anakinra for AS, 180–181
analgesics for AS, 165
ANKH genes, 33–34
ankylosing tarsitis, 100–103
ankylosis, 133
answer modalities for AS, 207–208
anti-$\alpha_4\beta_7$, 71
antibiotics
 clinical studies, 47–48
 for juvenile-onset spondyloarthritides, 102
 for reactive arthritis, 57–58
antidepressant therapy for AS, 165–177
anti-interleukin-12, 71
antirheumatic drugs
 Crohn's disease, 68, 69
 inflammatory bowel disease, 68, 69
 ulcerative colitis, 68, 69
anti-*Saccharomyces cerevisiae* antibody, 10, 67
anti-TNF-α-directed therapies. *See* TNF-α blockers/inhibitors
aphthous ulcerations, 67
5-ASA for AS, 168–169
ASCAs and Crohn's disease, 10
Assessments in Ankylosing Spondylitis (ASAS) Working
 Group, 154
axial involvement
 ankylosing spondylitis, 210
 clinical feature(s), 133
 Crohn's disease, 66
 inflammatory bowel disease, 66
azathioprine, 69
azithromycin for ReA, 56

B

bacteria in AS, 60–61
Bath Ankylosing Spondylitis Disease Activity Index (BASDAI),
 34, 54, 67, 84, 156
Bath Ankylosing Spondylitis Functional Index (BASFI),
 34, 54, 67, 85, 156
Bath Ankylosing Spondylitis General Index (BASGI), 67, 156
Bath Ankylosing Spondylitis Metrology Index (BASMI), 67
Bath Ankylosing Spondylitis Radiology Index (BASRI), 194
Berlin Enthesitis Index, 85
bisphosphonates for AS, 179–180
budesonide, 69

C

CARD$_{15}$
 ankylosing spondylitis, 33
 and Crohn's disease, 10–11, 68
 inflammatory bowel disease, 68
 ulcerative colitis, 68
cardiovascular disease
 ankylosing spondylitis, 146–147
 HLA-B27-associated cardiac disease, 82
career choices and AS, 216
cauda equina syndrome (CES), 200–201
celecoxib for AS, 162, 163
change vs. status scores for AS, 208–209
chemotherapy for ReA, 56
chest wall pain, anterior, 133
children. *See* Juvenile-onset spondyloarthritides
Chlamydia-induced ReA, 38, 39, 42
Chlamydia infection, 41
chlorambucil for uveitis, 113
chronic SpA, 57
 assessment of disease activity, 54
 ReA. *See* Reactive arthritis (ReA)
ciprofloxacin ReA, 56
classification criteria, 117–119, 132, 134, 138
 Amor criteria, 119, 138–139
 ankylosing spondylitis, 117–119, 135–138
 European Spondyloarthropathy Study Group criteria, 119, 139–141
clinical feature(s), 132–133
 ankylosis, 133
 axial involvement, 133
 chest wall pain, anterior, 133
 conjunctivitis, 111
 Crohn's disease, 66–67
 enthesitis, 133
 episcleritis, 111
 extraarticular features, 134
 eye disease, inflammatory, 111–113
 family studies, 134
 HLA-B27, 133–134
 inflammatory bowel disease, 66–67
 juvenile-onset spondyloarthritides, 95–97
 peripheral articular, 133
 sacroiliitis, 133
 scleritis, 111
 spinal pain, inflammatory, 133
 undifferentiated spondyloarthritis (uSpA), 78–85
 uveitis, 111
conjunctivitis, 107, 111
corticosteroids
 Crohn's disease, 68–69
 eye drops, 113
 inflammatory bowel disease, 68–69